EXOTIC
ANIMALS

A
VETERINARY
HANDBOOK

A collection of articles
from *Veterinary Technician*®

Published by Veterinary Learning Systems
Trenton, New Jersey

ISBN 1-884254-19-5

PREFACE

Practicing veterinarians are seeing increasing numbers of exotic pets, including birds, reptiles, ferrets, rabbits, and small rodents, for which owners are demanding quality veterinary care. Owner attachment to exotics can be as strong as to more traditional companion animal species and is not linked to purchase price, which can vary from a few dollars for a hamster to many thousands of dollars for a black cockatoo.

The role of trained veterinary technicians in an exotic pet practice is probably more important than in the standard small animal practice. Technicians and veterinarians can make a major impact on the well being of these animals by providing their owners with much-needed information. The caging and diet of exotic pets are often specialized, and owners need guidance on basic husbandry, which is so fundamental to preventive health care. Moreover, familiarity with the handling, restraint, and clinical techniques appropriate for the particular species is necessary to diagnose medical problems and administer treatment.

Finally, exotic pet medicine is interesting and challenging. No day is ever "routine"; I find that I am always learning new things. Examining differences between species often gives important insights into the similarities among species and the physical and physiological features that we take for granted.

This compilation of articles on the biology and medicine of exotic pets, drawn primarily from the pages of *Veterinary Technician*®, covers a wide variety of topics and is an important resource for veterinary technicians who work with exotic pets and their owners, as well as for anyone else who requires the fundamentals, no matter what their background. Additional articles from other sources have been added to present a more complete discussion of each species in the collection.

Elizabeth V. Hillyer, DVM

CONTENTS

ZOO AND WILDLIFE

GENERAL

FERRET PREVENTIVE MEDICINE AND CLINICAL TECHNIQUES

Elizabeth V. Hillyer, DVM
Oldwick, New Jersey

Of all the exotic pet species, ferrets are probably the most closely related to dogs and cats, both in terms of taxonomy and in terms of common disease problems. An understanding of basic ferret husbandry, preventive medicine, and clinical techniques should enable the small animal clinician to add ferrets to the roster of clinic patients.

MANAGEMENT

Housing.—Ferrets can be housed indoors or outdoors. Three important considerations related to their housing requirements are: 1) they do not tolerate heat, 2) they will chew rubber objects and develop gastrointestinal (GI) obstructions, and 3) they are escape artists.

Outdoor housing should include shelter from the wind, bedding to protect against cold, and, most importantly, shade from the sun and ventilation in summer. Ferrets that are housed indoors should be caged when the owners are away from home. Glass aquaria are not appropriate because of poor ventilation. The cage should include a sleeping area (carpeting is a good substrate), a litter pan, and containers for food and water. Ferrets tend to overturn their food and water bowls; therefore, the bowls should be tied down or weighted. A sipper bottle is an alternative for water.

Ferrets should always be supervised when out of the cage, and the house should be "ferret-proofed" by removing chewable objects, rubber especially, and closing off any small openings into walls or out of the house.

Diet.—Ferrets are carnivores with high protein (30% to 40%) and fat (20% to 30%) requirements. They can be fed free-choice on high-quality, dry cat foods or ferret foods. Dog foods are not appropriate for ferrets, nor are generic cat foods. Protein should come from animal, not plant, sources. Iams and Science Diet kitten chows are good choices; older ferrets (over 3 or 4 years of age) can be offered the adult cat foods. Many ferrets will enjoy daily bits of raw carrot or apple, cooked meat, raw liver, or the occasional raisin.

Ferrets develop their food preferences relatively early in life and may be very finicky about diet changes.

PREVENTIVE VETERINARY CARE

Restraint.—Most ferrets are easy to handle and do best with minimal restraint for the physical examination. For blood collection or treatments, a neck-scruff hold is most secure and also seems to have a calming effect. The ferret is held suspended vertically in the air by the neck scruff with legs dangling (e.g., for vaccines); or the ferret is scruffed and held on a table top with its hindquarters restrained also. Hindquarters should be restrained around the hips, not the feet, because ferrets will struggle if their rear legs are pulled out.

The (rare) aggressive ferret can be toweled, scruffed, and restrained, or tranquilized if necessary. Gloves are awkward for the handler and do not protect against bites.

Tranquilization.—The most rapid and safe "tranquilizer" is isoflurane gas (AErrane®, Anaquest, Madison, WI) administered by facemask in 0.5% increments until the ferret relaxes (usually at 2% to 2.5%). Induction and recovery are rapid, and outpatient blood testing or radiographs can be easily performed. Nausea is the most common side effect.

Injectable tranquilizers can be useful also but have the disadvantages of variable effect, frequently poor muscle relaxation, and prolonged recovery. Acepromazine is given at 0.1 mg/kg SQ. Tiletamine-zolazepam (Telazol® A. H. Robins Company, Richmond, VA) given at 2 to 8 mg/kg IM or low-dose ketamine (<20 mg/kg IM) usually gives poor muscle relaxation.

Vaccinations

Canine Distemper.—Ferrets are highly susceptible to the canine distemper virus, with close to 100% mortality after infection in unprotected ferrets. They should be vaccinated with a monovalent vaccine made from nonferret tissues; a good choice is one of chick embryo origin (Fromm-D®, Solvay Animal Health Inc., Mendota Heights, MN; or FERVAC-D, United Vaccines, Inc., Madison, WI). Kits should receive a series of boosters 2 to 4 weeks apart until 14 weeks of age. (Most ferrets purchased from pet stores come from large commercial breeders and have received one vaccine at about 6 weeks of age.) Thereafter, ferrets should be given a canine distemper vaccine once a year.

Ferrets do not need vaccines against other canine or feline diseases. They should never be given a multivalent vaccine, which may induce clinical disease problems.

Rabies.—Vaccination against rabies is recommended, particularly where the disease is endemic. There is one rabies vaccine (killed) approved for use in ferrets: Imrab® (Rhone Merieux Inc., Athens, GA), administered SQ at 3 months of age and then once a year.

Heartworm Disease.—Ferrets are susceptible to infection with *Dirofilaria immitis*. The infection is difficult to diagnose in ferrets, and none have been successfully treated for the disease; therefore, a preventive program is essential in endemic areas (for indoor ferrets also in high-risk areas). Ferrets are dosed with oral diethylcarbamazine DEC) at 5 to 11 mg/kg/day PO or ivermectin (Ivomec®, Merck & Co. Inc., Rahway, NJ) at 0.05 mg/kg PO or SQ once a month.

Testing for heartworm infection is difficult because most infected ferrets do not become microfilaremic. The ELISA tests for heartworm antigens are usually not sensitive enough to detect the low levels present in ferrets; however, the laboratory protocol for some can be amended to increase their sensitivity (contact the manufacturer for details).

Routine Testing

Juvenile Ferrets.—Routine testing for young ferrets includes a direct fecal, a fecal flotation, and screening for ear mites. GI parasites are uncommon, but coccidia, *Giardia*, and, rarely, roundworms can be seen. Treatment for these parasites is the same as for cats.

Ear mites are very common in ferrets, even in those from commercial breeding farms. Ferrets with ear mites should have a thorough ear cleaning; a small drop of Ivomec® can be placed in both ears (repeat in 2 weeks). Alternatively, an injection of Ivomec® (dose at 0.4 mg/kg SQ) can be given once and repeated in 2 weeks, but this seems to be less effective than topical ivermectin. Topical otic acaricide products may be difficult for clients to administer. Ferrets with refractory ear mite infections should receive whole body flea powdering or baths in addition to otic therapy.

Middle-age to Older Ferrets.—Insulinomas and adrenal tumors are very common in ferrets over 3 years of age. A good preventive health program should include routine screening for insulinoma, adrenal tumors, hairballs, lymphoma, and cardiac disease. Ideally, ferrets over 3 years of age should be examined twice a year, with laboratory testing and radiographs one to two times a year, depending on owner finances. Ferrets should be fasted for 4 to a maximum of 6 hours to detect susceptibility to hypoglycemia and to empty the GI tract of food—a significant amount of ingesta remaining in the stomach is suspicious for a hairball. Basic diagnostics include fasting blood glucose, whole body radiographs (to examine cardiac silhouette and stomach), and complete blood count (CBC) with differential.

CLINICAL TECHNIQUES

Diagnostic Testing.—Collecting blood from ferrets requires adequate restraint. Restraint options include: 1) isoflurane by facemask, 2) one or two able-bodied assistants, or 3) one assistant and a syringe of Nutri-cal® (Evsco Pharmaceuticals, Buena, NJ).

A small volume (up to 0.3 mL) of blood is easily collected from the cephalic or lateral saphenous vein using a Lo-dose® insulin syringe (27-gauge needle). Position of these veins and method of restraint are the same as for dogs and cats. A larger volume of blood is collected from the jugular vein using a 3-mL syringe with 22- to 25-g needle or butterfly catheter. The ferret is restrained at the edge of a table with its head held up vertically and the forelegs held down or, alternatively, on its back with the forelegs pulled back. In dorsal restraint, the ferret can be fed Nutri-cal®, a tasty treat that will distract most individuals. (A fasting blood glucose should be drawn before the Nutri-cal® gets too far into the ferret.)

The cranial vena cava is another site for blood collection in ferrets. This is a "blind" technique with potential for morbidity and should not be used if restraint is uncertain or if the ferret may have intrathoracic disease or a bleeding disorder. Necessary equipment includes a 25-g needle and 3-mL syringe. With the ferret restrained in dorsal recumbancy, the needle is inserted on the right or left side at the notch between the manubrium and the first rib and is directed at a shallow angle pointing toward the opposite hip. The needle is gradually advanced while applying gentle suction on the syringe until blood enters the hub. This technique is simple and rapid for collection of up to 3 mL of blood.

A sterile urine sample is collected by cystocentesis using a 25-g needle.

Chemical restraint is almost mandatory to obtain well-positioned radiographs of ferrets. Isoflurane is ideal for this purpose. The table top technique is used for ferrets in conjunction with exposure techniques adapted to their small size.

Treatment Techniques.—Ferrets are difficult to "pill," and oral medications are best given in liquid form or as the crushed pill mixed into Nutri-cal® or Isocal® (Mead Johnson Nutritionals, Evansville, IN). SQ and IM injections are given as in dogs and cats. Small-volume IV injections can be given into the cephalic or lateral saphenous veins using a Lo-dose® insulin syringe. Alternatively, caustic IV preparations can be given, with the ferret under isoflurane, into these veins using a small-gauge butterfly catheter.

Short indwelling 24-g IV catheters are easily placed in the cephalic or lateral saphenous veins. Isoflurane facilitates the procedure. Ferret skin is very tough; therefore, a small skin hole is made first by tenting the skin over the vein and inserting a 22-g needle through the skin, taking care to avoid the vein. The catheter is then passed through this opening. Jugular catheters are more difficult to place.

Endotracheal tube placement is facilitated by a small laryngoscope blade (Miller blade #0, North American Drager, Telford, PA). Small ferrets will take a 2.0 uncuffed tube, whereas large male ferrets may take a 3.0 cuffed tube.

Suggested Reading

1. Brown SA. Adrenal and pancreatic neoplasia. Proc North Am Vet Conf 1993;725-727.

2. Hillyer, EV. Ferret endocrinology. In: Kirk RW, Bonagura JD, eds. Current Veterinary Therapy XI. Philadelphia, Pa: WB Saunders Co, 1992;1185-1188.

3. Hillyer EV, Brown SA. Ferrets. In: Birchard SJ, Sherding RG, eds. Manual of Small Animal Practice. Philadelphia, Pa: WB Saunders Co, 1993 (In Press).

4. Rosenthal K. Ferrets. Vet Clin North Am Sm Anim Pract 1994 (In Press).

5. Silverman S. Diagnostic imaging of exotic pets. Vet Clin North Am Sm Anim Pract 1993; 23: 1287-1299.

Bone Marrow Depression Associated with Prolonged Estrus in the European Polecat or Fitch Ferret

Deborah Anne Martin, ACT
Animal Care Technology
St. Lawrence College, Saint-Laurent
Ontario, Canada

Ferrets have an interesting breeding pattern. They are seasonally polyestrous and mate and reproduce only during a specific period of the year (March to August).[1,a] The natural cycle likely developed to enhance the survival of the kits, which are usually born in the spring and summer.

The female ferret (Figure 1), or *jill*, is receptive to the male only when in estrus. Unlike dogs and cats, the male ferret, or *hob*, also has a breeding season. The testes are present in the scrotum only at that time; during July through December, the testes retract to the subcuticular caudoventral abdomen.[1] Even though the female ferret may be receptive to male advances and ready to mate, the male may be unable to make viable sperm when the testes are not in the scrotal sac. It has been shown that the cooler temperature within the scrotal sac is essential for spermatogenesis.[2]

Like other fur-bearing animals, a female ferret's estrous cycle is influenced by daylight hours.[2] As the daylight period lengthens, the brain responds by releasing follicle-stimulating hormone, which is necessary for the growth of the graafian follicles and the production of estrogens by the ovary.[2] In the female, signs of estrus include vulvar swelling (Figure 2) and I have noticed increased activity and sometimes better temperament. The female tends to be more playful and gives out an almost constant chirping or grunting sound while playing. Female ferrets are induced ovulators; if ovulation is not induced, a female may remain in estrus up to 120 days[3] or even as long as six months.[1]

In ferrets, bone marrow depression is the most common disease associated with prolonged estrus. Its incidence is reported to be greater than 50% in intact females that have not been bred during April through July.[1] The outcome may be fatal, despite attempted therapy.[3]

Bone Marrow

In young animals, the marrow exists as a richly cellular, highly vascularized connective tissue. As an animal ages, cellular marrow decreases in quantity, and is replaced by yellow marrow.[4] The cellular (active red) marrow persists in flat bones (ribs, pelvis, cranial bones), in short bones (vertebrae), and at the ends of long bones. The yellow nonproductive marrow occupies the shafts of the long bones and consists of fat cells, endothelial cells, and reticular cells.[5] The cellular marrow is capable of producing erythrocytes, thrombocytes (platelets), eosinophils, basophils, and neutrophils and is a minor production site for lymphocytes, plasma cells, and monocytes.[4] For effective hematopoiesis to occur, the relationship of the cellular to the nonproductive marrow must be stable and mutually compatible.[6]

Bone Marrow Depression

When bone marrow depression occurs, an abundance of inactive yellow marrow and almost no active red marrow are present. Excessive doses of estrogen given to dogs have been noted to produce the condition,[7] and similar effects have been seen in mice and rats.[8] An unspayed female ferret is particularly at risk because of her prolonged estrous

---

[a]The author has discovered that by changing the environment and sleeping pattern of her ferrets, their reproductive cycles can be altered. Breeders can thus lengthen or shorten estrous cycles to some extent to suit particular requirements.

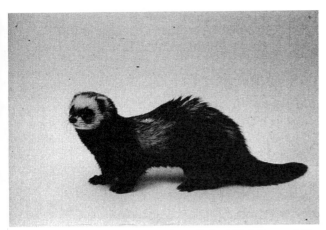

Figure 1—A typical fitch ferret. (From Ryland LM, Bernard SL, Gorham JR: A clinical guide to the pet ferret. *Compend Contin Educ Pract Vet* 5(1):26, 1983. Reprinted with permission.)

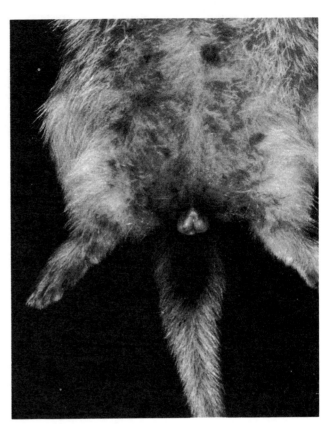

Figure 3—Shown is an estrous female that succumbed to bone marrow depression. Cutaneous petechiae, melena (staining tail), and alopecia are commonly seen. (From Ryland LM, Bernard SL, Gorham JR: A clinical guide to the pet ferret. *Compend Contin Educ Pract Vet* 5(1):31, 1983. Reprinted with permission.)

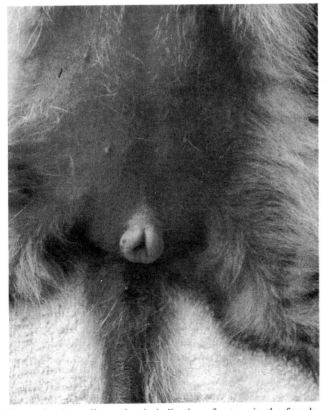

Figure 2—A swollen vulva is indicative of estrus in the female ferret. Alopecia of the ventral abdomen and tail is evident. (From Ryland LM, Bernard SL, Gorham JR: A clinical guide to the pet ferret. *Compend Contin Educ Pract Vet* 5(1):26, 1983. Reprinted with permission.)

cycle and high endogenous levels during the estrous period.[1] Bone marrow depression results in pancytopenia—lack of both white cells and red cells as well as platelets.[1] This in turn predisposes the animal to bacterial infections and hematologic disorders. When not bred, the female's vulva remains swollen (Figure 2); presumably the vagina's widened entrance, which is intended to aid the male in

mating, invites vaginal introduction of microorganisms. An extended estrous period takes its toll on a ferret's general body condition. It is a time of great stress, and an unbred female can easily lose up to 40% of her normal body weight.[1] Her depressed state also increases the chance of infection.

Clinical Findings

Clinical findings include signs of anemia, such as listlessness, depression, apathy, anorexia, and pale mucous membranes.[1,3] The lack of platelets often results in hemorrhages. Affected regions include mucosal surfaces (thrombocytopenic purpura) and subcuticular regions.[3] Melena may be present (Figure 3).[1] In two reported cases, a soft left protomesosystolic heart murmur was associated with the anemia.[3] Bilateral symmetrical alopecia is common.[1] Fever may occur associated with bacterial infection, raising the body temperature above the normal range of 38° to 40°C.[1] Development of shock as a sequela of septicemia or bacteremia may result in a core body temperature that is subnormal, however.[9] During the period of illness, pale mucous membranes and vulvar swelling are constant.[3]

Laboratory Findings

Laboratory findings include decreases in white cell count, red cell count, packed cell volume, and hemoglobin and a marked reduction in the platelet count (Table I). In short, they reflect the hypocellular bone marrow. The anemia is characterized as normochromic and normocytic, with a lack of regenerative response (extremely low numbers of or absent reticulocytes).[3] An occasional nucleated red blood cell detected in the peripheral blood in some cases was ascribed to release from sites of extramedullary hematopoiesis, such as the spleen.[3] Cases reported in the literature reveal low total plasma protein, despite dehydration—a factor attributed to the hemorrhages.[3]

Pathologic Findings

Pathologic findings parallel clinical observations. Necropsies have shown hemorrhages (petechiae to ecchymoses) observed in intestinal, cardiac, nervous, and urinary tissue.[3] Cutaneous petechiae may be evident (Figure 3).[1] Body tissues are generally pale.[3] In one case, multiple graafian follicles were detected on the ovaries.[3] Another case showed secondary bacterial bronchopneumonia.[3] The color of the marrow ranged from light tan to pale pink.[3] This fatty marrow floated in formalin.[1]

Histologic sections showed that the marrow was mostly yellow, or nonactive, and the red marrow was markedly reduced.[3] The few cells present in the marrow comprised lymphocytes, plasma cells, and hemosiderin-laden macrophages.[3]

Treatment

As already has been noted, bone marrow depression predisposes the female ferret to hemorrhage and secondary bacterial infection as a result of pancytopenia. Treatment is therefore directed toward correcting the underlying disorder, correcting the secondary problems, and to general supportive therapy. It is important that the ferret be treated as soon as any clinical signs are noted, as it has the best chance of cure with immediate therapy. If the animal is in adequate physical condition for surgery, immediate ovariohysterectomy is a logical approach to remove the underlying cause of the disorder. Often, though, by the time a ferret suffering from bone marrow depression is seen by a veterinarian, it is too late to perform surgery without great risk. In such circumstances, the veterinarian attempts to stabilize the animal's condition by treating the secondary problems and initiating supportive therapy until the ferret is strong enough to undergo surgery. Therapy may include blood transfusions, rehydration, and broad-spectrum antibiotics. In one case, the ferret recovered after a combination of ovariohysterectomy and 15 blood transfusions over a five-month period, in conjunction with doses of anabolic steroids and corticosteroids, force-feeding and oral vitamin supplementation.[8] In most instances, however, the prognosis is extremely poor.[1,3]

Because therapy is often unrewarding, prevention of the problem is encouraged. An owner who wants to breed a ferret eventually, although not during the animal's current estrus, can take the animal to a veterinarian for hormonal treatment to shorten the estrous period. By injecting 100 IU of human chorionic gonadotropin, which behaves like

TABLE I
Normal Blood Values Compared with Bone Marrow Depression Values for Ferrets

Parameter	Normal Range[1]	Depressed Value[3,a]
Hematocrit (%)	42–61	<10
RBCs ($\times 10^6/\mu l$)	6.8–12.2	<2.0
Platelets ($\times 10^3/\mu l$)	297–910	<20
WBCs ($\times 10^3/\mu l$)	4.0–19.0	<2.6
Hemoglobin (g/dl)	15–18	<3.5

[a]Depressed platelet value was derived from Reference 1.

luteinizing hormone and promotes ovulation,[1] the duration of estrus is decreased. Human chorionic gonadotropin should be given after the vulvar swelling reaches its full extent, typically about 10 days to 2 weeks after the onset of estrus.[1] If treatment is successful and ovulation takes place, the vulva should decrease to normal size and the estrous period should end in 20 to 25 days; the ferret then remains in anestrus for 40 to 50 days.[1] Megestrol acetate is sometimes used in ferrets and other species to delay or prevent estrus. It has been reported, however, that giving this drug may increase the risk of subsequent pyometra.[1]

An owner who does not wish to breed his or her ferret can elect ovariohysterectomy to prevent the bone marrow depression so commonly resulting from high circulating estrogens released by the ovaries. If ovariohysterectomy is considered out of the question, however, then an alternative is for the owner to locate a sexually mature male ferret and breed the female to him to forestall the onset of bone marrow depression.

Summary

Prolonged estrus is common in ferrets and is associated with a high incidence of fatal bone marrow depression characterized by nonresponsive anemia, thrombocytopenia, and granulocytopenia. Veterinary technicians who are aware of the dangers of prolonged estrus in ferrets can bring animals with clinical signs to the attention of the veterinarian for appropriate diagnosis and management.

REFERENCES

1. Ryland LM, Bernard SL, Gorham JR: A clinical guide to the pet ferret. *Compend Contin Educ Pract Vet* 5(1):25-30, 1983.
2. Roberts SJ: *Veterinary Obstetrics and Genital Diseases (Theriogenology)*. Ithaca, New York, S. J. Roberts, 1971.
3. Kociba GJ, Caputo CA: Aplastic anemia associated with estrus in pet ferrets. *JAVMA* 178:1293-1294, 1981.
4. Coles EH: *Veterinary Clinical Pathology*. Philadelphia, WB Saunders Co, 1974, p 15.
5. Benjamin MM: *Outline of Veterinary Clinical Pathology*. Ames, IA, Iowa State University Press, 1978, p 15.
6. Emerson LK: *Hematologic Diseases*. New York, Medical Examination Publishing Co, 1983, pp 59-69.

7. Halliwell REW: Steroid therapy in skin disease, in Kirk RW (ed): *Current Veterinary Therapy VI*. Philadelphia, WB Saunders Co, 1977, p 545.

8. Ryland LM: Remission of estrus-associated anemia following ova- riohysterectomy and multiple blood transfusions in a ferret. *JAVMA* 181:820-822, 1982.

9. Kirk RW, Bistner SI: *Handbook of Veterinary Procedures and Emergency Treatment*. Philadelphia, WB Saunders Co, 1981, p 55.

The Golden Hamster

Harry E. Stoliker, DVM
School of Veterinary Medicine
Purdue University
West Lafayette, Indiana

The golden, or Syrian, hamster, introduced into the United States during World War II, has gained in popularity as a research animal. The number of hamsters used annually in research is exceeded only by the number of rats and mice. The popularity of the golden hamster as a pet has also increased significantly over the years and, as a result, more and more of these caged pets are being presented to practicing veterinarians for treatment of various disease conditions. Animal health technicians working for practicing veterinarians are expected to know how to handle and restrain hamsters, collect blood samples, and administer medications orally and parenterally. Animal health technicians working in research facilities are also expected to know the clinical signs of common diseases of hamsters so that they can report deviations from normal. Table I is a listing of some general information and precautions concerning the hamster.

History

The golden, or Syrian, hamster is of the class Mammalia, order Rodentia, family Cricetidae, genus *Mesocricetus*, and species *auratus*. It originated from a single litter of eight caught near Aleppo, Syria in 1930. Four of the litter escaped, and one female was killed by its brother. The remaining three—one male and two females—produced a colony of 364 animals by the end of the first year of captivity. Descendants of these three littermates were first sent to the United States during World War II. In recent years, other hamsters have been imported, primarily for research purposes. Some golden hamster mutants kept as pets are the ruby-eyed, the long-haired, teddy (toy) bear, and hamsters of different-colored coats.

Research Uses

The cheek pouches of hamsters can be everted; this facilitates the study of microcirculation and the exposure of the cheek pouch surfaces to viruses, transplantable tumors, and carcinogens. Hamsters are also used in the study of nutrition, toxicity, chronic respiratory diseases, and dental caries.

Anatomy and Physiology

The sex of weanlings can be determined by comparing the anogenital distance (Figure 2). The distance is greater in males than in females. When viewed from above, the adult male posterior looks round because of the protrusion of the testicles, whereas the adult female's posterior appears square.

The life span of the hamster is usually two to four years. The female's milk is composed of 74% water, 12.6% fat, 9% protein, and 3.4% sugar. Hamster urine is cream colored and turbid due to crystalluria, and the pH is 8.0. Hamsters have a pouchlike area anterior to the stomach which contains microorganisms similar to those found in ruminants, and their utilization of dietary nitrogen is more like that of ruminants.

The dental formula for hamsters is

$$2 \left(I\, \frac{1}{1}\ C\, \frac{0}{0}\ PM\, \frac{0}{0}\ M\, \frac{3}{3} \right) = 16,$$

where I = incisors, C = canines, PM = premolars, and M = molars. The incisor teeth are nonrooted

---

Revisions by Elizabeth V. Hillyer, DVM

Originally published in Volume 2, Number 3, May/June 1981

TABLE I
SOME GENERAL INFORMATION AND PRECAUTIONS FOR HAMSTER CARE

Dos

Do empty hamster cheek pouches before the hamster is weighed (Figure 1).

Do always put the female in the male's cage for breeding.

Do warm a hamster slowly to insure that it is not hibernating if it appears to be dead.

Don'ts

Don't use the antibiotics that act primarily against gram-positive organisms, since they destroy the normal intestinal flora.

Don't feed a diet containing more than 5% crude fat.

Don't house adult hamsters together; this usually results in fighting and injury or death.

Don't leave a female with a male for breeding for more than one hour, because after breeding the female may attack the male.

Don't use wire-bottom cages for parturition and raising of the young.

Don't disturb females with young for at least three days after parturition.

Don't waken sleeping hamsters suddenly—they may bite.

and grow continuously. Incisor malocclusion and overgrowth can occur secondary to trauma or infection of the tooth. If overgrowth is occurring, the teeth can be cut with a pair of sharp nippers every three to six months. The molars are rooted and do not grow continuously like the incisors.

Hamsters sometimes go into hibernation; this appears to be a state of deep sleep. The hibernating hamster will curl up in a ball and may look dead. In this state, the body temperature drops to a few degrees above the ambient temperature. The respiration rate may decrease to less than one beat per minute,

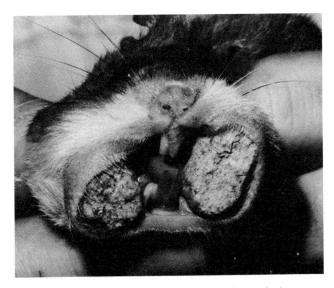

Figure 1—The cheek pouches should be emptied before the hamster is weighed.

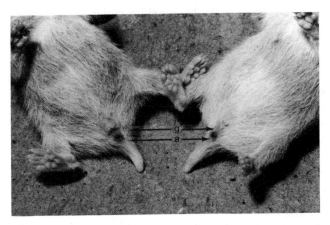

Figure 2—Sex can be determined by comparing the anogenital distance. The distance is greater in the male (*right*) than in the female (*left*). g, genital opening; a, anal opening.

and the heart rate is reduced to 4 to 15 beats per minute. Hibernation may last anywhere from a few minutes to seven days. If the ambient temperature drops to 4° or 5°C, some hamsters' metabolic rate starts to increase and they gradually awaken; others stay in hibernation and still others may die of cold. Slow warming of the hibernating animal will bring it out of this state.

Reproduction

Although hamsters may show evidence of sexual activity as early as 30 days of age, they are usually not bred until they reach 60 days of age, when the male weighs from 85 to 100 g and the female weighs between 95 and 120 g. The estrous cycle of four days duration starts at four to six weeks of age. Females are polyestrous year round and ovulate spontaneously. Ovulation occurs 8 to 10 hours postestrus. Ova implantation begins on day 5 and is completed by day 6 postbreeding.

Estrus usually occurs in the evening. It is characterized by a slight, mucoid, transparent vaginal discharge. The day after estrus, the vaginal discharge is thick, white, opaque, viscous, and more apparent in the morning. The appearance of this copious discharge indicates that estrus will occur again in three days. Females in estrus usually exhibit lordosis (a downward arching of the back with the tail pointed straight up in the air).

Breeding

Breeding usually occurs in the evening. In commercial operations, where males are usually kept separated from females, the females are placed in the male hamster cage for approximately 30 to 60 minutes. The hamsters must be watched to ensure that the female does not attack the male, since the female is the more aggressive of the species and may injure or kill the male.

In the home where pet males and females are housed together, breeding occurs spontaneously.

Hamsters are prolific breeders, so if the owner is not careful, he will soon have innumerable hamsters. The market for home-raised hamsters is very small, because most research hamsters have to be raised under exacting sanitary conditions that require special caging, air conditioning, food, and bedding to insure that they are as disease free as possible. Pet shops sometimes purchase the young from individual breeders. An outlet for the litters should be determined prior to breeding; otherwise—as with unwanted puppies and kittens—the humane shelter may be their final destination.

Pregnancy

On day 4 postbreeding, the vagina may be sealed by a sticky fluid which may be full of bubbles. The vaginal fluid may seem flocculent on days 5 and 6, changing to a waxy, mucoid consistency by day 10. Pregnant females gain weight steadily up to parturition. Pseudopregnant females gain weight up to day 5, and the estrous cycle resumes around day 9 postbreeding. The gestation period is 15 to 18 days, with an average of 16 days.

The litter size is usually from 5 to 10. Newborn hamsters weigh approximately 2 g, are hairless at birth, and have their eyes closed. The weaning age of hamsters is 28 days.

Mothers will frequently cannibalize their first litter. They generally raise a high percentage of the following litters, but they may cannibalize the pups if disturbed by loud noises, bedding changes, odors, etc. If the hamsters are housed in wire-bottom cages, cannibalism frequently occurs.

In commercial breeding operations, the breeding life of females and males are, respectively, one and two years. Retired breeders are usually sold for research purposes.

Temperament

Males are usually more docile than females, and they make better pets. Frequent handling, especially when the hamsters are young, makes them more tractable. If raised together, hamsters can usually be housed in the same cage, but as they grow older, they have a tendency to fight with each other. They should not be housed with other species of animals because fighting will invariably occur. Hamsters are very sensitive to loud noises, odor, changes in bedding, and the proximity to other animals, especially rats. When housed in the same room with rats, they frequently will not breed. The young are very playful, often wrestling, but their play may lead to injuries. They are very curious. If awakened suddenly out of a deep sleep and handled, they frequently bite.

Nutrition

To ensure adequate growth, hamsters should be fed a balanced commercial rodent diet containing not less than 24% crude protein. Food consumption of laboratory diets is 10 to 14 g/day. Many hamsters are given small amounts of lettuce, apple, or carrots once or twice a week. In the laboratory setting, any vegetables that are fed should be soaked in a chlorine solution (400 parts per million) for 30 minutes to prevent introduction of disease-producing organisms. An outbreak of tularemia causing 100% mortality in four- to six-week-old hamsters occurred in a breeding colony because of feeding contaminated, unwashed lettuce.

Pet hamsters should be fed a commercial pelleted diet. The diet can be supplemented with 10% to 20% treat foods, such as washed vegetables, fruits, seeds, crackers, and small amounts of cheese or cooked meat. Commercial rodent diets containing seeds should be avoided because hamsters tend to eat the seeds rather than the pellets, thereby consuming an unbalanced diet.

Water should be provided ad libitum. When on dry food, hamsters drink about 10 to 20 ml of water per day. Water intake decreases when the hamsters are fed fruits or vegetables containing large amounts of water.

Crude fat levels of about 5% are adequate. Fat levels of 7 to 9% in the diet have caused increases in the mortality rate. Increased levels of saturated fats in the diet cause hyperlipemia.

Housing

Hamsters are escape artists—they can get out of most cages if they do not have a secure lid. In commercial operations, plastic or metal boxes are usually employed. In the home, a cage made of glass (aquarium), hard plastic, or metal or a solid-bottom wire cage can be used. Hamsters will chew through wood and some soft plastic cages if they can find a spot that they can get their teeth into.

Ground corncobs or hardwood chips or shavings are suitable bedding materials. Hamsters may enjoy hard substances to chew on. Hardwood dolls can be purchased at lumberyards and cut into short pieces, or hardwood chew toys can be obtained from pet shops.

In commercial operations, hamsters are usually provided with 10 to 12 hours of light and 12 to 14 hours of darkness. Breeding colony rooms are maintained at temperatures of 72° to 74° F. The temperature in holding areas for nonbreeding hamsters is maintained at 69° to 71° F. The relative humidity is maintained between 40 and 60%. Having originated in the desert regions of Syria, hamsters can tolerate wide temperature fluctuations; the varying temperatures of the average household are well tolerated if the hamsters have adequate bedding to protect them from lower temperatures. The most suitable range of relative humidity for the hamster is not known, but since they are nocturnal desert animals, one can assume that they may not tolerate high humidity, especially when the ambient temperature is also high.

TABLE II
CLINICAL SIGNS AND ETIOLOGY OF SOME DISEASES OF HAMSTERS

Clinical Signs	Etiology
Diarrhea	Wet tail (*Campylobacter* spp.?), *Hymenolepis nana** (tapeworm), *Syphacia obvelata* (pinworms), *Salmonella* spp,* *Bacillus piliformis* (Tyzzer's disease), and cecal hyperplasia
Rectal prolapse	*Syphacia obvelata* (pinworms)
Intestinal prolapse	Proliferative ileitis, any cause of diarrhea
Constipation	*Hymenolepis diminuta* (tapeworm)
Pneumonia	Pneumonia virus of mice, Sendai virus, *Pasteurella pneumotropica*, *Diplococcus pneumonia*, *Streptococcus* spp, and *Mycoplasma pulmonis*
Hair loss, scaliness and small scabs	*Demodex aurati*, adrenal neoplasia, dermatophytosis
Hair mortality in the young	Wet tail, *Bacillus piliformis*, *Francisella tularensis*, and cecal hyperplasia
Abscesses, suppurative lesions of the skin and feet	*Staphylococcus aureus*
Rapid death	*Toxoplasma gondii*, trauma, cardiomyopathy, atrial thrombosis, chilling
No apparent signs (latent)	*Encephalitozoon cuniculi*, lymphocytic choriomeningitis
Alopecia	Dietary fat deficiency and hypovitaminosis A, low protein diet, adrenal neoplasia
Xerophthalmia	Hypovitaminosis A

*These diseases are zoonoses.

Health Problems

Iatrogenic Diarrhea

The normal intestinal bacterial flora is predominately gram-positive. Administration of antibiotics that act against gram-positive organisms, i.e., the penicillins, erythromycin, and lincomycin, can result in overgrowth of clostridial organisms, resulting in diarrhea and, usually, death.

Spontaneous Diseases

Hamsters kept under sanitary conditions and fed adequate diets have few spontaneous bacterial or viral infections. Spontaneous diseases that have been reported are (1) the zoonoses, tapeworms (*Hymenolepis nana* and *Hymenolepis diminuta*), salmonellosis (*Salmonella enteritidis* and *Salmonella typhimurium*), lymphocytic choriomeningitis, tularemia (*Francisella tularensis*), and toxoplasmosis (*Toxoplasma gondii*), and (2) nonzoonotic diseases, proliferative ileitis (wet tail), demodicosis (*Demodex aurati*), pinworms (*Syphacia obvelata*), pneumonia virus of mice, Tyzzer's disease

(*Bacillus piliformis*), encephalitozoonosis (*Encephalitozoon cuniculi*), pseudotuberculosis (*Yersinia pseudotuberculosis*), diplococcosis (*Diplococcus pneumoniae*), cecal hyperplasia (etiology unknown), *Pasteurella* pneumonia (*Pasteurella pneumotropica*), staphylococcosis (*Staphylococcus aureus*), streptococcosis (*Streptococcus* spp.), amyloidosis, polycystic disease, pregnancy toxemia, and, occasionally, neoplasms (the incidence is about 4%). The clinical signs and etiology of some hamster diseases are listed in Table II.

Amyloidosis and polycystic disease are age related. Glomerular amyloidosis has been reported to occur at the rate of 41.6% in 13- to 18-month olds and 82.2% in 19- to 27-month olds. The rate of generalized amyloidosis was 82% in the 19- to 27-month-old group, but this lesion was not found in younger animals. Polycystic disease was found in 57.5% of hamsters 1 to 27 months old and in 75.8% of the 13- to 17-month-old group. The cysts were found in the epididymis (47%), liver (42.5%), seminal vesicles (23.5%), pancreas (12.5%), renal pelvis (5.0%), adrenals (2.5%), esophagus (2.5%), uterus (4.3%), and ovaries (4.35%).

Hamsters, like dogs, can harbor demodectic mites without having clinical signs of infection. *Demodex*

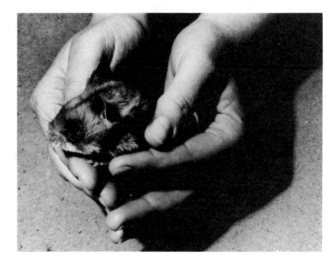

Figure 3—The hamster can be picked up by cupping the hands around it.

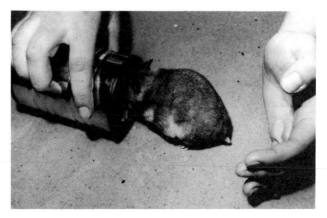

Figure 4—The hamster can be scooped into a tin can to pick it up.

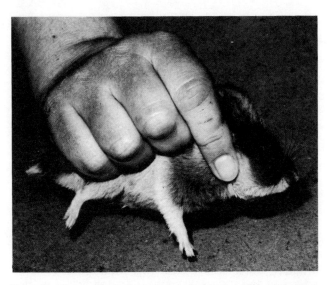

Figure 5—One method of restraining the hamster is by grasping as much skin as possible over the shoulders.

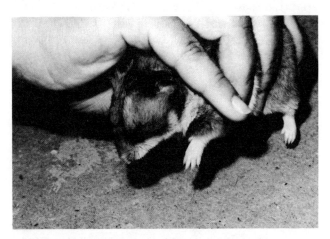

Figure 6—Another method of restraint is to grasp the hamster with the hand facing the rear of the body.

TABLE III

HEMATOLOGICAL AND BIOCHEMICAL VALUES IN NORMAL GOLDEN HAMSTERS

Test	Unit of Measurement	Value
HEMATOLOGY		
Erythrocytes (RBC)	$\times 10^6/mm^3$	4.0-10.0
Hemoglobin	g/dl	13.1-19.2
Hematocrit	%	39.2-58.8
Leukocytes (WBC)	$\times 10^3/mm^3$	5.2-10.6
Neutrophils	%	17.1-35.2
Eosinophils	%	0.22-1.54
Basophils	%	0.0-5.0
Lymphocytes	%	50.9-92.3
Monocytes	%	0.4-4.4
Sedimentation rate	mm/hr	0.3-0.96
BIOCHEMISTRY		
Platelets	$\times 10^3/mm^3$	300-573
Blood glucose	mg/dl	32.6-118
BUN	mg/dl	12-26
Calcium	mg/dl	7.4-12
Sodium	mEq/liter	106-146
Potassium	mEq/liter	4-6
Chloride	mEq/liter	86-112
Bicarbonate	mEq/liter	33-44
Phosphorus	mg/dl	3.5-8
Magnesium	mg/dl	2-3.5
Total protein	g/dl	4.3-7.7
Albumin	g/dl	2.6-4.1

aurati, which resembles the cigar-shaped *D. canis*, has caused lesions in aged hamsters. Its eggs are spindle shaped. *Demodex criceti*, which has a short, stubby body, produces oval eggs and lives in epidermal pits. It has not been reported to produce lesions.

Heavy pinworm infestations have been reported to cause rectal prolapse in hamsters.

Because of the hamster's susceptibility to many infections, it should not be housed with other species of animals in the laboratory, and care should be taken in the home so that it is not exposed to wild rodents, dogs, cats, or birds.

Restraint

In handling hamsters and administering treatment, they can be restrained in several ways. They can be picked up (1) by cupping the hands around them (Figure 3); (2) by scooping them into a tin can or paper cup (Figure 4); (3) by grasping as much skin as possible over their shoulders (Figure 5); (4) by grasping them with the hand facing the rear of the body (Figure 6); or (5) by placing the thumb and the index fingers around the neck, with the remainder of the fingers around the thorax.

Blood Collection

In the laboratory, cardiac puncture or periorbital bleeding from the orbital sinus are the methods of choice for blood collection. Approximately 2 ml of blood can be safely withdrawn via cardiac puncture from a 100-g hamster. Approximately 0.4 to 0.5 ml of blood can be obtained in plain or heparinized capillary tubes from the orbital sinus. These methods are used primarily in research animals.

Samples for routine hematology can be obtained by puncturing the dorsal or lateral surfaces of the tail or the paw pads or by clipping a toenail short enough to produce bleeding.

Normal blood values are given in Table III.

Administration of Medication

Oral medications are given in liquid form or as a crushed tablet mixed with a small amount of palatable paste, such as applesauce, jam, or smashed banana. The medication is administered using a tuberculin syringe (without needle) inserted in the side of the mouth and

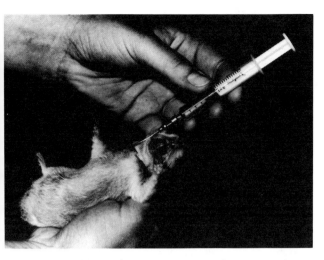

Figure 7—The holding technique in preparation for gavage is shown.

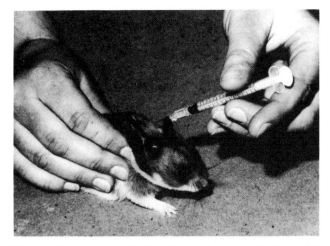

Figure 9—Subcutaneous administration can be done in the loose skin over the shoulders of the hamster.

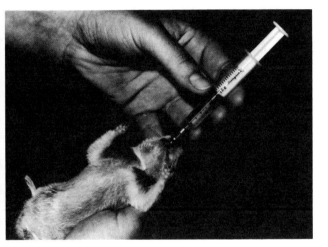

Figure 8—The instillation of fluids by gavage is shown.

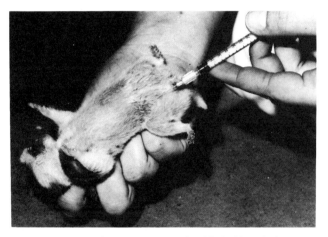

Figure 10—Peritoneal injections are made while holding the hamster's head down.

onto the tongue. The hamster can be held by the scruff of the neck or, if the animal is very tractable and enjoys the medication, in the palm of the hand.

One route of administration is by gavage, using a 1½ inch gavage needle with a ball on the tip. Figures 7 and 8 depict the holding technique in preparation for gavage and the instillation of fluids by gavage, respectively. Subcutaneous administration can be done in the loose skin over the shoulders of the hamster (Figure 9). Peritoneal injections are made while holding the hamster's head down (Figure 10), with care being taken not to insert the needle into the bladder or the viscera. Negative pressure should be applied to the syringe to insure that the needle is not in the intestinal tract. Intramuscular injections can be made into the muscle masses anterior and posterior to the femur. When entering the muscle mass posterior to the femur, the needle should be initially directed perpendicular to the surface until it has penetrated the skin; then it is directed parallel to the posterior surface of the thigh. Intravenous injections can be made into the femoral vein, but the animal must be completely immobilized for this procedure; anesthesia is usually required.

BIBLIOGRAPHY

1. Hoffman RA: Hibernation and effects of low temperature, in Hoffman RA, Robinson PF, Magalhaes H (eds): *The Golden Hamster: Its Biology and Uses in Medical Research*. Ames, IA, The Iowa State University Press, 1968.
2. Barthold SW, Jacoby RO, Pucak GJ: An outbreak of cecal mucosal hyperplasia in hamsters. *Lab Anim Sci* 28:723-727, 1978.
3. Brennan PC, Frits TE, Glynn RJ: *Pasteurella pneumotropica*: Cultural and Biochemical Characteristics, and its Association with Disease in Laboratory Animals. *Lab Anim Sci* 15:307-312, 1965.
4. Collins GR (ed): *Syllabus for the Laboratory Animal Technologist*. Joliet, IL, American Association for Laboratory Animal Science, 1972.
5. Dontenwill WHJ, Chevalier JJ, Harke HP, Lafreze U, Rechzeh G, Leuschnew F: Biochemical and hematological investigations in Syrian hamsters after cigarette smoke inhalation. *Lab Anim* 8:217-235, 1974.
6. Estes PC, Richter CB, Franklin JA: Demodectic mange in the golden hamster. *Lab Anim Sci* 21:825-828, 1971.
7. Ferm VH: The use of the golden hamster in experimental teratology. *Lab Anim Sci* 17:452-462, 1967.
8. Fisk CS, Wagner JE: Hamster enteritis, a review. *Lab Anim* 11:79-85, 1977.
9. Flatt RE, Kerber WT: Demodectic mite infestation in golden hamsters. *Lab Anim Dig* 4:6-7, 1968.
10. Flynn RJ: *Parasites of Laboratory Animals*. Ames, IA, The Iowa State University Press, 1973.
11. Gak JC, Graillot C, Truhaut P: Use of golden hamsters in toxicology. *Lab Anim Sci* 26:274-280, 1976.
12. Gleiser CA, Andrews EJ, Pick JR, Small JD, Weisbroth SH, Wescott RB, Wilsnack RE: *A Guide to Infectious Diseases of Guinea Pigs, Gerbils, Hamsters and Rabbits*. Washington, DC, Institute of Laboratory Animal Resources, National Academy of Sciences, 1974.
13. Gleiser CA, Van Hoosier GL, Sheldon WG, A polycystic disease of hamsters in a closed colony. *Lab Anim Sci* 20:923-929, 1970.
14. Gleiser CA, Van Hoosier GL, Sheldon WG, Read WK: Amyloidosis and renal paramyloid in a closed hamster colony. *Lab Anim Sci* 21:197-202, 1971.
15. Haberman RT: Spontaneous diseases and their control in laboratory animals. *Publ Health Rep* 74:165-169, 1959.
16. Haberman RT, Williams FP, Thorp WST, Identification of some internal parasites of laboratory animals. Public Health Service Publication, Washington, DC, 1958.
17. Hagen CA, Shefner AM, Ehrlich R: Intestinal microflora of normal hamsters. *Lab Anim Sci* 15:1835-193, 1965.
18. Harkness JE, Wagner JE: *The Biology and Medicine of Rabbits and Rodents*. Philadelphia, Lea & Febiger, 1977.
19. Hoffman RA, Robinson PE, Magalhaes H: *The Golden Hamster, Its Biology and Use in Medical Research*. Ames, IA, The Iowa State University Press, 1968.
20. Mortorana PA: The hamster as a model for experimental pulmonary emphysema. *Lab Anim Sci* 26:352-354, 1976.
21. *Nutrient Requirements of Laboratory Animals*, No. 10. Washington, DC, National Research Council, 1978.
22. Orsini MW: The external vaginal phenomena characterizing the stages of the estrous cycle, pregnancy, pseudopregnancy, lactation, and the anestrous hamster, *Mesocricetus auratus* (Waterhouse). *Proc Anim Care Panel* 11:193-206, 1961.
23. Pearson HE, Eaton MD: A virus pneumonia of Syrian hamster. *Proc Soc Exptl Biol Med* 45:677-679, 1940.
24. Perman V, Bergeland ME: A tularemia enzootic in a closed hamster breeding colony. *Lab Anim Sci* 17:563-568, 1967.
25. Renshaw H, Van Hoosier GL, Amend NK: A survey of naturally occurring diseases of the Syrian hamster. *Lab Anim* 9:179-191, 1979.
26. Small JD: Fatal enterocolitis in hamsters given lincomycin hydrochloride. *Lab Anim Sci* 18:411-420, 1968.
27. Soave OA: Diagnosis and control of common diseases of hamster, rabbits, and monkeys. *JAVMA* 142:285-290, 1963.
28. *Standard for the Breeding, Care and Management of Syrian Hamster*. Institute for Laboratory Animal Resources, National Research Council, National Academy of Sciences.
29. Williams CSF: *Practical Guide to Laboratory Animals*. Saint Louis, MO, The CV Mosby Co, 1976.

UPDATE

1. Harkness JE: Small rodents. *Vet Clin North Am [Small Anim Pract]* 24:89–102, 1994.

Laboratory Gerbils and Hamsters

Kay L. Stewart, RVT, LATg
Emily L. Johnstone, BS, RVT, LAT

Department of Biological Sciences
Freimann Life Science Center
University of Notre Dame
Notre Dame, Indiana

Veterinary technicians, whether working in biomedical research or in a veterinary practice, are likely to encounter gerbils and hamsters sometime during their careers. Because of their unique features, these species have become popular both as research tools and as pets. This article describes the maintenance and handling of gerbils and hamsters used for research; however, it also provides basic guidelines for those veterinary technicians who have contact with clients who own these species as pets.

History of Use in Research

Gerbils

Mongolian gerbils, also known as jirds, were first introduced into the United States in 1954 when Dr. Victor Schwentker obtained 11 breeding pairs from the Central Laboratory for Experimental Animals in Japan. Since then, gerbils have been used in various areas of research, including endocrinology, microbiology, and neurology.[1] Their docile and curious nature is just one of the characteristics that make gerbils appealing to the research scientist. Other favorable qualities include their low water consumption and low urine output, which make them easy to maintain; their high tolerance to temperature fluctuations; their ability to adjust to various diets; and their low incidence of naturally occurring diseases.

The major disadvantages to using gerbils in research are their quick, jerky movements, which make them difficult to catch, and their susceptibility to epileptiform convulsions.[2,3]

Hamsters

The species of hamsters most widely used in research is the Syrian hamster, also known as the golden hamster. As its name implies, this species was first obtained in Syria, where in 1930 a small litter was taken from a burrow. Golden hamsters were imported in 1938 into the United States, where they have become a valuable research animal for studies of dental disease, cancer, parasitology, and reproductive physiology. By 1971, hamsters had become the third most popular research animal, surpassed only by mice and rats.[4,5]

The unique anatomic and physiologic characteristics of hamsters appeal to research scientists. Other advantages of the use of hamsters include the short reproductive cycle and life span, relative freedom from spontaneous diseases, susceptibility to experimentally induced diseases, and acceptance of transplanted tissues and tumors because of its weak histocompatibility antigens.[5] The main disadvantage of using hamsters is that unpredictable and frequently aggressive behavior makes them difficult to handle.

Characteristics of the Species

Veterinary technicians working with gerbils and hamsters must familiarize themselves with the unique features of these species in order to distinguish normal behavior and appearance from clinical signs of disease. The spontaneous epileptiform seizures that normally plague as many as 20% of all gerbils can easily be mistaken for abnormal behavior by an inexperienced veterinary technician[2]; the distended cheek pouches that hamsters stuff with food or other materials (Figure 1) may appear to be abnormal facial growth.[6]

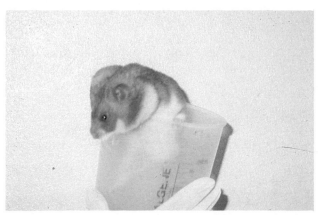

Figure 1—A hamster with cheek pouches that are stuffed with food can appear to have abnormal facial growth.

Although gerbils and hamsters seem very different, they share a few unusual characteristics. Both species have harderian glands, which are located behind the eyes, and scent glands located on the center of the surface of the abdomen on gerbils and on the flank area on hamsters.[7,8] The harderian glands produce pheromones that apparently play a role in sexual behavior, especially in gerbils; whereas the scent glands produce a secretion used to mark territories.[7,8] Because both species are resistant to radiation, they are ideal for radiobiological studies.[1,5]

The frequency of naturally occurring epileptiform seizures in gerbils has made them ideal subjects for neurologic studies; the frequent development of brain infarctions after unilateral ligation of the common carotid artery has made gerbils excellent models for studies of human cerebrovascular accidents or strokes.[8]

Because of the characteristics of their cheek pouches, hamsters are widely used in immunologic studies. The large cheek pouches are lined with buccal epithelium and are devoid of lymphatic glands and vessels; the pouches are therefore immunologically privileged areas that accept foreign tissue transplants that would normally be rejected. The immune system of hamsters has other characteristics that are atypical of other rodent species, including delayed cellular immunity (which is possibly caused by a short gestation period), lower response to certain antigens compared with that of other rodents, and absence of immunoglobulin D, which is one of the five described immunoglobulins.[5]

Because of their ability to develop dental caries similar to those that occur in humans, hamsters are commonly used in dental research. By providing hamsters with a defined diet and oral flora, the effect of such caries-inhibiting agents as fluorine can be tested.[5]

Hamsters hibernate at low temperatures (i.e., below 5 °C), although these conditions are not common in the controlled environment of a laboratory animal facility. Unlike other hibernating species, hamsters do not build up fat reserves before hibernation; if they do not awaken periodically to replenish their energy supply, they may starve to death.

Tables I and II present more detailed comparisons of the anatomic and physiologic features of gerbils and hamsters.

Sexing

The most common method of sexing rodents is by anogenital distance. In general, this distance is greater in males than in females—as much as two times greater in gerbils (Figures 2, 3, and 4). Because it can be difficult to determine the sex of an individual weanling, sexing these animals is most easily done by comparing several of the littermates.[2]

Other ways to sex gerbils include observing the darkened anogenital region of the scrotum in males, the larger body size of adult males, and the more pointed caudal end of males.[2] Hamsters can also be sexed by size; adult females are larger than males. Also, the caudal end of female hamsters is more pointed than that of males. The rounded look of male hamsters is attributable to the scrotum.

Handling and Restraint

Of the rodents most commonly used in research, hamsters tend to be the most difficult to handle, whereas gerbils are usually one of the easiest to handle. Both species, however, become well adjusted to restraint methods if handled routinely.

The restraint methods for gerbils are similar to those used for mice. To move a gerbil a short distance, grasp it by the base of the tail and gently lift it, taking precautions not to grasp near the tip of the tail because the skin around the tail can easily be stripped away. To restrain gerbils for injection or other procedures, either use the thumb and forefinger to grasp the skin at the base of the neck and lift into the palm of the hand or encircle the thorax with the thumb and finger (Figure 5).[8]

Whenever approaching gerbils, technicians should avoid sudden movements and loud noises in order to help prevent the onset of a seizure. Although some gerbils may still experience seizures even when they are not being handled, unnecessary excitement increases the potential for seizures.

Hamsters, which have a less predictable temperament, can be difficult to restrain. Because a hamster's tail is too short to grab, technicians must reach near the upper body and head to pick up a hamster. To lift a hamster, grasp the loose skin at the base of the neck (Figure 6) or surround the upper body with the thumb and fingers.[6] Care must be taken when holding hamsters by the scruff of the neck because they can still turn around and bite if not enough skin is grasped. Hamsters that are displaying obvious signs of aggression (e.g., teeth chattering, vocalization, or rolling onto their backs) can be picked up with the aid of a scoop or can.

Identification

To obtain data on laboratory animals, an accurate and understandable identification system must be established for each experimental animal or group of animals. A simple but impractical system is to house hamsters and gerbils

TABLE I

Comparison of Physiologic Data on Gerbils and Hamsters[9]

Feature	Gerbils	Hamsters
Birth weight (grams)	2.5–3	2
State of maturation at birth	Altricial	Altricial
Adult weight (grams)	Males 80–110; females 70–100	Males 85–130; females 95–150
Body temperature (°C)	35.8–39.0[a]	35.0–37.4[b]
Respiration rate (breaths/min)	90	90
Heart rate (beats/min)	360	275–425
Life span (years)	2–4	2–3
Daily food consumption (grams food/100 grams body weight/day)	5–8	10–12
Daily water consumption (ml water/100 grams body weight/day)	4–7	8–10

[a]96.4 °F–102.2 °F
[b]95 °F–99.3 °F

singly, using cage cards as the only identification system. Because of space limitations, however, most facilities try to house two or more animals together; a system to identify individuals therefore must be implemented. Temporary systems, such as hair clipping or dyes, can be used for short-term projects; but more permanent systems should be used for long-term projects. The best method of permanent identification for both species is the ear punch and ear notch system; the major disadvantage of this system is the possibility that ears may get torn during fights and the identification number may thus become difficult to read. Other types of permanent methods include toe punching (for small groups of animals) or ear tags.[2,4]

Management

Because of their social nature, gerbils seem to fare better when housed in pairs or in small groups. If introduced before sexual maturity, pairs or groups of either females or males are usually compatible. Overcrowding can lead to fighting among any combination of gerbils.

In general, hamsters can be housed in small groups. If fighting does occur, the remaining cagemates usually remain compatible if the aggressive animal is identified and removed.

If gerbils and hamsters are housed in groups, all cages should be observed daily for signs of fighting. The most common indications of fighting are sores or hair loss around the base of the tail, especially in males. Although overcrowding is usually the cause of aggression, some animals are naturally incompatible and should be housed singly.

How often the cages should be cleaned depends on the species, the cage population, the bedding material, and the ventilation system. Federal guidelines must also be considered, although they are often below the standards established by individual facilities.

TABLE II

Comparison of Anatomic Features of Gerbils and Hamsters[4,6,10,11]

Feature	Gerbils	Hamsters
Vertebral formula	C_7, T_{13}, L_6, S_4, Cx_{7+}	C_7, T_{13}, L_6, S_4, Cx_{13-14}
Dental formula	$2(I\frac{1}{1}, C\frac{0}{0}, P\frac{0}{0}, M\frac{3}{3})$	$2(I\frac{1}{1}, C\frac{0}{0}, P\frac{0}{0}, M\frac{3}{3})$
Number of toes	4 toes front 5 toes rear	4 toes front 5 toes rear
Number of mammary glands	8	12–17
Accessory sex glands	Ampullar glands, seminal vesicles, coagulating gland, prostate glands, Cowper's glands	Ampullar glands, seminal vesicles, coagulating gland, prostate glands, Cowper's glands

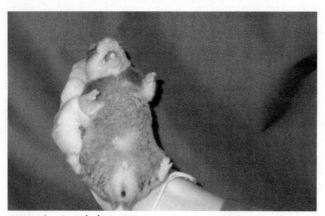

Figure 2—A male hamster.

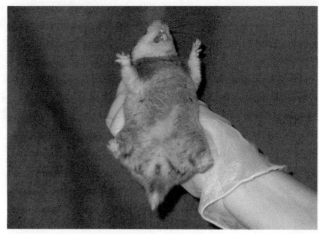

Figure 3—A female hamster.

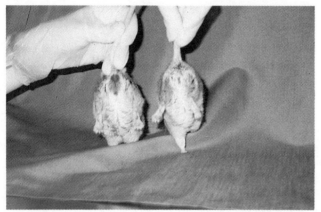

Figure 4—The male gerbil is on the left and the female gerbil is on the right. Note the darkened scrotal area of the male.

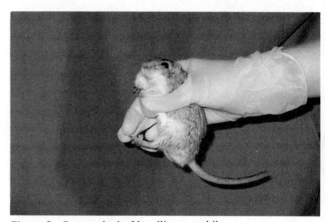

Figure 5—One method of handling a gerbil.

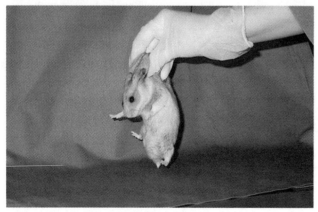

Figure 6—The proper way to lift a hamster by the scruff of the neck. Note the large amount of excess skin.

The absence of odor in the animal room should not be the determining factor in establishing guidelines for cage cleaning; a good ventilation system can mask an odor problem in a room. The odor within the animal cage itself should be the indicator of how often it needs to be cleaned. The odor in the cages is caused by ammonia, which is re-leased as urine evaporates. Increased ammonia levels can lead to serious health problems for the animals, potentially destroying an entire experiment.

Because of the high concentrating power of their kidneys, the resultant low urine output, and the low water content of their feces, gerbils require less frequent cage cleaning than most other rodents require. Considerations must be made, however, for cage population and environmental conditions (e.g., temperature and humidity); breeding cages with unweaned pups may need to be cleaned as often as every two or three days.[8]

Hamsters produce a highly alkaline urine that contains many crystals; their cages are therefore quickly soiled despite their habit of urinating only in one area of the cage. Their cages are also difficult to clean; most cages require an acid soak before regular cleaning.[8] Table III presents recommended environmental conditions for gerbils and hamsters.

Nutrition

Commercially prepared rodent feeds fulfill the basic nutritional requirements for gerbils; however, it may be necessary to supplement the hamster diet with additional vita-

TABLE III
Recommended Environmental Conditions
for Gerbils and Hamsters[4,8]

Conditions	Gerbils	Hamsters
Temperature (°C)	21–22[a]	20–24[b]
Humidity (%)	40–50	45–55
Light cycle	12 hours on/ 12 hours off	12 hours on/ 12 hours off
Ventilation (air changes/hour)	15–20	15–20

[a]70 °F–72 °F
[b]68 °F–75 °F

TABLE IV
Reproductive Data on
Gerbils and Hamsters[4,8]

Feature	Gerbils	Hamsters
Age of breeding onset (weeks)	10–12	6–7
Cycle length (days)	4–6	4
Gestation period (days)	24–26	15–18
Weaning age (days)	21	21
Breeding life span	1–2 years (4–10 litters)	1 year (5 litters)
Litter size	4–6	5–9

mins and minerals. Gerbils and hamsters can be given sunflower seeds in moderation, although such treats are not required. If sunflower seeds are readily accessible, gerbils will eat them exclusively; this behavior can lead to calcium deficiency and increases in body fat. Excessive amounts of dietary fat cause a buildup of fat around the ovaries of female gerbils; this buildup shortens the animal's reproductive life.

Muscular dystrophy caused by a vitamin E deficiency is possible in any hamsters that display general muscle weakness. Hamsters require higher dietary levels of such minerals as zinc, copper, and potassium than other rodents require; these minerals may need to be added to the basic diet.[5]

Manufacturers of animal diets should be consulted before any alterations in basic animal diets are made. Most diets are made to meet all nutritional requirements and can actually become nutritionally unbalanced if supplements are added. Table I presents daily feed and water requirements for hamsters and gerbils.

Breeding Systems

Before establishing breeding colonies of gerbils and hamsters, technicians must collaborate with investigators to ensure that all needs will be met. The type of colony (e.g., inbred or outbred) and the type of records to be kept must be established. Also, estimates of the ages and number of animals needed each week should be made. Once these guidelines have been set, efficient and productive breeding colonies can be established.

Gerbils intended for breeding should be paired just before sexual maturity (i.e., at approximately eight weeks of age). Gerbils are generally monogamous and rarely accept a new mate even after the old one is removed. Because males take an active part in rearing the young, they are usually left in the breeding cage at all times unless it is undesirable to breed a female during her postpartum estrus.[8]

Hamsters can be bred using various systems, including hand mating, sequential monogamous mating systems, or a harem breeding system. In hand mating, the male and female are placed together for a short period of time, usually 30 minutes, when the female is believed to be in heat. The pair should be closely observed; if the female is not in heat, she may fight with and may even try to kill the male. This system is used if the exact time of mating must be known.

In a sequential monogamous mating system, one male is rotated among seven females; each female is housed with the male for one-week intervals. Each time the male is reintroduced to the female, the pair should be closely observed for the first hour to ensure that the female accepts him. This system is cost-effective because it requires only a few males.

The harem system, in which three to five males are caged with 10 to 12 females, is commonly used to breed hamsters. The females are removed from the breeding cage on the seventh to tenth day to be housed individually until their litters are born and reared. This system is both cost-effective and time-effective. Its main disadvantages are the inability to keep accurate records and the increased incidence of fighting, especially among the females. Table IV presents specific reproductive data for gerbils and hamsters.

Conclusion

The popularity of gerbils and hamsters as research animals is increasing as investigators discover their value. These animals are also widely accepted as household pets. All technicians in research and clinical practices can have an impact on the health of these small mammals.

REFERENCES

1. Robinson DG Jr: Tumblebrook gerbils: 30th anniversary. *Gerbil Digest* 11(1):1–4, 1984.
2. Schaefers FF: The Mongolian gerbil, in Sapanski WB Jr, Harkness JE (eds): *Manual for Assistant Laboratory Animal Technicians.* Joliet, IL, American Association for Laboratory Animal Science, 1984, pp 198–205.
3. Robichaud D: Gerbils: The basic facts. *Vet Tech* 7(5):223–225, 1986.
4. VanHoosier GL Jr, McPherson CW: *Laboratory Hamsters.* Orlando, FL, Academic Press, 1987, pp 10–43, 61–70.
5. VanHoosier GL Jr, Ladiges WC: Biology and diseases of hamsters, in Fox JG, Cohen BJ, Loew FM (eds): *Laboratory Animal Medicine.* Orlando, FL, Academic Press, 1984, pp 123–132.

6. Williams CSF: *Practical Guide to Laboratory Animals*. St. Louis, The CV Mosby Co, 1976, pp 26–32.
7. Port CD: Anatomy, in Collins GR (ed): *Syllabus for the Laboratory Animal Technologist*. Joliet, IL, American Association for Laboratory Science, 1972, pp 111–114.
8. Holmes DD: The Mongolian gerbil in biomedical research. *Lab Anim Sci* 14(3):23–36, 1985.
9. Harkness JE, Wagner JE: *Biology and Husbandry in the Biology and Medicine of Rabbits and Rodents*. Philadelphia, Lea & Febiger, 1983, pp 25–32.
10. Robinson DG Jr: Reproduction in the Mongolian gerbil. *Gerbil Digest* 5(1):1–4, 1978.
11. Williams WH: *The Anatomy of the Mongolian Gerbil (Meriones unguiculatus)*. West Brookfield, MA, Tumblebrook Farm, 1974.
12. Stewart KL, Johnstone EL, Vecera JA: The laboratory mouse and rat. *Vet Tech* 9(5):264–272, 1988.

The Laboratory Mouse and Rat

Kay L. Stewart, RVT, LATg
Emily L. Johnstone, BS, RVT, LAT
June A. Vecera, RVT, LAT

Freimann Life Science Center
University of Notre Dame
Notre Dame, Indiana

Mice and rats are the animals most commonly used in biomedical research. Approximately 30 million to 40 million mice[1] and 10 million rats[2] are used annually; together they constitute 90% of the number of animals used in research each year.[3] Both species have been used in a wide variety of studies, ranging from the study of infectious diseases to the development of organ transplant procedures. The advantages of using mice and rats include their prolificity in breeding, short gestation periods and life spans, and manageability; the availability of inbred strains; and the large amount of data available for both species.[4,5] In this article, the general care and use of mice and rats in research will be described.

Strains of Mice and Rats

As mice and rats became more popular in research studies, investigators began to realize that they could genetically alter the animals through selective breeding to create animals that would yield more consistent and predictable results. The animals thus created have been termed *inbred strains*. The inbred strains are the result of at least 20 generations of consecutive brother × sister or parent × offspring matings. Inbred animals are genetically identical with respect to all highly heritable traits, such as blood type, tissue type, and biochemical properties. Therefore, tissue grafts from one animal, for example, will not be rejected by another animal within the same strain.[6]

Inbred strains must be carefully maintained and monitored to assure genetic purity and to detect any mutations that occur. Substrains do develop, however, as a result of the natural occurrence of mutations within the lines; this occurrence is referred to as *genetic drift*. A substrain will be unique to the breeding facility in which it develops.

When identifying an inbred strain, the substrain or the origin of the strain should always be given, because animals from the same strain but from different substrains may have enough genetic variance to affect a study.[6] Examples of strain and substrain designations are listed (see box—Strains of Mice and Rats).

Currently, there are more than 250 strains of inbred mice and more than 100 strains of inbred rats. New strains are constantly being developed. Mice that are genetically identical at all but one known locus on the chromosome (referred to as *coisogeneic* mice) have been developed to study the effect that that one particular gene has on an entire system. Inbred strains can be cross mated to form first-filial-generation, or F_1, hybrids. Hybrid mice are more vigorous than their inbred parents, yet they are still genetically identical. Thus, they are considered an important tool in many types of studies, especially immunologic studies.[6]

Although inbred mice have many advantageous characteristics, they do have some negative ones that limit their

Strains of Mice and Rats[7]	
Inbred Mice	**Outbred Mice**
AKR	Sencar
Balb/c	ICR
CBA/J	ND/4 Swiss
DBA	NIH Swiss
C57BL/10ScN	Swiss Webster
C57BL/6N	
Inbred Rats	**Outbred Rats**
Fischer	Sprague-Dawley (SD)
Lewis	Long-Evans (LE)
Copenhagen 2331	Wistar (WI)
Buffalo	
Brown Norway	
Spontaneous Hypertensive (SHR)	

use. Because they are inbred, they are much less vigorous than outbred mice. They are more difficult to breed; their average litter size is generally only half the size of that of outbred mice. Some inbred strains are very susceptible to various diseases and must be housed apart from other animals and even apart from other inbred strains. The decision of what strain of mouse or rat to use in a particular study must be made by a competent investigator or with the help of the breeding facility's veterinarian.[6]

Species Variations

Technicians working in laboratory animal medicine should be aware of the many anatomic differences between the various species with which they routinely work. Many species have unique features that may seem insignificant but can have a major influence on an experiment. Mice and rats, although similar in many aspects, have unique features that make them reasonable or unreasonable choices for specific research projects.

One of the distinguishing anatomic features of mice is that the bone marrow of the long bones is functional throughout their lives; whereas in rats and most other species, the marrow is replaced with fat in adulthood. Also, the mouse's thymus, unlike that of other species, does not regress with age. Another feature specific to mice is the presence of a brown fat gland, known as the *hibernating gland*. This light brown fatty tissue is found in various areas of the body, particularly between the scapulae, in the cervical region, within the thymus, and near the kidneys. Although this gland is considered an endocrine gland, there is no evidence that its secretions have hormonal function.[8]

In both mice and rats, the spleen size is greatly variable. It is common to see accessory splenic tissue in the pancreas

and in fat lobules of the mesentery in mice,[8] however, and not in rats.

The most obvious distinguishing feature of rats is that they lack a gallbladder. Instead, there are small tributary ducts that unite to form the bile duct.[8] More-detailed comparisons of the anatomic and physiologic features of mice and rats are presented in Tables I and II.[8,9]

Handling and Restraint

To avoid injury to themselves and the animals, technicians must learn the proper methods for restraining mice and rats. Both species will bite out of fear when improperly or roughly handled. When physically restraining a rodent, the handler must be firm, yet gentle. If held too loosely, the animal can get free or can bite; and if it is held too tightly, its air supply can be cut off, or other injury to the animal can result. The first time an animal is handled is usually the most difficult; once the animal has become accustomed to the handler and the types of restraint used, it learns to accept the routine.[10]

The common procedures that require restraint of the animals involved are injections, physical examinations, and blood sampling. For injections and physical examinations, physical restraint is all that is needed; whereas blood sampling usually requires chemical restraint.[1,10]

The method most commonly used for picking up a mouse or a rat is to lift it by the base of the tail. The use of this method should be limited to removing the animal from its cage to be placed into another cage or onto a nearby surface. The animal should not be held by its tail for a prolonged period of time because from this position it can swing up onto the handler's hand and can possibly bite. Also, care must be taken to grab the animal only near the base of the tail. If the animal is held by the tip of the tail, the sheath around the tail can slough, leaving the skin and vertebrae exposed.[1,10]

A mouse, because it is small, can easily be restrained with one hand, so that the other hand can be used to perform various procedures. To hold a mouse properly, the following steps should be taken: Pick up the mouse by the base of the tail and place it on a rough surface (cage top or wire mesh); gently pull back on its tail to cause the mouse to grab onto the surface (Figure 1); with the thumb and forefinger, grab the loose skin at the scruff of the neck (Figure 2); turn the hand so that the palm is facing upward; tuck the tail under the fourth and fifth fingers for additional control (Figure 3).[11]

Unlike the mouse, the rat usually requires two-hand restraint for total control. A common way to hold a rat is by grasping it around the thorax, just under the forelimbs. When attempting to pick up the rat in this fashion, the handler should first remove it from its cage by the base of the tail (Figure 4) and place it on a flat surface while maintaining a grip on the tail; the handler should then approach the rat from above and place a hand around the thorax. Care must be taken not to squeeze the rat's chest too tightly, be-

TABLE I

Comparison of Anatomic Features of Mice and Rats[8,9]

Feature	Mice	Rats
Vertebral formula	C7, T12–14, L5–6, S4, Cx27–30	C7, T13, L6, S4, Cx27–30
Dental formula	$2(I\frac{1}{1}, C\frac{0}{0}, P\frac{0}{0}, M\frac{3}{3})$	$2(I\frac{1}{1}, C\frac{0}{0}, P\frac{0}{0}, M\frac{3}{3})$
Number of toes	5 toes front / 4 toes rear	4 toes front / 5 toes rear
Number of mammary glands	5 pairs (3 pairs thoracic; (2 pairs abdominal)	6 pairs (3 pairs thoracic and 3 pairs abdominal, with a gap in the middle)
Accessory sex glands	One pair of prostate glands / One pair of seminal vesicles / One pair of bulbourethral glands / One pair of ampullary glands	Two pairs of prostate glands / One pair of seminal vesicles / One pair of bulbourethral glands / One pair of ampullary glands / One pair of coagulating glands
Type of uterus	Bicornuate with a single cervix	Bicornuate with separate cervices

cause it is easy to cut off the rat's air supply. The handler can then gain better control of the rat by grasping the tail with the other hand (Figure 5). Once the rat is secured, a second technician can give an injection or a physical examination or complete any other procedure.[2]

Most rats can be handled easily without injury to either the handler or the animal. On some occasions, however, it may be necessary to wear protective gloves (e.g., leather or wire-mesh gloves) to avoid injury. If gloves are necessary, the handler must be especially attentive to the amount of pressure applied to the rat's chest, because this is difficult to feel through protective gloves.

Commercial restrainers are available for restraining rats and mice. These devices usually allow access to either the head or the tail and to various areas along the body that are common injection sites. The advantage of such a device is

TABLE II

Comparison of Physiologic Data of Mice and Rats[1,10]

Feature	Mice	Rats
Birth weight (g)	0.5 to 1.5	5 to 6
State of maturation at birth	Altricial	Altricial
Adult weight (g)	Males: 20 to 40 / Females: 25 to 40	Males: 450 to 520 / Females: 250 to 300
Body temperature (°C)	36 to 38	35.0 to 37.5
Respiration rate (breaths/min)	94 to 163	70 to 115
Heart rate (beats/min)	325 to 780	250 to 450
Life span (years)	1.5 to 3	2.5 to 3.5
Food consumption (g/100 g body wt/day)	15	10
Water consumption (ml/100 g body wt/day)	15	10 to 12

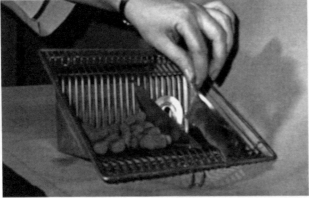

Figure 1—The first step in restraining a mouse is to lift it by the base of the tail and place it on a cage top, so that it will stretch out and grab onto the wires.

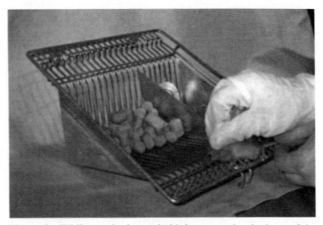

Figure 2—While continuing to hold the mouse by the base of the tail, the handler grasps the loose skin at the back of the mouse's neck.

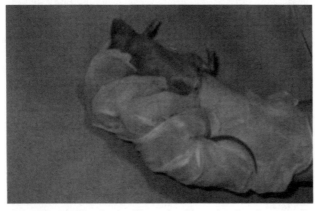

Figure 3—Finally, the handler turns his or her hand so that the palm is up and tucks the mouse's tail under the fourth and fifth fingers. (The mouse in Figures 1, 2, and 3 is an inbred mouse, a C_3H/HEJ.)

that it allows work to be accomplished by one person. Many times, however, it is more time-consuming to get the animal into the restrainer and contained properly than it is to use a two-person team.

Identification

Some type of animal identification system must be established for all research projects to assure that animals do not get confused with those from another study or with others within the same study. The cage card system is widely used, often in conjunction with another, more individualized system. The more commonly used permanent identification systems used on rodents are the ear punch system, the ear notch system, and a combination of both (Figure 6). Other permanent systems of identification include tail clipping and toe clipping. Dyes, hair clipping, or marking pens can be used to identify an animal temporarily.[1,10]

Male rodents can be distinguished from female rodents by the anal-genital distance. The anal-genital distance is greater in males than it is in females (Figure 7). To determine the sex of a particular rodent, it may be necessary to compare the rodent with another of the opposite sex.

Housing

The environmental conditions surrounding a laboratory animal can have a significant influence on the outcome of an experiment. Housing systems should be designed to provide comfort to the animal, meet federal guidelines, and reduce the number of unwanted experimental variables. The *housing system* includes the immediate environment—the cage, the rack that holds the cage, and the room in which the cage resides.[12]

Basic guidelines for optimum animal room conditions have been established by the federal government. Specifications have been made for lighting, ventilation, temperature, and humidity. The optimum lighting intensity for mice and rats is 75 to 100 foot-candles, on a cycle of 12 hours off and then 12 hours on. Ventilation is a major element of an animal's environment. It affects the regulation of temperature and humidity and the control of disease. The optimum ventilation is 15 to 20 air changes per hour. Thermostats should be set between 64° and 78°F with a variance of $\pm$ 2°F; and the humidity should be controlled to be within the range of 40% to 70%. Continual variance in any of these environmental parameters creates an unwanted variable in an experiment and could nullify experimental results.[1,10]

Nutrition

To obtain accurate results from experiments that involve animals, a scientist must start with healthy animals. Nutrition is vital to the health of experimental animals. Without proper diet, subtle physiologic changes can occur in the animals; such changes can negate an entire study.[13]

The most important nutrient for all species is water. Death can result from the loss of 10% of total body water. Thus, unless an experimental protocol states otherwise, mice and rats must have access to clean water at all times.[13]

Although dietary requirements depend on the physiologic status of the animal, in most circumstances commer-

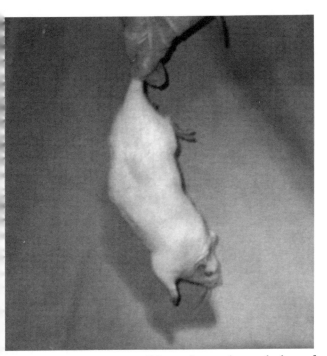

Figure 4—The proper way to lift a rat is to grab near the base of the tail, not the tip.

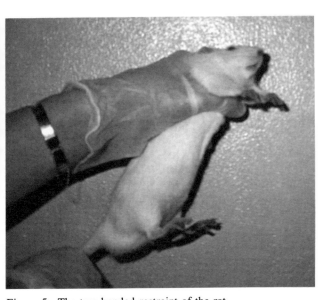

Figure 5—The two-handed restraint of the rat.

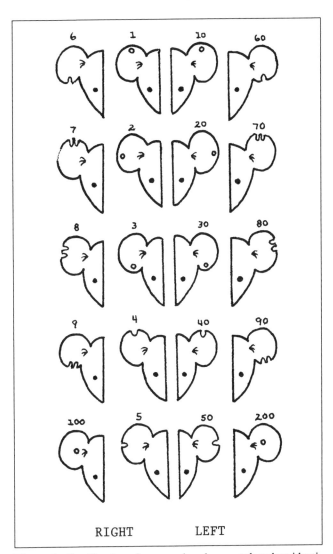

RIGHT   LEFT

Figure 6—Combination of ear-punch and ear-notch rodent identification system. By various combinations of notches and punches, rodents can be identified with a one-, two-, or three-digit number.

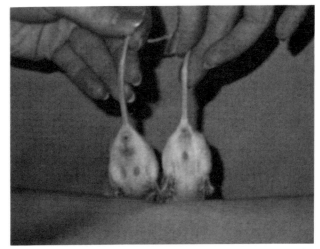

Figure 7—The anal-genital distance is the feature that distinguishes male rodents from female rodents. Shown above is a female mouse on the *left* and a male mouse on the *right*. Note that the anal-genital distance of the male is greater than that of the female.

cially produced feeds meet the nutritional needs of mice and rats. General rodent feed (e.g., Purina Rodent Laboratory Chow®—Ralston Purina) is designed to meet the dietary requirements of both mice and rats. It is formulated to reduce unwanted nutritional variables and will meet the needs of most experimental mice and rats with the exception of those being bred and those maintained in germ-free isolators. Special diets are commercially available for these animals with more particular needs. The feed used for breeders has an increased fat content; that used for axenic (germ-free) animals contains an increase of heat-

TABLE III
Reproductive Data of Mice and Rats[1,10]

Feature	Mice	Rats
Age at breeding onset (days)	50	65 to 110
Cycle length (days)	4 to 5	4 to 5
Gestation period (days)	19 to 21	21 to 23
Weaning age (days)	21 to 28	21
Breeding life span	8 mo (6 to 10 litters)	1.5 yr (7 to 10 litters)
Litter size	5 to 10	7 to 11

labile vitamins to allow the feed to remain nutritionally balanced after being steam sterilized.[13]

If experimental design requires the addition of other nutrients or an increase of those in the general formula, it is wise to consult with a feed manufacturer before altering the diet. Nutrient imbalances can be caused by altering specially formulated diets; such imbalances can endanger the health of animals.[13]

Breeding Colonies

The experimental requirements of a research facility may call for the establishment of an in-house breeding colony of mice or rats. The many benefits of having an in-house breeding colony usually outweigh the additional work and responsibility that it places on the facility's staff.

For an in-house breeding colony to be successful, there must be good communication between the technician that supervises the colony and the investigators that use animals from it. The colony should generate the minimum number of animals required to fulfill experimental needs. A surplus of animals results in having to euthanatize those not needed, and a shortage delays experimental procedures.

The major advantages of an in-house breeding colony include eliminating shipping costs; being able to provide investigators with a few animals at a time; being able to provide animals at various ages—from one-day-old pups to retired breeders; and the elimination of quarantine time. Some disadvantages to having an in-house breeding colony include the amount of time needed to maintain a well-run colony; the added care and recordkeeping required to maintain true inbred or true random outbred lines; and the additional monitoring required to maintain specific pathogen–free animals. When breeding in-house, to assure that proper genetic lines are being maintained, routine genetic monitoring should be done or animals should be routinely replaced by stock from a commercial breeder that does genetic monitoring of its colony.[6] The health of inbred animals should be checked by regular testing for common murine diseases. These tests can be done in-house with kits that are commercially available or they can be done by a commercial diagnostic laboratory. Investigators must be kept informed of any changes in the health status of the animals; these changes can introduce an unwanted variable into experiments.

The type of breeding systems used in a colony should be determined by the needs of the investigators. If exact records must be kept on each litter, then a monogamous system should be used. Also referred to as *intensive breeding*, this system involves the pairing of one female and one male for their entire breeding life. Advantages of this system are that it allows exact records to be kept; females can be bred on the postpartum estrus, which results in an increased frequency of litters; and it eliminates the females' fight for dominance, which occurs in other systems. The major disadvantage of a monogamous system is that it requires more males than other systems do.[1,10]

The other type of system that can be used is the polygamous, or harem, breeding system. By housing one male with two or more females, this system allows for maximum production of young with a minimum number of males. Keeping accurate records of each litter is not possible, however, unless the females are removed from the breeding cages before parturition. If the parturient female is left to deliver pups in the breeding cage, the other females will help in the rearing of the young, thus making it impossible to positively identify the real mother. By removing females from the breeding cage for parturition to aid in the recordkeeping, the chance for females to be bred during the postpartum estrus is eliminated, and the frequency of litters born to each female is reduced. Another disadvantage of the polygamous system is that the females in the breeding cage are in a constant battle for dominance, especially when they are returned to the cage after being removed to have their litters.[1,10]

When setting up the breeding cages, the animals to be mated must be properly selected: brother × sister matings for inbreds, and unrelated animals for outbreds. The intended breeders must be paired at the right age. If paired when they are too young, they may always be just cage mates and may never reproduce; if they are paired when they are too old, they may not accept each other. Specific reproductive data for mice and rats are presented in Table III.[1,10]

Conclusion

A brief overview of the many considerations that go into the daily maintenance of laboratory mice and rats has been presented. Technicians entering the field of laboratory animal science should review the literature available on laboratory animal medicine and should establish contacts with people in the field to expand their knowledge of laboratory animal medicine. Clear communication between technicians and the investigators whose animals the technicians are caring for is also very important to assure that the investigators' needs are being met.

REFERENCES

1. Leard BC: The mouse, in Sapanski WB Jr, Harkness JE (eds): *Manual for Assistant Laboratory Animal Technicians*, AALAS Publication 84-1. Joliet, IL, American Association for Laboratory Animal Science, 1984, pp 141–154.
2. Williams CSF: The rat, in *Practical Guide to Laboratory Animals*. St. Louis, The CV Mosby Co, 1976, pp 52–64.
3. Holden C: A pivotal year for lab animal welfare. *Science* 232:147–150, 1986.
4. Jonas AM: The mouse in biomedical research, in Gay WI (ed): *Health Benefits of Animal Research*. Washington, DC, 1987, Foundation for Biomedical Research, pp 1–20.
5. Gill TJ III, Harrington GM: The rat in biomedical research, in Gay WI (ed): *Health Benefits of Animal Research*. Washington, DC, 1987, Foundation for Biomedical Research, pp 31–40.
6. Laboratory animal management: Genetics. *Instit Lab Anim Resources News* 1(1):1979.
7. Harlan Sprague Dawley, Inc: *Laboratory Animal Price List 1987-88*. Indianapolis, IN, Harlan Sprague Dawley, July, 1987.
8. Port CD: Anatomy, in Collins GR (ed): *Syllabus for the Laboratory Animal Technologist*, AALAS Publication 72-2. Joliet, IL, American Association for Laboratory Animal Science, 1972, pp 111–114.
9. Jahn S: Advanced anatomy and physiology, in Stephans UK, Patton NM (eds): *Manual for Laboratory Animal Technicians*, AALAS Publication 84-2. Joliet, IL, American Association for Laboratory Animal Science, 1984, pp 13–65.
10. Stone J: The rat, in Sapanski WB Jr, Harkness JE (eds): *Manual for Assistant Laboratory Animal Technicians*, AALAS Publication 84-1. Joliet, IL, American Association for Laboratory Animal Science, 1984, pp 155–168.
11. Williams CSF: The mouse, in *Practical Guide to Laboratory Animals*. St. Louis, The CV Mosby Co, 1976, pp 41–51.
12. Inglis JK: *Introduction to Laboratory Animal Science and Technology*. Oxford, Pergamon Press Ltd, 1980, pp 7–33.
13. *Animal Diet Reference Guide*. St. Louis, Purina Mills, 1987, pp 4–8.

The Pet Guinea Pig

Margi Sirois, MS, RVT
Department of Animal Science
Camden County College
Blackwood, New Jersey

Guinea pigs (*Cavia porcellus*) are docile rodents that are popular as pets. They are more closely related to porcupines and chinchillas than to mice and rats. Their tranquil nature, relatively low cost, and ease of maintenance make guinea pigs excellent pets. They seldom bite or scratch, respond pleasantly to regular handling, and can be conditioned to squeal before such reward situations as the owner approaching the cage.

Although guinea pigs are generally hardy, poor husbandry practices will lead to immediate deterioration in health. A good husbandry program provides a system of housing and care that permits animals to grow, mature, and maintain good health. A thriving guinea pig has a higher resistance to disease than an unhealthy one does. Part of an owner's responsibility is to prevent the occurrence of disease and injury.[1]

The average life span of domesticated guinea pigs is three to four years. The most common pet variety is the English, or short-haired, guinea pig. Other varieties are the Abyssinian (with short, rough hair arranged in a rosette pattern) and the long-haired Peruvian. Because the varieties are often interbred, an abundance of colors and hair lengths is available[2] (Figure 1).

Handling and Restraint

Guinea pigs are easily frightened, make energetic attempts to escape being caught, and often struggle and squeal when handled. They can be lifted by grasping the trunk with one hand while supporting the hindquarters with the other hand (Figure 2). A pig must be handled gently because the lungs can be injured if the animal is grasped too firmly on the back. Support of the hindquarters is especially important when pregnant animals are being handled because it prevents struggling.[3]

Factors Predisposing to Disease

Housing and nutrition must be emphasized in the client education program, as these factors play important roles in disease predisposition. Guinea pigs are ordinarily quite vigorous but are extremely susceptible to environmental factors that reduce resistance to infection. These factors include poor sanitation, overcrowding, improper temperature and humidity control, and inadequate diet (particularly insufficient vitamin C).[1] Even a simple change in the location of a cage can cause some weight loss.

Illness might not be immediately obvious to an untrained observer. In general, healthy guinea pigs are tense, anxious, and alert. On the other hand, listlessness and leanness are unfavorable signs.[4]

Housing

Guinea pigs are not apt to climb and thus can be kept in open-top cages with sides at least 10 inches high.[1] A full-grown guinea pig requires approximately 101 square inches of floor space. A large aquarium is usually suitable. Solid floors with approximately two inches of bedding are difficult to clean but are preferred, especially for breeding animals. The bedding can be wood shavings or shredded paper. A box with a grid or mesh floor is easier to clean, but limbs are often broken if pigs that have not been raised on wire are then placed in housing with this type of floor.

Originally published in Volume 10, Number 1, January/February 1989

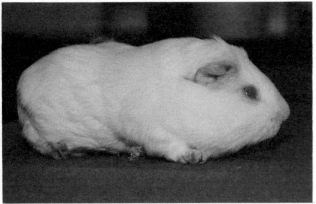

Figure 1A

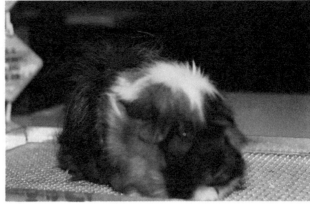

Figure 1B

Figure 1—The wide variety of hair color and length among guinea pigs includes (**A**) white short-haired guinea pigs and (**B**) tricolored Abyssinian guinea pigs.

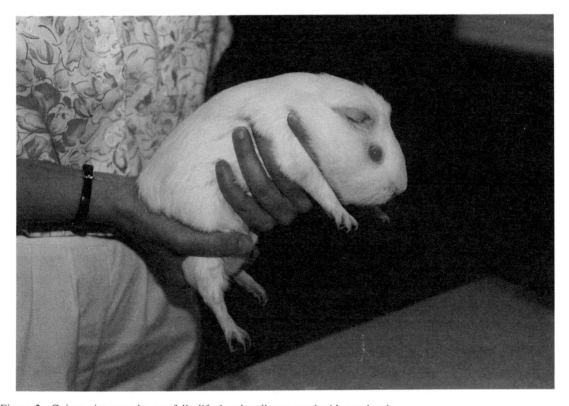

Figure 2—Guinea pigs must be carefully lifted and well supported with two hands.

If a young guinea pig must be put on mesh flooring, a piece of cardboard placed on the floor will ease the transition from a solid floor. By the time the animal has chewed up the cardboard and grown larger, it will have learned to walk safely on wire.[4]

Room temperature should be maintained between 65° and 75°F, and the cage should not be placed in direct sunlight. Guinea pigs kept singly in cages with wire floors require a higher room temperature than those kept in groups or in cages with solid sides and floors.[5] Ideal environmental humidity is between 45% and 55%. Temperature and humidity should be kept constant because guinea pigs are sensitive to extremes.

Adequate ventilation without excessive drafts should be provided. A simple method of air exchange is the use of a cage that has one or more wire-mesh sides. High temperature without adequate airflow predisposes to heat stress; low temperature and wet bedding predispose to pneumonia.[2]

Feeding and Nutrition

Feed is usually supplied ad libitum in a hanging feeder.

Porcelain bowls placed inside cages have been used, but this method allows feed to be contaminated with excreta. The preferred feed is pelleted and specifically labeled for guinea pigs. Like humans and monkeys, guinea pigs require a dietary source of vitamin C.[2] Rabbit feed looks like guinea pig chow but is lower in protein and lacks vitamin C. A guinea pig fed rabbit feed will demonstrate signs of vitamin C deficiency (scurvy) within two weeks.[1] It is important that the chow be no more than three months old (from time of manufacture) because vitamin C quickly loses its potency. The feed bag will normally be stamped with the date of manufacture[5]; feed should be purchased in small amounts to ensure its use within the three-month period.[6]

If there is doubt about the freshness of the feed, vitamin C should be supplemented directly. The preferred method of supplementation is mixing a small amount of L-ascorbic acid powder in the pet's water daily. Vitamin C can also be supplied in the form of such fresh vegetables as cabbage, kale, and carrots. These are relatively expensive sources of vitamin C. Some guinea pigs, however, will refuse to eat pelleted food if offered fresh vegetables. Lettuce in large amounts produces diarrhea and should be avoided.[7]

Like feed bowls, open water bowls usually become contaminated with excreta. An inverted bottle with a small sipper tube can be attached to the inside of the cage and suspended just above the bedding. Guinea pigs often play with the sipper tube, causing excessively wet bedding and wasted water; to alleviate this problem, a ball-bearing rather than a valveless sipper tube can be used.[6]

Guinea pigs often mix food and water in their mouths and then pass the mixture back into the sipper tube, causing a green discoloration of the water that resembles the color of algae.[2] The bottle and sipper tube should therefore be cleansed with each daily water change to avoid bacterial overgrowth in the bottle.

Reproduction

Guinea pigs are normally bred at three to five months of age. Females bred later often experience dystocia caused by fusion of the pubic symphysis.[2]

Sexing

In guinea pigs, unlike other rodents, anogenital distance is not an accurate method of determining sex. Instead, the guinea pig should be restrained and the shape of the external genitalia examined. The female's genital area appears Y shaped; the male's looks more like a straight slit. Gender can also be verified by exerting slight digital pressure cranial and caudal to the genital region; this pressure causes extrusion of the penis in males.[2]

Pregnancy and Parturition

The gestation period ranges from 63 to 70 days; average litter size is three to four (Table I). Most females come into estrus 2 to 15 hours postpartum; another mating is likely if the male remains in the cage. The young are born fully

TABLE I
Normal Physiologic Data for Guinea Pigs[7-9]

Parameter	Value
Gestation	63 to 70 days
Weaning age	21 to 28 days
Puberty	45 to 70 days
Breeding age	12 to 14 weeks
Life span	2 to 5 years
Water consumption	10 ml/100 g body weight/day
Food consumption	5 g/100 g body weight/day
Rectal temperature	100° to 104°F
Respiratory rate	110 to 150/min
Heart rate	150 to 160/min
Average adult body weight	
Male	900 to 1000 g
Female	700 to 900 g
Urine	Creamy white or yellow; thick, turbid
Feces	Dark green or brown; hard, cylindric pellets

haired and with eyes open. They can walk immediately after birth and will eat solid food within a few hours. Guinea pigs are usually weaned at 14 to 21 days by simply removing them from the mother. The young can reach puberty as early as four weeks of age. They should not be housed together after weaning because it is preferable that they not be bred for several months.[1]

Diseases Related to Poor Husbandry
Scurvy

As mentioned, when not provided sufficient amounts of vitamin C, guinea pigs quickly demonstrate deficiency. Clinical signs include prolonged periods of immobility, unthrifty appearance, distention around the joints, diarrhea, cutaneous sores, and anorexia. Patients often succumb to secondary infection before profound evidence of scurvy is apparent.[1]

Patients with signs of vitamin C deficiency should be given large amounts (20 to 50 mg/day) of ascorbic acid until recovery is evident. Vitamin C therapy should be considered in all guinea pigs that become anorectic from any cause. Guinea pigs usually enjoy the taste of ascorbic acid solution and will readily drink it from the end of a syringe or a glass dropper.[1]

Salmonellosis

Salmonellosis is a rare but highly fatal disease in guinea pigs. The most common source of infection is ingestion of contaminated feed, particularly green and leafy vegetables that have not been properly washed.

Clinical signs usually include anorexia; weight loss; light-colored, soft feces; conjunctivitis; and dyspnea. Positive diagnosis is subject to recovery of the organism from blood or feces. Because of its zoonotic potential and the difficulty of eliminating the organism, salmonellosis is usually not treated.[1]

Ulcerative Pododermatitis

Staphylococcus aureus is the primary causative agent of ulcerative pododermatitis in guinea pigs. A granuloma is present on the ventral surface of one or more of the patient's feet. The condition is also called bumblefoot and is comparable to that in poultry. Bumblefoot occurs most frequently in guinea pigs housed in cages with wire-mesh floors, particularly if the floors are rusted or soiled. Treatment involves removing the pigs to cages with clean, dry, soft bedding and giving antibiotics. Results are often discouraging because the inflammation is chronic and diffuse.[1,4]

Coccidiosis

Eimeria caviae is the usual causative agent of coccidiosis. The condition is normally nonpathogenic but rarely can cause colitis, diarrhea, and death. Because the sporulation time is 6 to 12 days, good sanitation disrupts the life cycle; prevention is thus uncomplicated. Clinical disease is rare. Diagnosis depends on isolation of the organism in feces. Sulfonamides given in the drinking water are effective if treatment is required.[4]

Trauma

In pet guinea pigs, the most common traumatic injury is fracture of the rear leg. The tibia is usually the bone involved. As mentioned, such fracture can occur when the pig catches a leg in wire flooring material. In addition, the fracture might result from the animal being dropped by a child. A simple, lightweight splint can be applied to provide support for the fractured bone.[7]

Ketosis

Ketosis is usually seen in well-nourished sows in late pregnancy, but it can occur in males or virgin females. The exact cause of ketosis is unknown, but a history of change in diet or housing is often noted.

Onset is acute. Patients demonstrate signs of lassitude and severe depression. Treatment consists of intravenous or intraperitoneal lactated Ringer's solution, calcium gluconate, or dextrose in conjunction with corticosteroids. The prognosis is poor.[1]

Alopecia

Diffuse alopecia over the flanks and back develops in all sows in late pregnancy. Thinning of hair occurs near the time of weaning during the transition from baby fur to adult hair.[7] Although the exact cause is unknown, alopecia is also apparently associated with stress conditions. Alopecia with a distinctive pattern or patch distribution can result from hair chewing, or so-called barbering. Animals can chew their own hair or that of a cage mate. The location of hair loss can provide a clue as to whether the loss is self-

inflicted or has resulted from barbering by a cage mate. Because pigs that barber themselves cannot reach the head or neck, these areas will not show evidence of hair loss.[3]

There is no specific treatment for alopecia other than the removal of an offending animal if hair loss resulted from barbering. When separation of the animals is impossible, providing good-quality hay might be a beneficial treatment for barbering problems by allowing the offending pig to chew and tug at something else as well as smaller pigs to escape by burrowing and hiding in the hay. Other measures to lower stress should also be taken.[1]

Preputial Infection and Vaginitis

Male guinea pigs sometimes develop preputial infections as a result of foreign material (e.g., bedding) becoming lodged in the preputial folds. Treatment consists of removing the particles and cleansing the area. Vaginitis in female guinea pigs is usually caused by entrapment of bedding in the vagina; a foreign-body reaction results. The problem is corrected by washing the area carefully and swabbing away the chips. It is usually helpful to place the patient on a different type of bedding until the area heals.[1]

Water Deprivation

Guinea pigs occasionally experience water deprivation even though an apparently adequate supply of water is present. Such deprivation occurs when (1) the pet is unfamiliar with or does not know how to manipulate the water-supplying device, (2) water devices are positioned too high or otherwise out of reach, (3) water is undrinkable because of impurities or odors in the device or in the water itself, (4) water devices or sipper tubes become unworkable because of air locks or lodged foreign material, or (5) territorialism on the part of dominant animals prevents less-aggressive individuals from drinking.[1]

Socialization

Because guinea pigs live in clans in the wild, domesticated pigs are generally more content when kept in pairs, especially if the owner is away for long periods. A single guinea pig, however, will thrive and develop a strong attachment to its owner if given an adequate amount of attention and affection. If two animals are kept, it is preferable that they be females, which are less likely to fight.[8]

Allergenicity

The guinea pig is among the worst animals for provoking allergic reactions in people. Children who are asthmatic or develop severe allergies should not keep guinea pigs as pets.[1]

Conclusion

Many practical reasons account for the popularity of guinea pigs as pets. They are inexpensive to purchase and maintain, have little odor, and are quiet and pleasant. The owner's attention to proper husbandry practices will lead to a rewarding relationship with the pet and assure it a long, healthy life.

REFERENCES

1. Holmes D: The guinea pig, in *Clinical Laboratory Animal Medicine.* Ames, IA, Iowa State University Press, 1984, pp 34-44.
2. Harkness JE, Wagner JE: *The Biology and Medicine of Rabbits and Rodents.* Philadelphia, Lea & Febiger, 1977, pp 14-16.
3. Arrington LR: *Introductory Laboratory Animal Medicine,* ed 2. Danville, IL, Interstate Printers and Publishers, 1978, pp 13-151.
4. Williams CSF: The guinea pig, in *Practical Guide to Laboratory Animals.* St. Louis, CV Mosby Co, 1976, pp 12-25.
5. Clifford DR: What the practicing veterinarian should know about guinea pigs. *VM SAC* 68:678-685, 1973.
6. Herrlein HG: *A Practical Guide on the Care and Use of Small Animals in Medical Research.* New City, NY, Rockland Farms, 1949, pp 49-54.
7. Wagner JE, Manning PJ: *The Biology of the Guinea Pig.* New York, Academic Press, 1976, pp 6-23.
8. Bielfeld H: *Guinea Pigs.* Woodbury, NY, Barron's Educational Series, 1983, pp 23-34.
9. Manning PJ, Wagner JE, Harkness JE: Biology and diseases of the guinea pig, in Fox JG (ed): *Laboratory Animal Medicine.* New York, Academic Press, 1984, pp 149-155.

An Introduction to Chinchillas*

Carol J. Merry, RVT, MS

Department of Health and Human Services

Public Health Service

Centers for Disease Control

National Institute for Occupational Safety and Health

Division of Biomedical and Behavioral Science

Physical Agents Effects Branch

Cincinnati, Ohio

Wild chinchillas were originally native to the South American countries of Peru, Bolivia, Chile, and Argentina. The animals were primarily found on the western slope of the Andes Mountains from sea level to 15,000 feet. The climate of the region is generally cool and

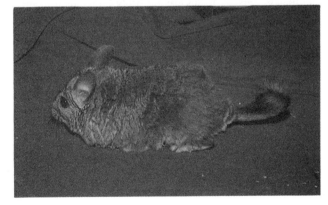

semiarid. Chinchillas were prized by the local Indian tribe, the Chinchas, who used the soft fur to

*The use of trade names in this article is for reference only and does not imply endorsement by the author, the Public Health Service, the National Institute for Occupational Safety and Health, or the publisher.

Originally published in Volume 11, Number 5, June 1990

adorn ceremonial apparel. The Chinchas were conquered by the Spaniards in the 1500s. The Spaniards coined the term *chinchilla*, or "little chincha."[1]

By the late 1800s, several million chinchilla pelts were being sent to Europe annually. The extensive hunting led to depletion of chinchillas in their native habitat; the animals are now practically extinct in the wild. As many as 90% of the remaining wild chinchillas exist on a 16-square-mile preserve in Chile.[2]

Chinchillas were brought to the United States by Mathias Chapman in February 1923.[3] Chapman established a small breeding colony; by the late 1940s, several ranchers were raising breeding stock descended from his original 11 animals. The first auction of pelts in the United States was held on June 21, 1954[4]; before this date, only breeding animals were marketed.

Today, there are chinchilla ranchers throughout the United States and Canada. Some ranchers raise a few individuals for breeding stock or the pet market; other ranchers manage thousands of animals, primarily for the fur trade. There are two generally recognized species: *Chinchilla brevicaudata* and *C. lanigera*. The latter species is raised in the United States.

Chinchillas are rodents with a single pair of incisors and four sets of molars. The teeth grow throughout life. The animals are most closely related to porcupines, guinea pigs (cavies), and agoutis. Chinchillas are described as resembling squirrels or giant gerbils; they have compact bodies, bushy tails, large eyes and ears, and long whiskers.

Adults weigh from 450 to 800 grams and are 25 to 35 centimeters long. Females are generally larger than males. The standard color is gray and ranges from very light to very dark. Selective breeding has produced mutant strains with beige, white, black, brown, silver, violet, or multicolored fur. Two common colors are pictured in Figure 1.

Chinchillas are herbivores. The young are precocial at birth. Breeders anecdotally report that the life span approaches 20 years. Chinchillas are gregarious, curious, and active. Although normally nocturnal, the animals are responsive to training and handling during the day. Vocalization includes a soft cooing sound of contentment, a bark of alarm or aggression, a spitting growl when very upset, and a doleful babylike cry when frightened or injured.

In recent years, the population of chinchillas in the United States has multiplied as a result of several developments. Fur ranchers that work cooperatively in large marketing groups have expanded production and stimulated demand for chinchilla as a luxury, ranch-raised fur. In addition, chinchillas are increasingly valuable as research subjects, particularly in otologic investigations.

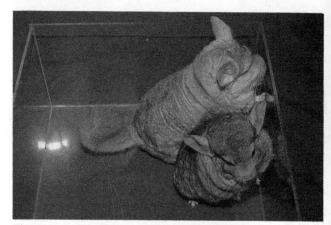

Figure 1—Beige and standard gray chinchillas.

Researchers can obtain inexpensive fur-chewing chinchillas from ranchers. The animals are hardy and convenient to house and work with in the laboratory. They are virtually odorless, and their dietary needs are easily fulfilled. Chinchillas have a charming, inquisitive temperament if handled gently. Their longevity makes them useful for long-term studies.

Of significance in auditory research, chinchillas have large bullae surrounded by thin bone that allows easy surgical access to the middle ear. The cochlea and surrounding structures are similarly accessible. Chinchillas have auditory sensitivity remarkably similar to that of humans.[5] Especially in studies of noise exposure and chemical ototoxicity, chinchillas offer a reasonable alternative to species that are more expensive or difficult to manage.

A new and burgeoning market for chinchillas as pets has also recently surfaced. The temperament and easy maintenance that make chinchillas attractive laboratory animals also endear them to the public.

Research chinchillas usually are fur chewers that are worthless to ranchers; discriminating pet owners, however, pay a premium for beautiful animals. In the midwestern United States, current pet prices for standard grays average $60 for males and more than $80 for females. The public is particularly attracted to the exotic mutant colors, which are rare and expensive. Veterinarians and technicians are increasingly asked to treat chinchillas and to offer advice on their care.

Care
Feeding

The natural diet of wild chinchillas comprises grasses and seeds. The animals have extremely large ceca, which assist in the digestion of roughage. Captive chinchillas should be fed high-quality pellets (e.g., ChinChow®—Ralston Purina or Provico®—Provico Feeds). Hay is given ad libitum. Loose timothy or similar grass is preferable, but cubed alfalfa is acceptable (Figure 2). Hay must be free of mold and insecticides.

Many chinchillas enjoy small supplemental feedings a few times a week. Such feedings can include one-quarter teaspoon (1 cc) of dry oatmeal, one or two raisins, a thin apple slice, a few sunflower seeds, or a carrot sliver. Excessive supplements can cause obesity, bloat, diarrhea, or other digestive upsets. Mineralized salt spools can be offered but are not necessary (Figure 2).

Chinchillas should be provided with objects on which they can gnaw and wear down their teeth. Suitable objects include a piece of white pine board, an untreated fruit-tree branch, or a commercially available chew block (blocks can be obtained from Blue Cloud Mineral Company, Saugus, California, or from Nutritional Research Associates, South Whitley, Indiana).

Water

Water, which should be always available, is best supplied by hanging bottles or continuous-drip systems. A chinchilla that has never accessed its drinking water this way should be closely observed to ensure that it is drinking from the bottle or drip outlet. It might be advisable to offer a water dish in addition to the bottle until the animal is secure in the new surroundings and is drinking well from the bottle.

Housing

In the wild, chinchillas live in burrows and rock crevices with a constant temperature of 10° to 13°C (50° to 55°F). Pet owners therefore should consider chinchillas to be caged indoor house pets. Adults can tolerate temperatures just above freezing but cannot survive in stagnant or drafty quarters. The animals are sensitive to heat and are stressed by temperatures hotter than 27°C (80°F). During moderate weather, owners can provide an outdoor hutch or run into which the pet is placed for a few hours each evening. Chinchillas seem to enjoy this outside exercise.

The ideal environment is a well-ventilated room with a temperature of 16° to 21°C (60° to 70°F), a humidity of 40% to 60%, and a 12-hour light-and-dark cycle. Cages with wire mesh bottoms are easy to clean, but some breeders and animal care personnel prefer solid-bottom cages bedded with white pine or hardwood chips (not cedar chips or sawdust). Solid bottoms are better for females with young; infants can be injured if their legs are caught in a mesh floor.

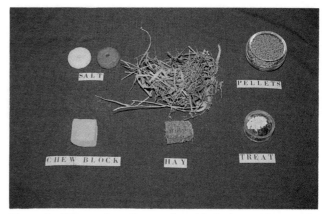

Figure 2—Salt spools, pellets, a chew block, hay, and treat mix are suitable dietary components.

Commercial cages vary in size. A cage that is 41 × 46 × 31 centimeters (16 × 18 × 12 inches) is adequate for a single chinchilla. A self-feeder for pellets and a water bottle should be attached to the cage. Cubed hay can be placed on the floor of the cage; if loose hay is provided, a hay rack is recommended. Exercise wheels are unnecessary.

Dusting

Chinchillas in the wild take frequent dust baths to help absorb skin oils before grooming. In captivity, periodic (several times weekly) dustings are required to maintain a good appearance. Sanitized chinchilla dust is available in grades ranging from extremely fine to slightly coarse (Blue Cloud Mineral Company). Talc and playground sand are not recommended. Cages can be equipped with custom dust bins that slide or tip in and out, or a pan filled with two to three centimeters of dust can be placed in the cage. Chinchillas will roll in the dust and fluff their fur for as long as an hour; the pan then can be removed (Figure 3).

Occasionally, dusting precipitates eye problems. In such cases, dust baths should be decreased or eliminated. Undusted chinchillas loose their fluffiness and develop matted fur; these conditions might not be significant, particularly in a research situation. Pet owners and breeders of show animals often offer dust daily.

Breeding

Chinchillas are mature at seven to nine months of age. Gestation is approximately 111 days, and the average litter contains two young (Figure 4).[6] The young are born precocial and fully furred. The eyes and ears are open, and teeth are present. Infants usually weigh 30 to 50 grams and are ready for weaning at six to eight weeks of age.

The external genitalia of males and females can be simi-

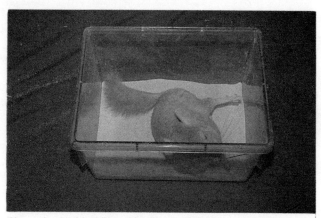

Figure 3—A chinchilla taking a dust bath.

lar in appearance. Male chinchillas have a larger genital papilla. Although there is no true scrotum, the abdominal testicles drop into the anal region during breeding. In females, the papilla is closer to the anus (Figure 5). In an anestrous or pregnant female, the vagina is tightly closed by a closure membrane; the anus and papilla thus appear to be adjacent.[7]

Commercial breeders use polygamous caging. One male has access to as many as five females. Adjacent pens of females have solid dividers and are interconnected in the back by a runway with adjustable doors into the pen of each female. When the doors are open, the male can come and go as it pleases. Each female wears a collar that prevents entry into the runway.

Chinchillas can be bred in pairs on a smaller scale. Animals should be introduced gradually because females can behave savagely toward strange males. Females discharge a vaginal plug after breeding. The plug can be a reliable indication that mating occurred.

Females undergo postpartum estrus within a few days after giving birth. Many breeders allow the male to have access to the mother and young for one week to encourage more breeding. A piece of polyvinyl chloride or metal pipe can be placed in the cage to allow the young to hide if the activity of the adults becomes too boisterous. In pair breeding, it might be unnecessary to remove the male from the cage. If the female continues to accept his presence, the male seldom bothers the offspring.

Common Ailments

Chinchillas are generally healthy. Poor husbandry and inadequate diet, however, are frequent sources of health problems. The following sections discuss common illnesses and offer recommended corrective actions.

Conjunctivitis

Conjunctivitis without clinical signs of upper respiratory infection is often caused by mechanical irritation of the

	1	2	3	4	5	6	7	8	9	10	11	12	13	14	15	16	17	18	19	20	21	22	23	24	25	26	27	28	29	30	31	
JAN.	**1**	**2**	**3**	**4**	**5**	**6**	**7**	**8**	**9**	**10**	**11**	**12**	**13**	**14**	**15**	**16**	**17**	**18**	**19**	**20**	**21**	**22**	**23**	**24**	**25**	**26**	**27**	**28**	**29**	**30**	**31**	
Apr.	21	22	23	24	25	26	27	28	29	30	1	2	3	4	5	6	7	8	9	10	11	12	13	14	15	16	17	18	19	20	21	May
FEB.	**1**	**2**	**3**	**4**	**5**	**6**	**7**	**8**	**9**	**10**	**11**	**12**	**13**	**14**	**15**	**16**	**17**	**18**	**19**	**20**	**21**	**22**	**23**	**24**	**25**	**26**	**27**	**28**	**29**	**30**	**31**	
May	22	23	24	25	26	27	28	29	30	31	1	2	3	4	5	6	7	8	9	10	11	12	13	14	15	16	17	18				June
MAR.	**1**	**2**	**3**	**4**	**5**	**6**	**7**	**8**	**9**	**10**	**11**	**12**	**13**	**14**	**15**	**16**	**17**	**18**	**19**	**20**	**21**	**22**	**23**	**24**	**25**	**26**	**27**	**28**	**29**	**30**	**31**	
June	19	20	21	22	23	24	25	26	27	28	29	30	1	2	3	4	5	6	7	8	9	10	11	12	13	14	15	16	17	18	19	July
APR.	**1**	**2**	**3**	**4**	**5**	**6**	**7**	**8**	**9**	**10**	**11**	**12**	**13**	**14**	**15**	**16**	**17**	**18**	**19**	**20**	**21**	**22**	**23**	**24**	**25**	**26**	**27**	**28**	**29**	**30**	**31**	
July	20	21	22	23	24	25	26	27	28	29	30	31	1	2	3	4	5	6	7	8	9	10	11	12	13	14	15	16	17	18		Aug.
MAY	**1**	**2**	**3**	**4**	**5**	**6**	**7**	**8**	**9**	**10**	**11**	**12**	**13**	**14**	**15**	**16**	**17**	**18**	**19**	**20**	**21**	**22**	**23**	**24**	**25**	**26**	**27**	**28**	**29**	**30**	**31**	
Aug.	19	20	21	22	23	24	25	26	27	28	29	30	31	1	2	3	4	5	6	7	8	9	10	11	12	13	14	15	16	17	18	Sept.
JUNE	**1**	**2**	**3**	**4**	**5**	**6**	**7**	**8**	**9**	**10**	**11**	**12**	**13**	**14**	**15**	**16**	**17**	**18**	**19**	**20**	**21**	**22**	**23**	**24**	**25**	**26**	**27**	**28**	**29**	**30**	**31**	
Sept.	19	20	21	22	23	24	25	26	27	28	29	30	1	2	3	4	5	6	7	8	9	10	11	12	13	14	15	16	17	18		Oct.
JULY	**1**	**2**	**3**	**4**	**5**	**6**	**7**	**8**	**9**	**10**	**11**	**12**	**13**	**14**	**15**	**16**	**17**	**18**	**19**	**20**	**21**	**22**	**23**	**24**	**25**	**26**	**27**	**28**	**29**	**30**	**31**	
Oct.	19	20	21	22	23	24	25	26	27	28	29	30	31	1	2	3	4	5	6	7	8	9	10	11	12	13	14	15	16	17	18	Nov.
AUG.	**1**	**2**	**3**	**4**	**5**	**6**	**7**	**8**	**9**	**10**	**11**	**12**	**13**	**14**	**15**	**16**	**17**	**18**	**19**	**20**	**21**	**22**	**23**	**24**	**25**	**26**	**27**	**28**	**29**	**30**	**31**	
Nov.	19	20	21	22	23	24	25	26	27	28	29	30	1	2	3	4	5	6	7	8	9	10	11	12	13	14	15	16	17	18	19	Dec.
SEPT.	**1**	**2**	**3**	**4**	**5**	**6**	**7**	**8**	**9**	**10**	**11**	**12**	**13**	**14**	**15**	**16**	**17**	**18**	**19**	**20**	**21**	**22**	**23**	**24**	**25**	**26**	**27**	**28**	**29**	**30**	**31**	
Dec.	20	21	22	23	24	25	26	27	28	29	30	31	1	2	3	4	5	6	7	8	9	10	11	12	13	14	15	16	17	18		Jan.
OCT.	**1**	**2**	**3**	**4**	**5**	**6**	**7**	**8**	**9**	**10**	**11**	**12**	**13**	**14**	**15**	**16**	**17**	**18**	**19**	**20**	**21**	**22**	**23**	**24**	**25**	**26**	**27**	**28**	**29**	**30**	**31**	
Jan.	19	20	21	22	23	24	25	26	27	28	29	30	31	1	2	3	4	5	6	7	8	9	10	11	12	13	14	15	16	17	18	Feb.
NOV.	**1**	**2**	**3**	**4**	**5**	**6**	**7**	**8**	**9**	**10**	**11**	**12**	**13**	**14**	**15**	**16**	**17**	**18**	**19**	**20**	**21**	**22**	**23**	**24**	**25**	**26**	**27**	**28**	**29**	**30**	**31**	
Feb.	19	20	21	22	23	24	25	26	27	28	29	1	2	3	4	5	6	7	8	9	10	11	12	13	14	15	16	17	18	19		Mar.
DEC.	**1**	**2**	**3**	**4**	**5**	**6**	**7**	**8**	**9**	**10**	**11**	**12**	**13**	**14**	**15**	**16**	**17**	**18**	**19**	**20**	**21**	**22**	**23**	**24**	**25**	**26**	**27**	**28**	**29**	**30**	**31**	
Mar.	20	21	22	23	24	25	26	27	28	29	30	31	1	2	3	4	5	6	7	8	9	10	11	12	13	14	15	16	17	18	19	Apr.

Figure 4—A gestation chart for chinchillas. The numbers in boldface represent the date of conception. The probable date of birth, 111 days later, is directly below. (From Houston JW, Presturich JP: *Chinchilla Care*, ed 4. Los Angeles, Borden Publishing Co, 1962, p 43. Reproduced with permission.)

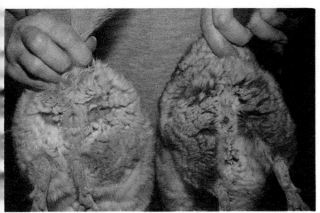

Figure 5—A comparison of male and female genitalia. The male is on the right.

eyes. Such irritation can result from dust baths, dirty bedding, or poorly ventilated quarters. Improved husbandry, cessation of dust baths for a few weeks, and brief therapy with ophthalmic ointment usually resolve the problem. Obtaining a culture from the affected eye might demonstrate a bacterial organism, which should be tested for sensitivity to appropriate antibiotic agents.

Enteritis

Enteritis usually can be traced to poor management. Soft or liquid feces or an abrupt absence of feces might be the first clinical sign. Patients can be listless and dehydrated. Occasionally, a chinchilla is found dead and the diagnosis is based on necropsy. Fecal cultures from affected animals often produce an overgrowth of such organisms as *Pseudomonas*, *Pasteurella*, *Proteus*, *Salmonella*, and *Escherichia coli*.[8] *Pseudomonas* infections evidently are particularly common.

Treatment is difficult because of the acute onset and rapid death associated with enteritis. Antibiotic therapy (based on sensitivity testing of cultured organisms) and fluid replacement are the primary forms of treatment. Oral sulfonamides and chloramphenicol palmitate are readily accepted by chinchillas but must be judiciously administered because the agents can suppress normal gut flora.

For patients that are undergoing antibiotic therapy, breeders often recommend daily feeding of one teaspoon of flavored yogurt (with active cultures) to help replenish favorable gut flora. Most chinchillas quickly learn to accept yogurt and eat it readily from a spoon. Providing a second water bottle filled with an oral electrolyte solution (e.g., Pedialyte®—Ross Laboratories) might be beneficial.

Less commonly reported gastrointestinal problems include parasitic infestation with *Giardia*, coccidia, or tapeworms.[9] These parasites are rare in properly managed herds.

Hair Rings

Male chinchillas can accumulate a ring of hair around the penis and under the prepuce. If not removed, this hair affects breeding ability and can lead to irritation, infection, and severe damage to the penis. Males should be checked for this condition at least four times per year. Hair rings are removed by applying a sterile lubricant to the penis and prepuce and gently rolling the ring off the penis.

Dental Problems

The incisors and molars of chinchillas grow throughout life. Severe dental problems can develop in animals that are deprived of chew blocks and other gnawing material or that have malocclusion. The teeth can curl outward into the cheek spaces or, in extreme cases, can grow inward and upward into the palate.

The tooth roots can penetrate the bony ocular orbits and produce so-called weepy eyes. Patients with this condition have difficulty eating and frequently are thin and untidy in appearance. Crooked incisors can be trimmed with guillotine-type nail trimmers. Malocclusion of the molar surfaces is difficult to treat. Affected chinchillas are unsuitable as pets and are usually pelted by fur ranchers as quickly as possible.

Fur Chewing

Fur chewing is the curse of the chinchilla industry. A lion's mane appearance is often produced when all of the fur within reach on the lower body has been chewed short (Figure 6). Fungal cultures and microscopic examinations are invariably negative.

There are many popular theories but scant documented research concerning the cause of fur chewing. It has been suggested that the vice is induced by boredom or stress. Loud noises, improper diet, stagnant quarters, and small or dirty cages have been incriminated. The fact that fur chewing sometimes seems to be transmitted from mother to offspring might indicate that the behavior is learned.

One theory suggests that the syndrome is caused by a fur-breakage fungus that has not yet been isolated. In the 1960s, this idea was promoted among breeders by Ethel M. Shaull. Dr. Shaull determined that "normal" chinchillas sometimes became fur chewers when housed in proximity to chewers.[10] In addition, chewers treated with captan or other fungicides frequently regrew their fur, at least temporarily. Some ranchers thus add fungicides to the dust

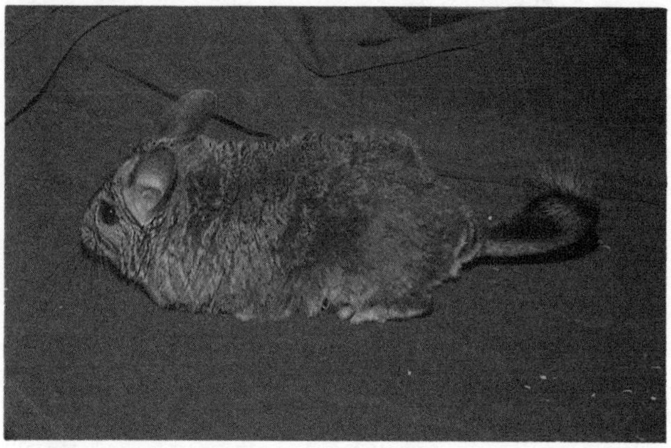

Figure 6—A fur chewer.

bath material at periodic intervals.

According to another hypothesis, fur chewers might have abnormal adrenal glands or hypophyses. One researcher used histologic examination to demonstrate hyperplasia of the hypophysis and fatty degeneration of the adrenal cortex in fur chewers.[11] Another study considered histologic indicators, isotope tracers, and plasma chemistry in fur chewers. There was evidence of increased thyroidal and adrenocortical activity, but it is unclear whether this activity was a cause or an effect of the syndrome.[12]

More documented research is needed. Ranchers rigorously cull fur chewers from their stock. Although such chinchillas might not be objectionable for research, the motley appearance makes them undesirable as pets.

Clinical Information
Anesthesia

In a clinical setting, chinchillas usually respond well to inhalation anesthesia via masking as well as to parenteral (intramuscular) anesthesia. Halothane, halothane combined with nitrous oxide, and methoxyflurane have been successfully used to maintain an adequate plane of anesthesia for surgery.

The head of the patient can be inserted into a small cone to facilitate delivery of the gas. The animal can also be placed in a small induction chamber until sedation is sufficient to allow masking. Application of an appropriate eye ointment is recommended to prevent drying of the ocular membranes by the air and gas flow. As an alternative, anesthesia can be induced with an injectable agent, such as ketamine hydrochloride (10 mg/kg); the patient can then be masked until a stable plane of anesthesia is achieved.

For the sake of quick immobilization, short procedures, or convenience, it might be preferable to achieve anesthesia via intramuscular injection. Ketamine hydrochloride combined with acepromazine maleate or with xylazine hydrochloride has been noted to be safe and effective.[13] Ketamine hydrochloride can be administered alone for short (20-minute) procedures. For longer procedures, a mixture of ketamine hydrochloride and xylazine hydrochloride is useful. A dose of 20 to 30 mg/kg of ketamine hydrochloride and 1.5 mg/kg of xylazine hydrochloride can be administered intramuscularly. This dose provides as much as two hours of adequate anesthesia and requires a four- to six-hour recovery period.

A stock bottle containing 10 cc of ketamine hydrochloride (100 mg/ml) plus 2.5 cc of xylazine hydrochloride (20 mg/ml) can be prepared in advance. The dose can be calculated by multiplying the weight of the patient (in kilograms) by 0.375 for 30 mg/kg or by 0.275 for 20 mg/kg. For a one-hour procedure, a 600-gram chinchilla can thus be given 0.600 kg × 0.275 mg/kg, or 0.17 cc, of the mixture. The dose is best administered in the upper thigh muscle with a 25-gauge needle mounted on a 1-cc tuberculin syringe. If necessary, anesthesia can be prolonged by giving ketamine hydrochloride at 25% to 50% of the original dose.

To dry mucous secretions, atropine (at 0.05 mg/kg, or weight [in kg] × 0.1) can be administered 15 minutes before the induction of anesthesia. When ketamine hydrochloride is used, eye ointment is applied because the patient's eyes will remain open and unblinking. The use of a warming pad is recommended to maintain the body temperature of sedated patients. A convenient pad that requires no power supply is the Deltaphase® Isothermal Pad (Braintree Scientific). Such pads are activated by immersion in warm water or by heating in a microwave oven.

Hematology

It is difficult to draw blood from chinchillas. For anesthetized patients, especially those undergoing terminal procedures, cardiac puncture is effective. In diagnosing an animal that is awake, toe clipping or foot puncture (with a lancet or sterile needle) provides enough blood for a microhematocrit, differential slide, or Unipet® (Becton Dickinson) white blood cell count. The femoral vein can be used. The leg veins, tail veins, and ear veins are generally difficult to use.

The cranial sinus of a chinchilla is located at the confluence of the sagittal cranial suture and the two bullae. This sinus is an accessible site for obtaining large quantities of blood (0.5 to 1.0 cc) during chronic procedures.[a]

[a]Boettcher FA, Bancroft BR, Salvi RJ: Personal communication, State University of New York at Buffalo, 1989.

TABLE I
Reported Chinchilla Blood Values[a]

	Researcher						
Parameter	Newberne[14]	Casella[15]		Kraft[16]		Strike[17]	
Number of animals	12	—	8	10	5	41	52
Sex	—	Male	Female	Male	Female	Male	Female
Age (years)	—	1	1	1.5 to 4.0	1.5 to 4.0	1.8	1.8
Red blood cells ($\times 10^6/\mu l$)	6.93	8.75	7.69	9.45	10.67	7.25	6.60
White blood cells ($/\mu l$)	9,300	9,633	9,633	11,539	11,300	7,610	7,990
Percentage of total white blood cells (%)							
Neutrophils	45.0	30.0	23.0	27.3	37.1	42.2	44.6
Lymphocytes	51.0	64.0	73.0	68.5	59.0	54.7	53.6
Monocytes	1.0	4.0	2.0	1.6	1.4	1.3	1.2
Eosinophils	2.0	1.0	1.0	2.6	2.3	0.9	0.5
Basophils	0	1.0	1.0	0.0	0.0	0.9	0.4
Hemoglobin (g/dl)	13.2	13.0	13.0	12.8	13.5	11.7	11.7
Platelets ($\times 10^3/\mu l$)	—	—	—	—	—	254	298
Blood sampling	Ear Vein	—	—	Ear Vein	Ear Vein	Cardiac Puncture	Cardiac Puncture

[a]Data compiled by Douglas W. Stone, DVM, Department of Animal Laboratories, Ohio State University.

Simple Averages from Data

Red blood cells	8.19
White blood cells	9,572
Neutrophils	36%
Lymphocytes	60%
Monocytes	2%
Eosinophils	1%
Basophils	1%
Hemoglobin	12.7

TABLE II
Chinchilla Serum Chemistry Values[18]

Parameter	Range
Blood glucose (mg/dl)	60 to 120
Serum urea nitrogen (mg/dl)	10 to 25
Cholesterol (mg/dl)	40 to 100
Total plasma protein (g/dl)	5 to 6
Albumin plasma protein (g/dl)	2.5 to 4.2
Aspartate transferase (units/dl)	15 to 45
Alanine transferase (units/dl)	10 to 35
Alkaline phosphatase (units/dl)	3 to 12
Calcium (mg/dl)	10 to 25
Phosphorus (mg/dl)	4 to 8
Sodium (mEq/L)	130 to 155
Potassium (mEq/L)	5.0 to 6.5
Chloride (mEq/L)	105 to 115

The normal packed cell volume of a chinchilla is approximately 40%. The blood volume ranges from 40 to 65 ml/kg. Other standard blood values appear in Table I. Table II lists serum chemistry values. Additional normal values for chinchillas include the following: the rectal temperature is 37° to 38°C (99° to 100°F); the resting respiratory rate is 45 to 65 breaths/min; and the resting heart rate is 150 beats/min.

Urinalysis

The urine of chinchillas, like that of other herbivorous animals, is normally alkaline and contains varying amounts of calcium carbonate crystals. The results of a typical urinalysis using a dipstick (N-Multistix®—Miles Laboratories) are depicted in the box, "Normal Chinchilla Urinalysis."

The microscopic examination can demonstrate varying amounts of amorphous debris and tiny crystals. White and red blood cells are not normally present. Casts are rare. In a clean-catch sample, few bacteria should be present. A few squamous epithelial cells are normal; the presence of cells is especially likely in females, which occasionally shed many epithelial cells.

Normal Chinchilla Urinalysis

Color	Yellow to slightly amber
Turbidity	Usually cloudy
pH	8.5
Protein	Negative to trace
Glucose	Negative
Nitrates	Negative
Ketones	Negative
Bilirubin	Negative
Urobilinogen	0.1 to 1.0 mg/dl
Blood	Negative
Specific gravity	Often exceeds 1.045

Conclusion

Chinchillas have become animals that veterinarians and technicians can expect to encounter. The ranch-raised fur market, the pet industry, and research institutions recognize that chinchillas are valuable and desirable. Veterinarians and technicians therefore can benefit from a familiarity with the basic characteristics, husbandry, and medical management of these animals. Such information is particularly useful to veterinary personnel in private pet practices and research laboratories.

Acknowledgments

The author thanks Douglas W. Stone, DVM, of the Department of Animal Laboratories, Ohio State University, for supplying written and verbal information that was valuable in the preparation of this article. Unpublished general data concerning chinchillas were provided by Michael Rudnick, PhD, MD. Special appreciation is expressed to Linda Carr and Judy Curless for typing and proofreading the manuscript.

■

REFERENCES

1. Houston JW, Presturich JP: *Chinchilla Care*, ed 4. Los Angeles, Borden Publishing Co, 1962, p 15.
2. Cubberly P: Last refuge for wild chinchilla protected. *Focus* 10(6):5, 1988.
3. Zeinert K: *All About Chinchillas*. Neptune City, NJ, TFH Publications, 1986, pp 11–16.
4. Bowen EG, Jenkins RW: *Chinchilla: History, Husbandry, Marketing*. Westerville, OH, Shoots Chinchilla Ranch, 1988, p 10.
5. Henderson D, Hamernik RP: Evoked-response audibility curve of the chinchilla. *J Acoust Soc Am* 54(4):1099–1101, 1973.
6. Houston JW, Presturich JP: *Chinchilla Care*, ed 4. Los Angeles, Borden Publishing Co, 1962, p 43.
7. Hafez ESE: *Reproduction and Breeding Techniques for Laboratory Animals*. Philadelphia, Lea & Febiger, 1970, pp 209–223.
8. Kraft H: *Diseases of Chinchillas*. Neptune City, NJ, TFH Publications, 1987, pp 106–107.
9. Stampa S, Hobson NK: Control of some internal parasites of chinchillas. *JAVMA* 149:929–932, 1966.
10. Shaull EM: Fur quality and fur breakage in the chinchilla. *Chinchilla World* 37(2):9, 1988.
11. Kraft H: *Diseases of Chinchillas*. Neptune City, NJ, TFH Publications, 1987, p 127.
12. Vanjonack WJ, Johnson HD: Relationship of thyroid and adrenal function to "fur chewing" in the chinchilla. *Comp Biochem Physiol [A]* 45:115–120, 1973.
13. Hargett CE, Gautier IM: *Comparison of Three Anesthetics for Chinchilla*. Fort Rucker, AL, Army Aeromedical Research Laboratory, 1988, pp 1–22.
14. Newberne PM: A preliminary report on the blood picture of the South American chinchilla. *JAVMA* 122:221–222, 1953.
15. Casella RL: The peripheral hemogram in the chinchilla. *Mod Vet Pract* 44:51, 1963.
16. Kraft VH: The morphological blood picture of the chinchilla villigera. *Blut* 6:386–387, 1959.
17. Strike TA: Hemogram and bone marrow differential of the chinchilla. *Lab Anim Care* 20:30–38, 1970.
18. *The Care of Experimental Animals: A Guide for Canada*. Ottawa, Ontario, Canadian Council on Animal Care, 1969, p 438.

The Origin and Care of Mongolian Gerbils in Captivity— Part I

Mikel Lynn Parkhurst, RVT
Rabbit Hill Farm
Red Oak, Texas

In 1984, the population of pet rabbits and rodents was nine million in only 2.1% of U.S. households.[1] Since then, the rodent population has continually been increasing; and the need to educate technicians about rodent care has become more apparent.

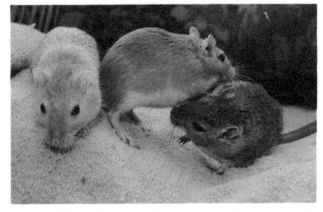

The unique anatomy and physiology of rodents further substantiate that need. Caring for rodents

Originally published in Volume 12, Number 10, November/December 1991 in a research facility with controlled conditions and constant supervision is much different than caring for rodents in a companion animal environment.

Origin

Gerbils are in the order Rodentia,[2] which is one of 17 that make up the class Mammalia, that is, animals that have hair and suckle their young. Rodentia is the largest of all mammalian orders and contains 1800 or more groups. Gerbils are in the suborder Myomorpha, which is divided into nine families. The family Cricetidae (rodent family) comprises five subfamilies, one of which is Gerbillidae and comprises all gerbils.[3] This group contains more than 80 species,[3] each having a common name based on either its locality or some of its distinguishing physical features (i.e., sand rats, fat-tailed mice, naked-soled gerbils, Jerusalem gerbils, and Mongolian gerbils).[4]

The term rodent is derived from *rodo*, which is Latin for gnaw.[2] All rodents share a common characteristic: their incisors grow continually. The two upper incisors overlap and barely touch the two lower incisors to facilitate very efficient chiseling action.[2] Rodents are able to gnaw through telephone cables, concrete, wood, and thin metals.

Rodents have been very successful in surviving; their population has been kept in balance by humans, snakes, lizards, hawks, owls, foxes, cats, wolves, and wild dogs.[2]

The gerbil's natural habitat extends throughout most of Africa, into parts of Europe, and across Asia into Mongolia and China.[3] Gerbils tend to live in arid areas and have adapted in several ways to the scarcity of water. They burrow and cover the entrance to their tunnels during the hottest part of the day, thereby keeping moisture in the burrows and affording protection against dehydration. Because temperatures fall rapidly in the desert, seeds and vegetation become covered with dew, which serves as a vital source of fluids[3] stored in the gerbil's fatty cell layers.[4] During the winter, gerbils living in the northern desert are not hibernators in the strict sense but instead become less active and rely mostly on food stored in or near their burrows.[4] One species, the great gerbil (*Rhombomys opimus*), has been known to store as much as 130 pounds of food in a special chamber in its burrow.[4]

The Mongolian Gerbil

The Mongolian gerbil (*Meriones unguiculatus*), or clawed jird, is the most common gerbil found in the United States. It was discovered by Pere David, a French missionary, during the 1860s; he also made the giant panda known to the western world. Some of these wild gerbils were

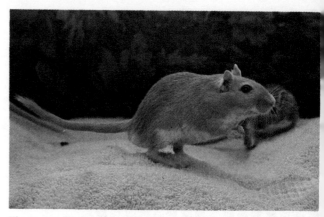

Figure 1—Adult male cinnamon gerbil with white-tipped tail.

caught and sent to Japan, where they were bred freely.[3] They were then given to scientists in the U.S.; Dr. Victor Schwentker established them at Tumblebrook Farm (West Brookfield, Massachusetts) as research animals in 1954.[3,5]

The Mongolian gerbil is native to the deserts of Mongolia and northeastern China. As the gerbil's use in research increased, so did its popularity as a pet. Gerbils are burrowing social animals with cycles of activity: burrowing, eating, gnawing, playing, and grooming are alternated with periods of rest or sleep. In captivity, a gerbil's circadian rhythm consists of activity during the day and night, with a peak in the middle of the dark cycle (midnight). Gerbils consume equal amounts of food and water during the day and night.[5]

Anatomy

Mongolian gerbils are ratlike in appearance except for their longer and more powerful hindlegs, which aid in jumping or hopping.[4] The ability to leap instantly in any direction except backward (even the poorest jumper can leap at least a few feet per jump) enables gerbils to survive predation by birds and snakes, which are the main predators of Mongolian gerbils.[4] Unlike true rats, whose principal means of locomotion is running, gerbils tend to hop or jump. This action keeps the gerbil off the hot desert sand as much as possible.[4] Also unlike rats, gerbils have a tuft of fur on the tip of the tail (Figure 1) that is usually lighter or darker than the rest of the body; this may serve to confuse predators. The tail helps provide balance when the gerbil is standing on its hindlegs or jumping.[3] Like some lizards, a gerbil can lose part of its tail and survive; however, it will not regenerate.[3]

Gerbils have an extremely keen sense of hearing because of their well-developed auditory or otic bullae (section of skull that houses the brain's acoustical center).[4] The ears of

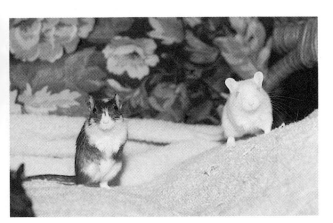

Figure 2A

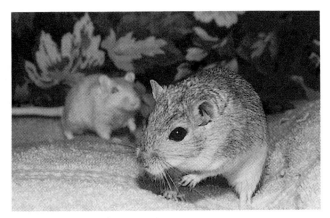

Figure 2B

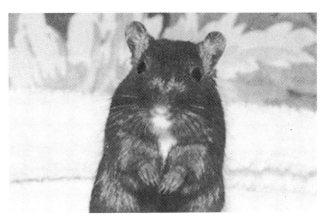

Figure 2C

Figure 2—(**A**) Albino male *(right)* and piebald male. (**B**) Agouti male *(right)* and cinnamon male. (**C**) Adult black male. The albino and the cinnamon have ruby red eyes.

Physiology

Like many rodents, gerbils depend on bacterial action in the intestinal tract for vitamin B synthesis; they therefore practice coprophagy. Gerbils are frequently reported to have lipemia,[1] probably as a result of diet; the chance of developing lipemia is increased by feeding high-fat chows or sunflower seeds. Even diets with fat levels of 4% to 6%, however, can lead to lipemia; high serum cholesterol levels of 1590 mg/dl have been reported by feeding rodent diets plus 1% cholesterol.[1]

Gerbil blood has several characteristics not found in the blood of other rodents.[1] For example, some of the red blood cells of each sex of gerbil have distinct polychromasia and basophilic stippling[1,6] (Table I) not found in the blood of other rodents. The packed cell volume, hemoglobin concentration, total white blood cell count, and circulating lymphocyte count are higher in male gerbils than in females.

Mongolian gerbils exhibit epileptiform seizures ranging from hypnotic to convulsive states. Any stress, including a change in the environment, can cause a seizure. The potential for seizures is greater for newly acquired gerbils; however, they spontaneously recover within 24 hours. Gerbils suffering a seizure should be left alone.

Behavior and Reproduction

In the wild, gerbils live in underground tunnels that have a main chamber with simple connecting chambers or more complex tunnels with numerous chambers, including a special chamber for food storage.[2] Wild gerbils are not known to be carnivorous and rarely are cannibalistic. Mongolian gerbils are not known to be carnivorous in the wild, al-

the Mongolian gerbil are moderate in size, whereas those of smaller species appear larger in proportion to the head size. The vision of Mongolian gerbils is equally well developed,[3] as the eyes are positioned to provide a wide field of vision and have the ability to detect the slightest movement nearby.

The coat color of the wild Mongolian gerbil is agouti; each hair has a white base, a yellow center band, and a black tip. In captivity, mutations have produced various coat colors (Figure 2), such as black, albino, white, dark-tailed white, cinnamon, Canadian white spot (agouti or black), piebald, magpie, lilac, blue, cream, gray agouti (very rare), dove, silver, and sable.[3] No doubt other color forms will be introduced in the future.

The body weight of mature Mongolian gerbils may exceed 100 grams.[5] The average body weights of males and females are 80 to 90 grams and 70 to 80 grams, respectively. The combined length of the body and tail varies from 21 to 24.5 centimeters. At birth, the tail measures approximately 25% of the body length; at maturity, the length of the tail is approximately 90% of the length of the body.[5]

TABLE I
Physiologic Values for Gerbils[1]

Characteristic	Value	Characteristic	Value
Adult body weight		Blood volume	66–78 ml/kg
Male	65–100 grams	Erythrocytes	$8\text{--}9 \times 10^6/\mu l$
Female	55–85 grams	Reticulocytes	21–54/1000 RBC
Birth weight[a]	2.5–3.0 grams	Stippled red blood cells	2–16/1000 RBC
Body temperature	37.0°C to 38.5°C	Polychromatophilic red blood cells	5–30/1000 RBC
Karyotype	44		
Sex chromosomes		Hematocrit	43% to 49%
Male[6]	2 (XX)	Hemoglobin	12.6–16.2 mg/dl
Female[6]	2 (XY)	Leukocytes	$7\text{--}15 \times 10^3/\mu l$
Food consumption	5–8 g/100 g/day	Neutrophils	5% to 34%
Water consumption	4–7 ml/100 g/day	Lymphocytes	60% to 95%
Vaginal opening	41 days	Eosinophils	0% to 4%
Breeding onset		Monocytes	0% to 3%
Male	70–85 days	Basophils	0% to 1%
Female	65–85 days	Platelets	$400\text{--}600 \times 10^3/\mu l$
Estrous cycle	4–6 days	Serum protein	4.3–12.5 mg/dl
Gestation period		Albumin	1.8–5.5 mg/dl
Nonlactating	24–26 days	Globulin	1.2–6.0 mg/dl
Lactating	27–48 days	Serum glucose	50–135 mg/dl
Postpartum estrus	Yes	Blood urea nitrogen	17–27 mg/dl
Litter size	1–12[b]	Creatinine	0.6–1.4 mg/dl
Weaning age[c]	20–26 days	Total bilirubin	0.2–0.6 mg/dl
Litters per year	7 average	Cholesterol	90–150 mg/dl
Respiration rate	90 breaths/min	Serum calcium	3.7–6.2 mg/dl
Oxygen use	1.4 ml/g/hr	Serum phosphate	3.7–7.0 mg/dl
Heart rate	360 beats/min		

[a]Depends on litter size.
[b]Twelve is the exception, and the dam usually has difficulty.
[c]I prefer weaning at four to five weeks of age.

though they have been known to destroy small litters and to rebreed[4]; there may be a selective advantage in the wild.[1] In captivity, gerbils may devour their young if the environment is stressful.[4]

Gerbils live in colonies. A typical colony may comprise as many as three males and as many as seven females in addition to juveniles. Because an established group will not tolerate newcomers, a high degree of inbreeding would be expected; studies of captive stock, however, show a unique system that avoids inbreeding. An adult female travels to other colonies, mates with a male of that colony, and then returns to her colony to later give birth and rear the young.[3] If pet gerbils are paired, breeding will occur regardless of whether they are related.

The gestation period for nonlactating females is 24 to 26 days but can be as early as 21 days. The gerbil's estrous cycle is four to six days; estrus lasts about 24 hours.[1] Sixty percent of female gerbils have a postpartum estrus within 18 hours of parturition.[1] If this occurs, implantation is delayed and gestation therefore prolonged. Otherwise, the female could produce more young while still nursing a litter. The gestation period for lactating females is increased by up to two days for each young nursed.

Husbandry

Mating and parturition usually occur during the dark cycle. Impending parturition is easy to detect, as the female will become more active about four days before parturition and then undergo a drastic decrease in activity and assume a ball-like position two to three days before partition. Movements by the unborn pups are apparent; their activity increases as parturition nears.

Approximately four days before parturition, the female's cage should be thoroughly washed; bedding and nesting material should be fresh and dry. If parturition occurs before the cage is cleaned and the parents are unaccustomed to frequent handling, the cage should remain undisturbed until the pups are two weeks old; if the parents are accustomed to being handled, the owner can probably clean the cage a few days after parturition. Otherwise, the mother could neglect or even eat the young. I have found, however, that pet gerbils that are handled frequently are more likely to let the owner handle the young without negative results. The cage should be placed in an area where little or no traffic is present. The room environment should be softly lit in the light cycle and dark in the dark cycle.

When the female gives birth, she spreads the hindlegs and assumes a ball-like position, tucking the head between the hindlegs. As the pup appears in the vaginal opening, the female pulls the pup out by using her teeth and forepaws. Gerbil pups are born helpless with their ears and eyes sealed (altricial young) and hairless (Figure 3). The ears open in approximately five days, the eyes open in 16 to 17 days (as late as 19 days), and the hair appears in six days (as early as three days).[1] The pups are usually weaned at 21 days,[1] but I prefer four to five weeks.

Neonates can be sexed; but because of the sensitive nature of the mother, it is not advisable. Males do not have teats. Females have four pairs of teats: two thoracic and two inguinal. If gerbils are weaned at four to five weeks, they can be sexed at that time. Males have a greater anogenital distance (10 mm) than do females (5 mm). The dark scrotal sacks of males can also be seen at this age. To avoid overpopulation and inbreeding, weanlings of the same sex should be housed together. Care should be taken to avoid overcrowding.

Socialization

There is some indication that males housed together fight more often; however, in my experience fighting has not been a problem, regardless of gender, as long as enough space is provided and the individuals are housed together before eight weeks of age. Fighting between individuals (male and female, male and male, female and female) may occur if they are introduced to one another after eight weeks of age.

If the mother has a cagemate, male or female, it can remain in the cage with the mother and pups; gerbils exhibit cooperative behavior by watching out for each other's young. If more pups are not wanted and the cagemate is a male, however, it should be removed for 48 hours to avoid

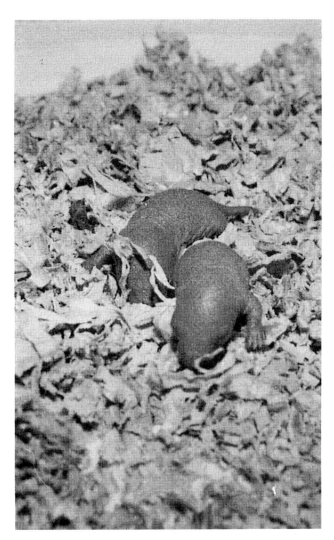

Figure 3—Three-day-old gerbil pups. Note that hair is beginning to show.

postpartum pregnancy; if both the male and female continue to show interest in breeding, the male can be removed for another 24 hours and returned. The cagemate should not be removed for more than two weeks because the aggressive nature of the female with the pups may make her react to the former mate as a stranger.

Gerbils are social animals and should always be kept in pairs—never alone. Gerbils that are paired at six to eight weeks of age will probably bond for life. They reach sexual maturity at 10 to 12 weeks of age. If a breeding pair is obtained, the male can be neutered to avoid overpopulation. Gerbils breed year-round and have a reproductive life ranging from 15 to 20 months. Their life span is between four and five years.

The gerbil's territorial and colonial nature evidently is governed by a chemical mechanism.[4] Mongolian gerbils of both sexes, as well as most other gerbil species, have a midventral abdominal pad comprising large sebaceous

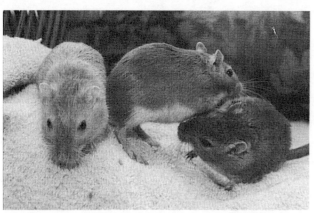

Figure 4—Agouti male (*right*) greeting a cinnamon male (*center*) by sniffing the scent gland.

glands.[1] The glands contain an oily behavior-mediating substance known as pheromone (most animals produce one or more types of pheromones that govern a variety of behaviors).[4] Pheromone plays a significant role in mate and offspring identification. Research has shown that there are chemical differences among the scent substances of individual gerbils of the same species[4] (Figure 4). Dominant and subordinate individuals can be identified by observing the marking behavior when this gland is used. Males that mark objects more often than other males are more dominant and probably more fertile. The scent gland is not the cause of dominance or fertility; however, the gland is controlled by gonadal hormones, which contribute to increased fertility.[7]

Another form of cooperative behavior in gerbils is displayed by thumping of the hindlegs. The precise reasons for thumping remain unknown, but the behavior has been observed in numerous situations.[4] Gerbil colonies tend to be in close proximity, and a gerbil from one colony will warn surrounding colonies of impending danger by thumping its feet. Thumping has also been observed in individuals just before fighting, with the result being one gerbil retreating from the other. Various sequences of thumping and more aggressive thumping on the part of a given indi-

vidual may be distinguishing the more dominant gerbil; the message seems to be clear to the subordinate gerbil. Thumping has also been observed in mating rituals. Females thump when they are in estrus, and males thump before and after mounting the female. The male must mount at least five times before ejaculation can occur; thumping by the male in what appears to be a hypnotic state before each mount seems to be necessary for ejaculation to occur.

Gerbils learn quickly—in some situations, 10 times faster than rats.[5] Maze performance is poor because gerbils are overly curious. Gerbils are easy to keep and train, so easy that the U.S. Federal Aviation Agency (FAA) has invested money in a program aimed at training gerbils to sniff out bombs at airports.[4] I have one gerbil that learned its name because I spoke the name each time I entered the room; the gerbil now does vertical loops when I call its name.

Acknowledgments

I greatly appreciate the assistance of Sandy Johnson, DVM, East Lake Veterinary Clinic, and Tony Myers, DVM, Forest Clinic, Dallas, Texas, who reviewed this manuscript before submission for publication, and the editorial assistance of Allison Esposito.

■

REFERENCES

1. Harkness JE, Wagner JE: *The Biology and Medicine of Rabbits and Rodents*, ed 3. Philadelphia, Lea & Febiger, 1989, pp 1, 34–40, 61, 73–76, 85–86, 95–97, 139, 164, 198–199.
2. Barrie A: *Gerbils as a New Pet.* Neptune City, NJ, TFH Publications, 1990, pp 5–9, 34.
3. Alderton D: *A Petkeeper's Guide to Hamsters & Gerbils.* Morris Plains, NJ, Tetra Press, 1986, pp 34–35, 42–47.
4. Ostrow M: *A Complete Introduction to Gerbils.* Neptune City, NJ, TFH Publications, 1987, pp 13–14, 23–26, 44, 52–57.
5. Gerbil care and maintenance. *Gerbil Digest* 2(2):1–4, 1975.
6. Viegas-Pequignot E, Benazzou T, Dutrillaux B, Petter F: Complex evolution of sex chromosomes in Gerbillidae (Rodentia). *Cytogenet Cell Genet* 34:158–167, 1982.
7. Pendergrass M, Thiessen D, Friend P: Ventral marking in the male Mongolian gerbil reflects present and future reproductive investments. *Percept Motor Skills* 69:355–367, 1989.

The Origin and Care of Mongolian Gerbils in Captivity— Part II

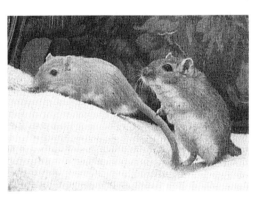

Mikel Lynn Parkhurst, RVT
Rabbit Hill Farm
Red Oak, Texas

During the past decade, the popularity of pet rodents and rabbits has been increasing on a steady basis. The advantages of educating technicians about rodent care have become more apparent with this growing trend. Part I of this two-part presentation examined the origin of Mongolian gerbils as well as their anatomy, physiology, behavior and reproductive habits, husbandry, and socialization tendencies. In Part II, the housing, bedding, and nutritional needs of Mongolian gerbils are reviewed as well as diseases specific to this group of rodents.

HOUSING

Several types of containers are suitable for gerbils. Factors to consider when selecting a container include safety, intrusion, and anti-escape mechanisms. The floor of a container should be solid and free of sharp or abrasive corners. Owners should be advised that gerbils can chew through paper, cardboard, plastic, and thin metals.

If a wire-bottom cage is used, the cage sides should be solid. Because gerbils are natural burrowers, their claws are worn down by constant digging. Use of an all-wire cage may minimize digging behavior, thereby allowing the claws to grow too long; long claws make food handling difficult. Instead, I prefer glass or Plexiglas® housing. Plexiglas® houses are easy to clean and maintain the gerbil in a safe environment.

Mature gerbils should be housed with a minimum floor space of 230 cm² (36 inches²) per gerbil. A breeding pair requires an area of 1300 cm² (180 inches²). The cage sides should be high enough to accommodate hanging water containers; gerbils should not be given water in open containers, such as bowls.

Improper housing is the primary reason that a gerbil escapes into the home environment. Gerbils should not be underestimated; their curiosity and persistence encourage escape attempts. Gerbils rarely stray more than 50 feet from their burrows[1]; paired gerbils may escape together. If the gerbils are a breeding pair, retrieval is essential to avoid uncontrolled reproduction.

The environment within a cage is very important; the temperature may not be the same as that of the room, especially in glass or Plexiglas® cages. Leaving the cage in direct sunlight is dangerous to the animal. Even though gerbils in their natural homeland can withstand temperatures colder than freezing and in excess of 100°F (37.8°C), caged gerbils are not so adaptable.[1] To survive extreme temperatures, the wild gerbil burrows into a cooler or warmer place. In a caged environment, gerbils become uncomfortable in temperatures hotter than 35°C (95°F).[2] Their ability to tolerate heat decreases as humidity increases. Humidity should be greater than 30% but lower than 50%. When the humidity is higher than 50%, a gerbil's coat begins to mat and look rough. Gerbils are usually housed at temperatures between 18°C and 29°C (65°F to 85°F), with a temperature of 22°C (72°F) being the usual compromise.[2] A thermometer should not be left inside the gerbil cage; gerbils are good chewers—so good that it is illegal to keep gerbils as pets in California because of the potential for crop destruction.[2]

BEDDING

Numerous bedding materials are available, but not all materials are suitable for gerbils. Pine and cedar shavings are appropriate. Materials for nesting also should be available. All gerbils naturally nest, regardless of whether they are male or female; the nesting behavior does not occur just during parturition. Cloth materials should be avoided because gerbils devour some of the material while they shred it. Paper towels, empty paper towel rolls, and empty wrapping paper rolls are all appropriate. Nothing toxic, however, should remain on the nesting material. Because most cardboard rolls are held together by nontoxic glue, usually of animal origin, their use is acceptable and even provides extra protein. Alfalfa is another appropriate nesting material in addition to being a good source of food.

Gnawing material should also be provided. I have found that construction shims (pine or cedar) are an excellent source of gnawing material. They are inexpensive and can be obtained at a local lumberyard. Only tree limbs from trees that have not been sprayed or treated with toxic material should be used.

The bedding material should be fresh and dry. Stale bedding can cause excess dust to accumulate and a condition called *sore-nose*.[2] Sore-nose, or nasal dermatitis, is common in gerbils and is associated with excessive accumulation of porphyrins around the nasal area (see the section on Diseases).

If food and water are given in proper amounts, bedding usually does not need to be changed for several weeks. If the cage needs to be changed more frequently, the gerbils are probably being overfed, a water bottle is leaking, or a gerbil is ill. Low urine output and dry fecal matter lead to less odor and a cleaner environment.

FOOD

Rodents consume more seed grown in the United States than is exported to other countries.[3] Because gerbils are granivorous or herbivorous, they should be fed wholesome, fresh, clean, nutritious, palatable food. Pet gerbils are affected more frequently than laboratory gerbils by nutritional deficiencies, probably because of owner lack of knowledge of nutrition. In addition, research facilities can obtain prepared chow specifically formulated for gerbils.

Gerbils should be fed ad libitum using feeders or a ceramic dish. If plastic dishes are used, the gerbil will probably eat the dish too. Rabbit chow (nonmedicated) is a good source of food if it is mixed with other foodstuffs. The exact proportion of each amino acid in the protein building blocks needed for gerbils is unknown.[1] Therefore, variety is the key to a healthy diet. Although sunflower seeds are high in fat and low in calcium and should be fed in small quantities as treats only, sunflower seeds apparently boost milk production in lactating females.

Alfalfa is good for lactating females, not only for milk production but, as mentioned, for nesting material. The alfalfa should be purchased in small quantities for gerbils kept in small numbers; otherwise, the alfalfa can become stale, which may result in diarrhea. Small animals can expire quickly because they dehydrate quickly when diarrhea is unnoticed by an owner who is unaware of the clinical signs of diarrhea.

Preparation of Soaked Seeds and Sprouts[3]

Soak fresh seed in warm water for 12 hours. Rinse the seed and store in a warm, dark area for 24 hours. Small shoots should appear. Wash the sprouts.

Note: Because the protein and vitamin content of seeds is extremely high, feeding seeds is especially recommended for pregnant and pup-rearing females.

Dry Foodstuff Mixture

Rabbit chow (nonmedicated)	36%
Corn (whole or cracked)	18%
Oats (crimped or rolled)	18%
Canary seed	11%
Milo	9%
Pigeon feed	7%

Wheat germ can be supplemented to the diet every other day or so (because wheat germ must be refrigerated, do not blend in with above mixture). Bonemeal or powdered milk also can be added for lactating females.

With the growing popularity of gerbils as pets, more commercially packaged food mixtures are becoming available. Most of these mixtures are nutritionally sound. Some, however, contain too many sunflower seeds, which can lead to obesity and malnourishment.

Fresh vegetables should also be included in a gerbil's diet. Fresh vegetables are a good source of essential minerals, such as calcium, potassium, phosphorus, iron, and zinc, as well as of trace minerals, such as manganese and magnesium. Green vegetables provide a variety of necessary vitamins, including vitamin A, a majority of the vitamin B complex, and vitamin C. Fresh vegetables also provide gerbils with much of the cellulose they require for proper digestion. Gerbils can be given store-bought or home-grown lettuce, cabbage, kale, broccoli, and celery if the vegetables have been washed and towel-dried thoroughly. Root vegetables, such as carrots, turnips, and beets, are good for a gerbil's diet. Soaked seeds and sprouts also are a favorite among gerbils, and they are especially nutritious for pregnant and pup-rearing females (see Preparation of Soaked Seeds and Sprouts).[3] If vegetables are not home-grown or purchased, weeds from the yard are sometimes acceptable; however, I advise against using weeds unless they are free of insecticides, pesticides, and excrement.

Regardless of whether vegetables are home-grown or store-bought, care must be taken not to leave uneaten vegetables in the cage for more than a few hours, as bacteria can invade the vegetables and cause decay; if decayed vegetables are eaten by the gerbil, repercussions ranging from mild diarrhea to death can occur. Because gerbils bury their food, the owner should be cautioned to look under bedding for uneaten vegetables.

If gerbils are kept in large numbers, a diet can be mixed by the owner. The feed store is a good source for a dry food mixture (see Dry Foodstuff Mixture). Vegetables and treats, such as sunflower seeds, should only be fed occasionally at owner discretion.

Because gerbils are predisposed to high cholesterol and lipemia,[2] diet is a crucial factor in maintaining minimal fat and cholesterol levels.

Nutritional imbalances may appear as weight loss or failure to gain, hair loss, anemia, deformed bones, or central nervous system abnormalities.[2]

WATER

Gerbils have a large adrenal weight–to–body weight ratio that contributes to their unique water-conserving capabilities. In the wild, gerbils obtain all their water from food. In captivity on a diet of dry foodstuff, gerbils do not obtain water from their food. Contrary to popular belief, gerbils must be provided with fresh, clean water at all times. If fresh vegetables are fed on a regular basis, gerbils can obtain the water they require from the vegetables; however, I recommend providing water along with vegetables to be safe.

Selection of a water container is important. The best arrangement is a container that can be placed on the outside of the cage with the drinking tube extending into the cage. The rubber stoppers used in some water containers are readily eaten by gerbils if the containers are hanging from the inside of the cage. The consequences of eaten rubber stoppers are numerous; for example, the now-exposed water container allows entrance by nursing pups. Once a pup is inside the tube, it will be unable to turn around and escape, causing it to suffocate. If a plastic cage is used, a hole can be drilled through the side and the end of the sip-

History Protocol[2]

Animal involved
  Species and strain
  Sex
  Age
  Source (how obtained)
  Breeding status
Environment
  Cage type and location
  Type of feeder and water bottle
  Bedding material
  Sanitation level
  Waste disposal
  Other species in the colony
  Disturbances within the colony
  Recent changes or introduction of new
    animals
  Light cycles
  Ventilation
  Room temperature
  Ventilation
  Humidity

Diet
  Source
  Composition
  Storage
  Dietary supplementation
  Recent dietary changes
Health
  Previous diseases
  Previous treatments
  Breeding record
  Quarantines
Owner complaints
  Onset of signs
  Progression of signs
  Number of gerbils exposed
  Morbidity and mortality in the colony
  Ages and sex of gerbils affected in the
    colony
  Apparent clinical signs on presentation

per tube placed through the hole with the larger tube (which contains the water) hanging on the outside of the cage. Water containers must be checked frequently to ensure that they are working properly, as they can easily malfunction because of the vacuum within which they work. Hanging the water container outside the cage also eliminates water spilling into the bedding and food, thus creating an ideal environment for bacterial growth.

Common signs of dehydration are overactivity within the first 24 hours of inadequate water intake; a dull haircoat; nonpliable skin; dry and red mucous membranes of the nostrils, mouth, and anus; decreased dry food intake; and decreased urine and feces production.[4] One of the most common causes of cannibalism among gerbils is food or water deprivation.[2]

DISEASES

When a gerbil is presented to a veterinary facility, a history must be taken. The history protocol provides good guidelines to care (see History Protocol).[2] There are various diseases that plague gerbils, although gerbils are resistant to many diseases that affect other rodents. The signs and causes associated with some conditions are listed in Table I.[5]

The following sections review some conditions that are common in a gerbil population.

Nasal Dermatitis. Frequently called sore-nose, nasal dermatitis is a common problem that is associated with accumulation of porphyrins around the nasal area. Porphyrins are secreted by the harderian glands, which are located behind the eyes.[2] Porphyrins are highly irritating if allowed to accumulate on the external nares and can result in bacterial infection. *Staphylococcus* is frequently isolated from the affected area. Stress can also cause increased secretion of porphyrins by the harderian glands. The condition often occurs in weanling gerbils. Except for association with porphyrins, the primary cause of nasal dermatitis is unknown. In weanling gerbils, I have minimized frequency of the condition by weaning at an older age (four to five weeks) after ensuring that the mother is not pregnant. In the 125 adult gerbils I house, I have eliminated nasal dermatitis by reducing stress and providing suitable bedding. Conversely, I have induced nasal dermatitis by inadvertently introducing stress. If nasal dermatitis is suspected, cleaning the nose, providing suitable bedding, and eliminating stress in the early stage usually avoid bacterial infection. If the gerbil stops eating or assumes a depressed posture with matted coat, it should be presented to the veterinarian.[2]

TABLE I
Common Clinical Signs Presented by Mongolian Gerbils

Signs	Causes
Bleeding; large areas of skin appear damaged (H_2O_2 can be used for minor cuts)	Injuries caused by fighting, particularly during mating period; introduction of new gerbil
Diarrhea or loose droppings; noninfectious must be distinguished from infectious	Feeding excessive amounts of green foodstuff
Hunched posture and reluctance to move; fur in poor condition and held away from the body; diarrhea	Protozoal parasite causing coccidiosis; bacterial infection causing Tyzzer's disease
Skin irritation, hair loss, scabs	Lice and mites, such as *Demodex,* spread by contact with infected individuals and their surroundings
Hair loss in circular pattern; center of lesion dry and scabby	Fungal disease; such as ringworm (spores can survive for long periods)
Bald areas on head, tail, or sides of body; must be distinguished from ringworm and other parasitic conditions	Fur chewing, self-inflicted or by member of group; environmental stress and/or lack of suitable chewing material; presence of exercise wheels (tails can be pulled off if caught in the wheel)
Threads of saliva around mouth	Dental malocclusion, especially of the incisor teeth
Kinked tail	Genetic; other physiologic abnormalities (do not breed animal)
Seizures	Inherited trait seen in most Mongolian gerbils

Cutaneous or Subcutaneous Swelling. Abscesses or neoplasms are most often the cause of swellings.[2] Tail and perianal abscesses are most common because of frequent biting at these sites. Neoplasms of the skin are relatively common among gerbils. The midventral scent gland in gerbils is often mistaken as abnormal and is a common location for abscesses.

Nasal Discharge and Dyspnea. A nasal discharge is associated with heat stress, allergy, or respiratory infection.[2] Pneumonia is frequently seen in gerbils with dyspnea. Fluid in the thoracic cavity or diaphramatic hernias may also cause dyspnea.

Ocular Discharge. Gerbils may have primary conjunctivitis, dacryoadenitis, or ocular infection secondary to systemic disease.[2] Dust can cause excessive lacrimation and produce red (porphyrin-containing) tears associated with nonspecific stress.

Neuromuscular Signs. Torticollis-otitis media, otitis interna, or encephalitis may cause head tilt.[2] Gerbils have an apparent resistance to otitis media, a common and debilitating condition in other rodents and in young humans. Such resistance may be associated with the gerbil's relatively high resistance to pathogens and with ear drainage that is superior to that in other rodents.[2]

Incoordination and Convulsion. Epileptiform seizures in gerbils are quite phenomenal.[2] The types of seizures are hypnotic, cataleptic, or convulsive episodes with a variable threshold for onset. In the wild, seizures have a protective effect; a carnivorous predator is unlikely to consume a seemingly sick animal. Encephalitis, poisoning, toxemias, and trauma can also produce convulsions.[2]

Prevention of epileptiform seizures can be achieved by frequent handling beginning when the gerbil is young, avoidance of undue stress or startling the animal, and not changing environments too frequently.[6] Some strains of gerbils are more prone than others to seizures. Research toward developing gerbils that do not seizure is in progress. Anticonvulsant drugs may cause fatalities and are contraindicated.

Sudden Death. Chilling or overheating, septicemia, streptomycin, toxicity, starvation or dehydration, neoplasia, or trauma can cause sudden death in gerbils.[2]

Tyzzer's Disease. Tyzzer's disease, caused by *Bacillus piliformis* infection,[2] is the most common disease of gerbils. This acute, highly fatal disease is presented most often in weanling animals, but adults may also be affected. Poor environmental sanitation, stress of shipping, immunosuppressors, and crowding contribute to development of the disease. Chronically infected animals exhibit weight loss and rough haircoat; eventual death is typical. In more acute cases, there may be edema, congestion, hemorrhage, and focal ulceration of the intestine. In weanling or stressed animals, the disease is acute and enzootic and causes rough haircoat, lethargy, and death within 48 to 72 hours. There is no good screening test for Tyzzer's disease. An ELISA has been developed for detection of anti–*Bacillus piliformis* serum antibodies in rabbits and could be applied to detect serum antibodies in rodent species.

Neoplasia. Spontaneous neoplasia has been reported in approximately 24% of gerbils older than two years of age; the incidence increases with age.[2] Neoplasms in gerbils cover a wide range of types, with tumors of the female reproductive system being the most common. Fluid-filled cysts on the female reproductive system have been mistaken for tumors; the cysts have been confirmed at necropsy. These cysts have been successfully drained; although recurrence is most likely, the cysts can be drained repeatedly, thereby prolonging the gerbil's life span.[a] Adrenal adenomas and adenocarcinomas are also common. Neoplasms of the skin include basal cell carcinomas, melanomas, sebaceous adenomas, and squamous cell carcinomas and are often found in association with the midventral scent gland.[2]

Miscellaneous. Incisor malocclusion, neoplasia, and enteric disease are among several factors leading to progressive weight loss and death. Food and water deprivation are among the most common causes of precipitous weight loss and death in gerbils. Food or water deprivation is difficult to establish in a history; the usual cause is negligence in making food and water accessible.[2]

RESTRAINT

Gerbils are not known for biting; but when they do bite, it can cause serious injury. Gerbils may bite when they are in pain or startled. The technician should first introduce his or her hand into the gerbil's cage and allow the gerbil to investigate the new handler. After a few minutes, the gerbil can be handled more confidently and successfully if sound restraining techniques are used.

Gerbils are restrained by grasping their loose dorsal skin.[4] The gerbil first should be placed on a flat surface. The technician can then gently press down against the gerbil's back while keeping the fingers straight. The fingers and thumb should then curl around the opposite sides of the gerbil, with as much skin as possible being grasped. The skin against the abdomen and thorax should be taut, but the restraint should not interfere with breathing. This type of restraint is good for handling gerbils that bite, dosing with oral medication, examining the ventral scent gland, administering intraperitoneal injections (premedicating for surgery), and examining the head region.

When moving a gerbil from one place to another, the base of the tail should be grasped with the handler's thumb and index finger while the body is being supported with

the palm. Gerbils will jump when they are in unfamiliar surroundings; by holding the base of the tail, the gerbil is secured and cannot jump. When grasping the tail, the tail should not be held distally. A gerbil may shed its tail if it is pulled too hard; this is a survival mechanism.

BLOOD COLLECTION

Orbital sinus bleeding is usually the method of choice for small rodents.[2] Rodents are routinely anesthetized for orbital bleeding. The rodent is held on a flat surface in lateral recumbency. A microhematocrit tube is rotated and positioned caudally and medially at the angle or medial canthus of the eye into the orbital sinus. When blood flow ceases or the amount required is obtained, the tube is withdrawn. Eye trauma, harderian gland lesions, and nasal hemorrhage may occur with this technique. With care and experience, the technique can be performed with minimal stress and the ruptured vessels will repair quickly.

Blood can also be collected from the tail vein.[2] Warming the tail first will increase blood flow, and the vein will be easily detected.

Total blood volume is approximately 6% of the body weight.[2] As much as 25% of the total blood volume can be collected in a two-week period. Replacement of blood volume with fluids (0.9% saline) should be considered. With gerbils, microanalytic methods should be used to minimize the blood volume that must be withdrawn.

ANESTHESIA

Nocturnal species have a prolonged anesthetic sleep when anesthetized in the afternoon because the hepatic metabolism is at its lowest point. Even though gerbils are not true nocturnal animals, consideration should be taken depending on the individual gerbil's habits. The type of bedding that is used should also be considered when anesthetizing gerbils. Cedar and pine beddings induce hepatic enzymes and therefore decrease anesthetic time.[2]

Various preanesthetics should be used with caution, if they are used at all. Acetylpromazine and chlorpromazine lower the seizure threshold in gerbils. Ketamine hydrochloride (40 mg/kg intramuscularly) can be used as an induction agent for methoxyflurane but is not the drug of choice; diazepam (10 mg/kg intraperitoneally) can be substituted for ketamine hydrochloride. Diazepam and halothane work well together. Pentobarbital sodium (6% solution) given at 0.01 ml/10 g (60 mg/kg) intraperitoneally can induce surgical anesthesia for 30 to 45 minutes. This anesthetic has a ceiling dose of 6 mg; however, hypothermia is a major concern.[7] Isoflurane has also been used successfully in gerbils.

[a]Myers T: Personal communication, Dallas, TX, 1991.

The danger involved in the use of gas anesthetics in small animals, such as gerbils, is greater for the personnel involved in the procedure because most veterinarians use cones or masks rather than endotracheal tubes. Scavenger systems are hard to use with cones or masks in small animals because the cones or masks must be alternately administered and withdrawn to maintain a constant surgical plane. Because of this difficulty, scavenger systems are not properly used with gas anesthetics in small animals, thereby posing a threat to veterinary personnel involved with the procedure. Safety precautions should be followed accordingly.

Gerbils should be monitored carefully during anesthesia and kept warm after surgery. Heating pads and lamps should be avoided; isothermic pads are safer. Hot water bottles filled with warm water can also be used. Gerbils can be burned if the pads or hot water bottles are overheated.

ORAL VERSUS INJECTABLE MEDICATION

There is controversy about the use of oral medication in gerbils. Because of the destructive nature of oral antibiotics to digestive microflora, oral medications (if they are used) should be used cautiously in all animals that depend on bacterial action in the intestinal tract for vitamin B synthesis. Neomycin is especially harmful and should be avoided.[b] Streptomycin (50 mg/55 to 65 g body weight) apparently causes high mortality (80% to 100%)[8] in gerbils and should never be administered.

CONCLUSION

For many years, children have been the principal owners of gerbils; but small pets are becoming more popular in general. Rodents, especially gerbils, seem to be a pet of the future. Technician knowledge of the care and handling of gerbils is therefore essential.

ACKNOWLEDGMENTS

I greatly appreciate the assistance of Sandy Johnson, DVM, East Lake Veterinary Clinic, and Tony Myers, DVM, Forest Villa Animal Clinic, Dallas, Texas, who reviewed this manuscript before submission for publication, and the editorial assistance of Allison Esposito.

■

REFERENCES

1. Ostrow M: *A Complete Introduction to Gerbils.* Neptune City, NJ, TFH Publications, 1987, pp 13-14, 23-26, 44, 52-57.
2. Harkness JE, Wagner JE: *The Biology and Medicine of Rabbits and Rodents,* ed 3. Philadelphia, Lea & Febiger, 1989, pp 1, 34-40, 61, 73-76, 85-86, 95-97, 139, 164, 198-199.
3. Barrie A: *Gerbils as a New Pet.* Neptune City, NJ, TFH Publications, 1990, pp 5-9, 34.
4. Stark DM, Ostrow ME (eds): *Assistant Laboratory Animal Technician.* Cordova, TN, American Association for Laboratory Animal Science, 1989, pp 48-49, 66.
5. Alderton D: *A Petkeeper's Guide to Hamsters & Gerbils.* Morris Plains, NJ, Tetra Press, 1986, pp 34-35, 42-47.
6. Cutler MG, MacKintosh JH: Epilepsy and behavior of the Mongolian gerbil: An ethological study. *Physiol Behav* 46:561-566, 1989.
7. Muir WW III, Hubbell JAE: *Handbook of Veterinary Anesthesia.* St Louis, CV Mosby, 1989, pp 253-256
8. Russell RJ, Johnson DK, Stunkard JA: *A Guide to Diagnosis, Treatment and Husbandry of Pet Rabbits and Rodents.* Edwardsville, KS, Veterinary Medicine Publishing Co, 1981, p 40.

[b]Johnson S: Personal communication, Dallas TX, 1991.

Nutrition and Pet Rabbits

Susan Donoghue, VMD
Nutrition Support Services, Inc.
Pembroke, Virginia

Domesticated rabbits can be great pets. Naturally quiet yet alert and inquisitive, they come in a variety of sizes, colors, and appearances. Short haired or long haired; large, medium, or small sized; erect eared or lop-eared—all make fine companions. Some pet rabbits are kept outdoors in hutches; others are kept indoors, trained to use a litter box, and given the run of the home.

Although owners are usually responsible and well-meaning, the nutritional needs of pet rabbits are sometimes not met. Owners that are familiar with the feeding of dogs and cats may lack understanding of the needs of nonruminant herbivores. A veterinary technician's counsel of rabbit owners about diet may prevent nutritional disease. In addition, the technician's experiences with rabbit nutrition are applicable to hospital care because sick rabbits that are presented to veterinary hospitals may require nutrition support.

Nutritional Problems
Supermarket Diets

Pet rabbits that are fed only foods from supermarkets are at risk for malnutrition. Individual foods for humans are not complete and balanced as are many commercial diets for animals. Most human foods lack one or more essential nutrients; humans achieve nutritional completeness by selecting a variety of foods and by taking supplements (e.g., multivitamin pills). Owners often fail to achieve such balance for their rabbits.

Most technicians know of house rabbits that are fed produce and cereals. Much of the produce commonly fed to rabbits is low in calories and deficient in several essential nutrients (Table I). Many cereals (e.g., granola) contain too much fat (for rabbits) and too few essential nutrients, such as calcium. Almost all supermarket foods, even those labeled "high fiber," contain an inadequate amount of fiber for rabbits.

Fiber

Gastrointestinal disease caused by low fiber intake may be the most prevalent feeding problem in house rabbits.

Rabbits have a simple stomach and a specialized lower bowel. They are hindgut fermenters, as are other companion animals (e.g., horses and iguanas), but have special adaptations. Large fiber particles quickly transit the ileum and colon; fine low-fiber particles travel backward (via reverse peristalsis) from the colon into the cecum for fermentation.[1] Cecal fermentation yields short-chain volatile fatty acids (propionate, butyrate, and acetate) that are absorbed and used for energy.

The fiber residue is excreted as hard fecal pellets. The nonfiber portions are excreted and consumed (coprophagy) and are referred to as soft feces or night feces. Compared with hard feces, soft feces contain less fiber and more water, protein, volatile fatty acids, vitamins, and minerals.[1] Coprophagy is normal in rabbits and, incidentally, in hares, lemmings, and koalas.

Rabbits that are fed low-fiber diets may be presented with signs of gastrointestinal disease, such as diarrhea or constipation. Some patients exhibit such behavioral signs as hair chewing. Many are very sick and anorectic.

Improving Supermarket Diets

Supplements can be added to supermarket foods to increase fiber and to improve levels of calories, calcium, and other essential nutrients. Such diets are difficult to balance without training in ration formulation, however. A diet change is usually safer, cheaper, and more convenient for owners.

Diets of hay, commercial rabbit food, and treats usually ensure nutritional completeness and adequate fiber intake. These diets are considered in more detail here.

Finding Fiber

High-fiber plant foods, referred to as roughages or forages, include fresh grasses and legumes, hay, pellets, and cubes. Forage in pellets and cubes has been chopped into small pieces and then compressed. Research in cattle suggests that grinding and pelleting forage increases food intake and utilization of digestible energy.

TABLE I
Calorie and Nutrient Contents of Supermarket Foods[a]

Food Item	Energy (kcal/g as fed)	Protein	Fat	Nonfiber Carbohydrate	Fiber	Calcium	Phosphorus
				(% dry-matter basis[b])			
Romaine lettuce	0.18	21	5	56	11	1.1	0.4
Spinach	0.26	36	3	48	7	1.0	0.6
Dandelion greens	0.44	18	5	61	11	1.2	0.4
Beet greens	0.24	24	3	51	14	1.3	0.4
Alfalfa sprouts	0.39	37	4	39	12	0.2	
Carrots	0.42	9	2	82	8	0.3	0.3
Granola	4.5	11	18	70	1	0.1	0.3
Puffed oats	4.0	16	7	74	2	0.1	0.5
Flaked bran	3.3	13	2	82	4	0.1	0.5
Bran and fruit cereal	3.1	10	1	84	4	0	0.6

[a]Pennington JAT, Church HN: *Bowe's and Church's Food Values of Portions Commonly Used*. Philadelphia, JB Lippincott Co, 1985.
[b]Water contents vary greatly.

In herbivores, fiber aids gut motility and water balance and yields calories via fermentation. Herbivores generally prefer and maintain better gut motility and function with long-stem fiber (found in hays, fresh forage, and coarsely chopped cubes) rather than short-stem fiber (found in meals, pellets, and, recently, some small cubes).

Hay can be purchased from feed stores and farms. Alfalfa cubes are readily available from pet shops but are relatively expensive. The cubes also can be purchased from feed stores in 50-pound (22.7-kg) bags and stored in metal trash cans in a cool, dry room. Such a purchase is suitable for a large rabbitry, but consumption is too slow if 50 pounds of cubes are fed to a few rabbits—vitamin A activity is diminished. This loss of activity is the primary nutritional change that is likely to cause a clinical problem.

For pet rabbits, product quality and owner convenience may be the primary determinants of the form of roughage selected. Suburban owners may find small bags of pellets or cubes easier to manage than hay bales. Forage need not be of the highest quality if the remaining diet of commercial pellets and treats is of superior quality.

Commercial Diets

Rabbit pellets are designed to be complete feeds (Table II). Such diets are formulated to provide all nutrients and fuel sources necessary to meet the particular requirements at a given stage of the animal's life cycle. Pellets are easy to store and feed, can be offered free choice, and minimize waste. They contain 12% to 28% crude fiber and 14% to 19% crude protein. Occasionally, commercial diets cause nutritional problems.

At the North American Veterinary Conference in Orlando, Florida, in January 1992, vitamin A deficiency was described in an unpublished report of a rabbitry that fed pellets composed of old alfalfa hay. Carotene, the precursor of vitamin A, is lost as hay ages; the pellets in question were made from two-year-old hay. The purchaser should look for pellets that are bright green; brown pellets may contain scant carotene. Rabbits that are deficient in vitamin A exhibit increased mortality, poor reproduction, birth deformities, and (in erect-eared rabbits) drooping ear tips.

In another rabbitry, vitamin A intoxication was diagnosed.[2] The problem was caused by errors in pellet preparation—10 times the recommended level of vitamin A was added inadvertently. Clinical signs of vitamin A intoxication are similar to those of vitamin A deficiency: poor reproduction and birth defects. Despite occasional problems with commercial feeds, rabbit pellets are the safest and most convenient way to provide balanced and complete nutrition to pet rabbits.

Snacks

Supermarket produce and cereals make fine treats and snacks for pet rabbits. Small amounts of greens, vegetables, cereals, and low-fat snacks (e.g., rice cakes) are well accepted by rabbits. Owners should be counseled to limit snack feeding and to ensure that most of the daily food consumed is pellets and forage.

Snacks offered should be fresh and washed. Produce must be free of foreign objects (e.g., plastic twist ties and rubber bands) and washed thoroughly before feeding.

TABLE II
Examples of Forages and Rabbit Feeds

Food Item	Energy (kcal/g as fed)	Protein	Fat	Nonfiber Carbohydrate	Fiber	Calcium	Phosphorus
				(% dry-matter basis[b])			
Alfalfa hay[a] (sun-cured early bloom)	1.50	18	3	46	23	1.4	0.2
Timothy hay[a] (sun-cured, midbloom)	1.64	9	3	51	31	0.5	0.2
Clover[a] (red, fresh)	0.46	21	3	42	26	1.7	0.4
Alfalfa meal[a] (dehydrated, 15% protein)	1.50	17	3	41	29	1.4	0.2
High-fiber pelleted diets[b]	1.80	16	2	44	28	—	—
Pelleted diets for growth and reproduction[b]	2.40	19	2	50	20	—	—
Pelleted diets for all life stages[b]	2.20	16	2	49	22	—	—

[a]Committee on Animal Nutrition: *United States–Canadian Tables of Feed Composition*, ed 3. Washington, DC, National Academy Press, 1982.
[b]Data are calculated from guaranteed analyses on labels.

Feeding Management

Rabbits adjust their food intake according to the energy content of the diet.[1] For example, when a diet is changed from low-energy supermarket produce to high-energy pellets, fewer pellets (than produce) are consumed. Pet rabbits may overeat, however, and obesity can be a problem. It is usually controlled by adding high-fiber, low-energy coarse hays to the usual diet.

Depending on their size, age, environmental temperature, reproductive status, and health, rabbits consume approximately 150 to 400 calories (kcal) of metabolizable energy (ME) daily.[3] Energy needs are determined by calculating basal metabolic rate (BMR = $70 \times$ body weight in kg$^{0.75}$) and then multiplying by a maintenance factor (1.5 for adults with limited activity; 2.0 for growth).

Dry feeds, such as pellets and hay, contain approximately 1.5 to 2.5 kcal of metabolizable energy per gram (43 to 71 kcal per ounce). A healthy, three-year-old, male house rabbit that weighs two kilograms (4.4 pounds) thus requires approximately 175 kcal daily, or approximately four ounces of pellets. If the pet is very active or the house is cold, more calories are needed.

Water is provided by sipper-tube bottles or bowls and must be clean and wholesome. Rabbits drink approximately 5 to 10 milliliters per 100 grams of body weight daily.[4]

Nutrition Support

Sick rabbits that are presented to veterinary hospitals may need nutrition support. Such common disorders as hairballs and respiratory disease lead to anorexia. In order to avoid catabolism of vital tissue protein as a result of low calorie intake, nutrition support is recommended.

Selecting Diets for Sick Rabbits

Enteral diets, or slurries made with enteral diets, may be fed to rabbits via syringe or nasogastric tube. In selecting ingredients for rabbits and other herbivores (unlike ingredients for carnivores), it is necessary to look for products with less fat and protein and more complex carbohydrates and fiber.

Although enteral diets fed to sick rabbits provide needed calories and nutrients, none is ideal for hindgut fermenters. The enteral diets are made for humans. Even less acceptable are products made specifically for dogs and cats; these products contain more fat and protein, relatively few carbohydrates, and no fiber.

Enteral diets are relatively isosmolar (300 mOsm/kg) or hyperosmolar (greater than 400 mOsm/kg). Feeding isosmolar enteral diets can begin with minimal dilution for the first few meals. Feeding hyperosmolar diets begins with a 50:50 dilution with water to avoid stomach upset.

Although ideal for humans, enteral diets contain relatively high fat and low fiber levels for rabbits. Most of the fiber-containing enteral diets use soy polysaccharide to provide approximately 2 to 10 milligrams of fiber per milliliter. Alfalfa hay, by comparison, has 200 milligrams of long-stem fiber per gram; the fiber in enteral diets is of insufficient quantity and less-than-ideal physical form. Nevertheless, enteral diets provide a useful adjunct to medical and surgical care and save the lives of anorectic patients.

Slurries

Enteral diets may be blended with other ingredients to increase fiber and palatability. Two successful ingredients are yogurt and alfalfa meal.

A recipe used successfully in sick rabbits by Julie Langenberg, VMD, at the School of Veterinary Medicine of the University of Wisconsin-Madison consisted of the following: a commercial enteral diet (8 ounces; 227 grams), low-fat fruit yogurt (8 ounces; 227 grams), and alfalfa meal (4 tablespoons; 54 grams). This mix provides approximately 8% crude fiber, 1.1 kcal/ml, 17% protein (on a dry-matter basis), 8% fat, and approximately 60% carbohydrate. The alfalfa meal increases fiber (although not long-stem fiber) in a form that is more appropriate for rabbits. The diet can be fed via syringe or tube and can be managed easily by owners.

The three-year-old, male house rabbit, when sick, requires approximately 160 ml/day of slurry to meet its need for 175 kcal daily. Nutrition support would entail 20 milliliters administered four times daily for the first day, followed by 30 milliliters four times daily for the next day and then 40 milliliters four times daily.

REFERENCES

1. Partridge GG: Nutrition of farmed rabbits. *Proc Nutr Soc* 48:93–101, 1989.
2. DiGiacomo RF, Deeb BJ, Anderson RJ: Hypervitaminosis A and reproductive disorders in rabbits. *Lab Anim Sci* 42:250–254, 1992.
3. National Research Council: *Nutrient Requirements of Rabbits.* Washington, DC, National Academy Press, 1977.
4. Harkness JE: Rabbit husbandry and medicine. *Vet Clin North Am Small Anim Pract* 17:1019–1044, 1987.

Bibliography

Harkness JE, Wagner JE: *The Biology and Medicine of Rabbits and Rodents*, ed 3. Philadelphia, Lea & Febiger, 1989.

Dr. Donoghue, Series Editor of CLINICAL NUTRITION, is a Diplomate of the American College of Veterinary Nutrition and a founder of Nutrition Support Services in Pembroke, Virginia. Dr. Donoghue developed the first full-time nutrition support service in a veterinary hospital at the University of Pennsylvania from 1986 through 1988. She has authored more than 50 articles on nutrition in veterinary journals. Authors who are interested in contributing to CLINICAL NUTRITION are invited to contact Dr. Donoghue at Nutrition Support Services, Route 1, Box 189, Pembroke, VA 24136; 703-626-3081 (fax 703-626-3564).

Husbandry
of the Rabbit—Part I

Janet Amundson Romich, DVM, MS
Madison Area Technical College
Madison, Wisconsin

Laura Ayers, CVT
National Wildlife Health Laboratory
Madison, Wisconsin

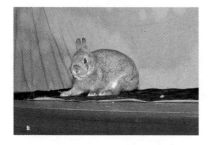

Since the time of the monks in the Middle Ages, rabbits have been caged to be used as a source of food and fur production. Today, because of their ease of care and quiet nature, rabbits have gained popularity as domesticated pets. There are several breeds of rabbits that vary greatly in size and in the ratio of body surface to body weight. Rabbit breeds are usually grouped according to size. Dwarfs, standards, and giants are the three major groups; however, specialty groups also exist. Small breeds (under two kilograms) include the Dutch belted and Netherland dwarf (Figure 1). Medium breeds (two to five kilograms) include the Angora, Californian, New Zealand, chinchilla, and rex. Large rabbits (more than five kilograms) include Flemish and checkered giants. Lop-eared rabbits (Figure 2) are considered a specialty group. These rabbits have long, draping ears. There are four types of lop-eared rabbits based on size (from smallest to largest): Holland, mini, French, and English. In general, the smaller the rabbit, the earlier the onset of sexual maturity and the greater the caloric requirement per unit of weight.

Anatomy and Physiology

Rabbits have well-developed sensory systems to prevent capture and destruction by predators. The most noticeable external characteristic of rabbits is their long ears. The ears gather sound and are an easily accessible blood collection site because of the presence of readily visualized vasculature. Some believe that the ears also serve as a thermoregulatory organ; however, most mammals have internal methods of thermoregulation via the hypothalamus. The eyes of rabbits are well adapted. Rabbits have a field of vision that is approximately 170° for each eye. Rabbits also have a wide, panoramic field of vision created by the lateral positioning and prominence of the eyes; a small binocular field to the rear; and a small area of overlap in the front due to the small nasal area. These adaptations give the rabbit an advantage in escaping predators. Rabbits also have a well-developed nictitating membrane. During sleep or anesthesia, this fold moves from the medial canthus across the cornea to protect the eye. Rabbits have pupillary dilatation that is extremely light sensitive (about eight times as sensitive as that of humans). This type of dilatation helps rabbits to detect slight changes in their environment. Rabbits have a cleft upper lip and an undivided lower lip that form a relatively small external mouth opening. The external nares are ovoid shaped and merge with the cleft in the upper lip.

Rabbits are fairly delicate animals. Only eight percent of the body weight of a rabbit is skeleton. The vertebral formula for rabbits is $C_7 T_{12} L_7 S_4 Cd_{16}$, but 13 thoracic vertebrae are present in some animals. Rabbits have powerful hindquarters that are adapted for jumping. Proper restraint of the hindquarters is essential in rabbits to prevent injury.

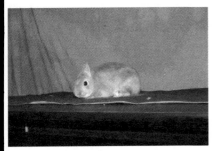
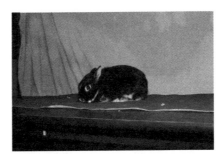
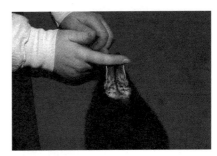

Figure 1A   **Figure 1B**   **Figure 1C**

Figure 1—Netherland dwarf rabbits. (**A**) Netherland dwarf with a solid color pattern (orange). (**B**) Netherland dwarf with a martin color pattern. The body color of rabbits with the martin color pattern differs from the color on the feet, ventral abdomen, and the triangle behind the ears. A black silver martin (black = body color; silver = tip color) is shown. (**C**) Triangular area behind the ears of a Netherland dwarf rabbit with the martin color pattern.

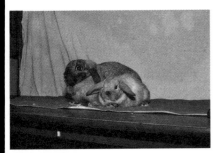
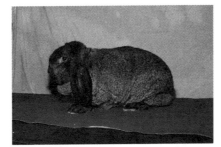
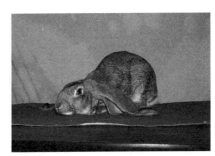

Figure 2A   **Figure 2B**   **Figure 2C**

Figure 2—Lop-eared rabbits. (**A**) The Holland lop is the smallest lop-eared rabbit. This rabbit has a color pattern known as sooty fawn. The term *sooty* derives from the gray tipping pattern that resembles soot. Fawn, a light tan, is the primary body color. An adult and a four-week-old are shown. Notice how the color intensifies as the animal ages. (**B**) French lop-eared rabbit that is larger than the Holland lop. This rabbit is steel colored, termed for its deep gray color with dark tipping on individual hairs. (**C**) English lop-eared rabbit. This type of lop-eared rabbit has the largest ear span. The color of this English lop is known as an agouti color pattern.

Some differences occur in regard to the internal organs of rabbits. The heart of the rabbit is smaller than the heart of other mammals; the right atrioventricular valve is a bicuspid instead of a tricuspid; the liver has four lobes; the pancreas is diffuse; the simple stomach lacks specialized regions and is thin-walled and large; the cecum is large, thin-walled, and (when coiled with its termination) is a thick-walled vermiform process.

The rabbit is a monogastric herbivore that is also coprophagic; therefore, gastrointestinal adaptations are important in understanding nutrient requirements. Hindgut fermentation of plant material is accomplished via adaptation of the large intestinal group of the rabbit. Two types of feces are passed in rabbits. The type most commonly passed is round and firm. The other type is known as night feces or cecotrophs. Cecotrophs are soft, wet stools of cecal origin that are a source of B vitamins and protein. Cecotrophs are ingested by the rabbit (usually directly from the rectum) to provide the rabbit with B vitamins and protein. Anorexic rabbits

should thus be supplemented with B vitamins. Rabbits cannot vomit, and this is important to remember when histories are taken.

Sexual maturity occurs earlier in females than in males and earlier in small breeds than in large ones. Small breeds can be bred at four to five months of age. Giant breeds are not ready to be bred until 9 to 12 months of age. Rabbits do not exhibit obvious, reliable external signs of estrus. Behavioral changes and a turgid vulva in rabbits during estrus may be noticed by some observant owners. Male rabbits have a hairless scrotum and do not have a glans penis. The testes descend at about 12 weeks of age. Male rabbits, or bucks, do not have nipples. The inguinal canals remain open for life. This is important to remember when rabbits are neutered. If a rabbit is neutered via open castration, the inguinal ring or tunic area needs to be closed to prevent herniation of the intestine. The estrous cycle of the female rabbit is irregular. There is a 4- to 17-day period of receptivity with one to two days of inactivity interspersed. Females, or does, are induced ovulators, and ovulation occurs 10 to 13 hours after breeding. The gestation period is 30 to 33 days. Pseudopregnancy can occur and generally lasts 15 to 17 days.

In the final days of gestation, the doe builds a nest from bedding material or hair from her dewlap, thighs, and abdomen. Young rabbits are born hairless, blind, and deaf. Sexing young rabbits may be difficult because the anogenital distance varies only slightly between females and males. Does will eat the placenta and still-born offspring, and cannibalism may be observed; therefore, external noise and handling should be kept to a minimum after a litter is born. Typical litter size is 4 to 10 kits. Does are infrequent nursers and only feed the kits once or twice daily. Weaning usually occurs at six to eight weeks.

Many people believe that rabbits only have two large buck teeth. The dental formula actually is I 2/1, C 0/0, P 3/2, M 3/3 for a total of 28 teeth. Rabbits have open-rooted teeth that grow continuously; therefore, teeth should be periodically examined to ensure that they are properly aligned to wear each other down. If the teeth are too long, they should be trimmed in an appropriate manner.

Rabbits have unique physiologic values (see the box). The blood of the rabbit (Figure 3) and granulocyte morphology varies from other mammals. The rabbit heterophil or neutrophil (also known as the pseudo-eosinophil or amphophil) resembles the eosinophil of other species. The granules of the neutrophil are diffusely pink and may be either fine or round. Eosinophils of rabbits have granules that are round, larger, and much more brightly eosinophilic than those of neutrophils. Lymphocytes, monocytes, and basophils of rabbits are similar in morphology to other mammals. High lymphocyte numbers (30% to 70%) may be normal in rabbits. Leukocytosis is uncommon in rabbits with an infection. Elevations in the number of heterophils may be evident during infectious disease. The erythrocyte morphology of the rabbit is similar to other mammals with anucleated, biconcave, and disklike erythrocytes. The only difference in erythrocyte morphology of the rabbit is that the red cell morphology looks like a regenerative response because there is a vast variation in cell size. Hemostatic cells are similar to platelets of other mammals. The mean corpuscular volume of the rabbit is 65 to 72 femtoliters, and the normal packed cell volume is 36% to 48%.

The urine of rabbits is turbid and varies in color from clear to deep orange or reddish brown. The variation in the urine color is caused by the variety of diets fed to

Physiologic Values for Rabbits[a]

Body temperature	38.0°C–39.6°C
Life span	5–6 years
Heart rate	130–325 beats/min
Respiratory rate	32–60 breaths/min
Erythrocytes	$4–7 \times 10^6/\mu l$
Hematocrit	36%–48%
Hemoglobin	10.0–15.5 mg/dl
Leukocytes	$9–11 \times 10^3/\mu l$
Neutrophils	20%–75%
Lymphocytes	30%–80%
Eosinophils	0%–4%
Monocytes	1%–4%
Basophils	2%–7%
Platelet	$250–270 \times 10^3/\mu l$
Serum protein	5.4–7.5 g/dl
Albumin	2.7–4.6 g/dl
Globulin	1.5–2.8 g/dl
Serum glucose	75–150 mg/dl
Blood urea nitrogen	17.0–23.5 mg/dl
Creatinine	0.08–1.8 mg/dl
Total bilirubin	0.25–0.74 mg/dl
Serum lipids	280–350 mg/dl
Phospholipids	75–113 mg/dl
Triglycerides	124–156 mg/dl
Cholesterol	35–53 mg/dl
Serum calcium	5.6–12.5 mg/dl
Serum phosphate	4.0–6.2 mg/dl

[a]Values listed are only approximate and may not represent the normal range in a given population. Information on specific species can be located in various reference publications.

rabbits (i.e., feeding too much alfalfa in the form of pellets and blocks may result in increased calcium levels in the urine, thus, the urine may appear cloudy white) or by porphyrin pigments present in the urine, which cause the reddish brown coloration. Because rabbits are herbivores, the urinary pH is alkaline and ranges from 8.0 to 9.0. Urine is the major route of calcium excretion in rabbits; therefore, crystals occur commonly in rabbit urine. The most frequently encountered crystals in rabbit urine are triple phosphate, calcium carbonate monohydrate, and anhydrous calcium carbonate.

General Care

Rabbits may be housed inside or outside. Adult rabbits should be individually housed in hutches or suspended wire cages that are structurally sound, provide

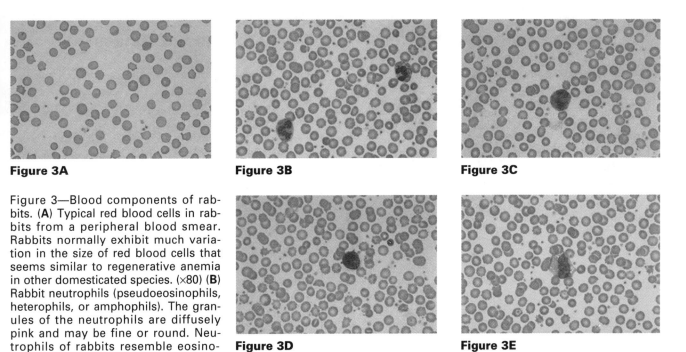

Figure 3A

Figure 3B

Figure 3C

Figure 3D

Figure 3E

Figure 3—Blood components of rabbits. (**A**) Typical red blood cells in rabbits from a peripheral blood smear. Rabbits normally exhibit much variation in the size of red blood cells that seems similar to regenerative anemia in other domesticated species. (×80) (**B**) Rabbit neutrophils (pseudoeosinophils, heterophils, or amphophils). The granules of the neutrophils are diffusely pink and may be fine or round. Neutrophils of rabbits resemble eosinophils of other species (×80). (**C**) Rabbit eosinophil with granules that are round, larger, and much more brightly eosinophilic than those of the neutrophils (×80). (**D**) Rabbit basophil. It is similar to the basophils of other mammals with round, dark granules (×80). (**E**) Rabbit monocyte. It is similar to the monocyte of other mammals with a large nucleus and vacuoles in the cytoplasm (×80). (Courtesy of Linda Sullivan, DVM, School of Veterinary Medicine, University of Wisconsin, Madison, Wisconsin)

protection from predators and adverse environments, are of adequate size, are easily sanitized, and are equipped with hopper feeders and sipper tube water bottles. The size of the pet rabbit determines the housing needs. Large rabbits should have a minimum of five square feet of space. Medium rabbits should have four square feet, and small rabbits should have three square feet. Cages should be at least 14 inches high. Wire mesh is generally recommended because it can be easily sanitized. Wire mesh openings should be 1 inch × 2 inches on the sides and ½ inch × 1 inch on the floor.

Rabbits that are indoor pets can be litter trained, and a litterbox can be kept inside the cage or in an appropriate location in the house. Indoor rabbits should be caged when left unattended. The material used in the box should contain a substance that is both absorbent and, if eaten, digestible. A paper organocellulose product is available as well as a compressed wheat grass product that is superior to other materials often used. Cedar and pine shavings are often used but are not recommended. Cedar can cause respiratory problems; pine is not absorbent and can lead to urine scalding. Cat litter can stick to the perineal area or feet and cause dermatologic problems for pet rabbits. Regardless of the bedding substrate used, it needs to be changed frequently to prevent urine scald or ammonia inhalation.

The most common behavioral problem in pet rabbits is chewing. Provision of digestible litter material, high-fiber diet, and safe chew toys may be helpful. Rabbit-proofing a house in which a rabbit is allowed to roam freely is essential to prevent injury from electrical cords and possible toxins in the environment. Unsupervised exercise is not recommended.

Another important consideration when housing a rabbit is ambient temperature. Ambient indoor temperature should remain between 40°F and 80°F; ideally, rabbits should not be housed outdoors if temperatures are above 85°F. Rabbits can tolerate cool temperatures better than warm temperatures. Excessively warm temperatures can result in heat prostration; decreased fertility may result if shade or a cooler environment is not provided. Incubators are rarely used for sick rabbits because of the heat intolerance of the species. The ideal temperature for rabbits to be housed is 60°F. If outdoor housing is chosen, the enclosure must have a shaded area that allows the rabbit to avoid direct sunlight if the temperature is too warm as well as an enclosure where the animal can shelter itself from the elements. Most breeders and pet enthusiasts have a separate housing area that is attached to the hutch. This facilitates easier cleaning and allows the rabbit to spend time on a floor with a smooth surface instead of the wire mesh. Time spent off the wire mesh

Rabbit Emergencies

Persistent choking or wheezing
Difficulty in breathing
Sudden weakness or lethargy
Not eating for 24 hours (especially if weak or depressed)
Watery diarrhea
Persistent or bloody diarrhea
Loss of use of any limb
Fractures in which blood is present or bones are
  protruding
Uncontrolled bleeding
Large lacerations
Coma
Seizures
Head trauma that accompanies lethargy or depression
Animal bites
Eye injuries

Signs of Illness

Hair loss (possibly caused by mutilation or infection)
Chronic intermittent diarrhea
Anorexia (see in 24 hours if appetite does not return)
Fractures
Periodic weakness (may indicate systemic disease)
Periodic salivation or pawing at the mouth (teeth should
  be checked)
Lumps or bumps on the skin
Chronic coughing
Unusually aggressive behavior
Small lacerations or signs of injury
Persistent scratching
Ear infections and head tilt
Lethargy, depression, changed attitude
Pus or thick crusts around the eyes or nose
Broken teeth

helps alleviate sore hocks in rabbits. In cool weather, grass hay should be added to the housing area to provide insulation for the rabbit. Daily changing of this hay is optimum for good sanitation.

Although rabbits are lively and affectionate pets, they are also delicate and may require special care. Technicians should be trained to respond to the common concerns of rabbit owners. Technicians and owners should be well informed about specific emergencies and signs of illness (see the boxes) that affect rabbits to ensure proper care, treatment, and prevention of such episodes in the future.

Restraint

Caution should be used whenever a rabbit is restrained. If the animal struggles, the lumbar portion of the spine can fracture or luxate. Gloves should not be used when handling rabbits because they do not allow for adequate control and may frighten rabbits. Rabbits should *never* be grabbed by the ears. The environment in which the rabbit is restrained should be made as calm and comfortable as possible. Rabbits are very sensitive to loud noises and odors and do not like slippery surfaces. A towel or mat should be used on the examination table. This may make the rabbit feel more secure, allow for solid footing, and prevent scrambling. The amount of restraint depends on the procedure. Physical examinations require minimum restraint whereas oral examinations require maximum restraint.

Rabbits that are carried a short distance can be scruffed by the neck and supported with the other hand on the rear quarters (football hold). Rabbits can also be cradled in the arms when scruffed by the neck and supported by the rear legs with the free hand. The head of the rabbit should face the crook of the arm. Allowing a rabbit to hide its face tends to relax some animals. The best and safest way to move a rabbit a long distance is to use a carrier or a box. Rabbits are great chewers and should not be left unattended in carriers for long periods of time.

Placing rabbits on their backs may be helpful for trimming nails and cleaning ears. The animal can be placed on its back and held firmly between the legs of a technician that is sitting. The rabbit is positioned with the back legs closest to the technician. Stroking the abdomen may help to calm the rabbit. Hypnosis of rabbits has also been used for minor procedures, such as toenail clipping, injections, and radiography. The rabbit is restrained on its back (eyes covered or uncovered) in a V-shaped rack or in the crook of the arm. The belly is gently stroked until the rabbit relaxes. Breathing will slow from approximately 51 to 21 breaths per minute.

Injections

Subcutaneous injections can be given in the neck, flank, or back area of the rabbit. Intramuscular injections can be given in the thigh, gluteal, or lumbar muscles. The same precautions to prevent nerve injury in other species should be used.

Intravenous injections can be given in the marginal ear vein or the cephalic vein. Intravenous injections given in the ear vein may result in skin sloughing when administered by untrained personnel; therefore, the cephalic vein may be the best choice. Any vein used for blood collection can be used for intravenous injection; however, sedation may be required. A 25- or 27-gauge catheter is recommended; however, butterfly catheters may be easier to use than needles.

Medicating

Medicating rabbits orally can be accomplished by pushing the pill into the interdental space, and the rabbit will generally chew the pill. Rabbits have large cheek pouches; therefore, it is imperative to make sure they are ingesting the medication. Pills that are crushed and mixed in liquid or administration of a drug suspension may be superior to giving pills to ensure that the rabbit receives the entire dose. Medication can be placed in the feed or water of most rabbits. Adding molasses or jam may be necessary to disguise the flavor of some medications. Because it is also difficult to distinguish whether the rabbit has taken the entire dose with this method, administering medication via a drug suspension is the optimum method.

If the rabbit needs to be orally medicated, a feed or flexible tube that is 2.0 to 3.5 millimeters in diameter can be used. A section of hard plastic hose or a wooden dowel should be used to keep the animal from chewing the tube.

A curved-tip, 12-cc syringe with the tip cut halfway off can be gently pushed into the interdental space. The syringe should be pointed backward in the mouth and only inserted far enough to allow liquid in the oral cavity.

Blood Collection

The blood volume of rabbits is approximately 5.5% to 6.5% of their body weight. Calculation of appropriate volumes before blood collection is important. If the rabbit is healthy and nonanemic, 5 to 7 ml/kg is the maximum amount of blood that should be collected at one time.

The marginal ear vein (located on the convex surface of the ear) is generally used to collect a blood sample in laboratory rabbits. A rabbit restraint box is by far the easiest way to restrain the rabbit for one-person collection. The veins in the ear are very delicate and can tear or collapse very easily. It may be helpful to shave the area, disinfect with alcohol, apply petroleum jelly or xylene, distend the vein with digital pressure at the base of the ear, nick the vein with a scalpel or needle, and collect the blood into a pipette or tube. Xylene can be irritating and should be removed with alcohol after blood collection. The central artery of the ear (also on the convex surface of the ear) can also be used for blood

collection. A 27- or 25-gauge needle or butterfly catheter and a syringe can be used to collect up to 3 cc of blood. In general, the ear vein is not used to collect larger volumes of blood in pet rabbits due to the risk of thrombosis and necrosis of the ear tips.

The cephalic vein can be used for collection of a small volume of blood (<0.3 ml); however, it is difficult to get a nonanesthetized rabbit to hold its foot still for a long period of time. Small amounts of blood can be taken from a nail trim; however, this is not generally recommended because it makes the rabbit afraid to have its feet handled. Other available sites are the saphenous, femoral, penile, and sublingual areas.

Jugular veins of the rabbit can also be used as a site for blood collection (sedation may be helpful). The rabbit should be restrained like a cat for jugular blood collection. In females with large dewlaps, jugular blood collection is difficult. If intravenous catheters are placed for blood collection, it may be helpful to nick the skin with an 18-gauge needle initially and then thread the catheter. Fluid therapy is 100 ml/kg/day. The dose is usually divided twice or three times a day and administered either subcutaneously or intravenously.

Anesthesia

Rabbits are anesthetic risks and require specialized anesthetic techniques. Extreme care should be taken whenever a rabbit is anesthetized. Variation of response is a factor when any animal is anesthetized. Specific factors, such as age, sex, strain, weight, health, and nutritional status should be taken into account. It should be noted that the ingesta-filled ceca can cause falsely elevated body weight values in rabbits. In addition, duration of anesthesia effects can be longer in animals anesthetized in the afternoon due to changes in hepatic metabolic activity evident in nocturnal animals.

Fasting rabbits before anesthesia administration is controversial. Rabbits do not vomit, and it takes approximately three days to clear the gastrointestinal tract of ingesta; therefore, fasting is usually not needed. Most practitioners, however, fast rabbits two to eight hours before anesthesia is given.

Atropine can be given subcutaneously at 1 to 3 mg/kg if desired; however, it should not routinely be given without just cause. Some rabbits possess an enzyme that may interfere with the response to atropine. This enzyme potentially can degrade atropine and make the administered dose ineffective. Acepromazine maleate at 1 mg/kg or diazepam 5 to 10 mg/kg can be used as a tranquilizer. Ketamine hydrochloride alone provides poor analgesia and skeletal muscle relaxation in rabbits.

The drug, however, can be used for restraint at a dose of 20 mg/kg. A combination dose of intramuscular diazepam (5 to 10 mg/kg) given 30 minutes before intramuscular ketamine hydrochloride (25 mg/kg) is adequate for such things as dental procedures. Animals that may be subjected to foreign matter entering the airways should be intubated because their reflex mechanism is maintained but not reliable.

Isoflurane is the ideal inhalant anesthetic gas available at this time. Isoflurane inhalant anesthesia is recommended because it causes good relaxation, quick induction, and recovery. Rabbits should be induced at 2% to 3%. Induction should be raised slowly to 5% then maintained at 2.5% to 3%. Mask induction is suggested for rabbits that are not intubated on a routine basis and for short procedures (less than 20 minutes). Methoxyflurane is hepatotoxic and should not be used in rabbits. Halothane may result in cardiopulmonary problems in rabbits.

Endotracheal intubation can be difficult in rabbits because of the long distance from the incisors to the epiglottis, the sharp teeth, and the small mouth. If this method is chosen, a tube that is 3.5 millimeters or less in diameter is suggested (tube size depends on the size of the rabbit). This procedure is superior to mask anesthesia because of the decreased exposure of gas to clinic personnel, decreased anesthetic risk, and improved patient monitoring. The extended time spent attempting intubation, however, may lengthen anesthesia time. Although endotracheal intubation has its benefits, veterinarians must access whether the increase in anesthetic time is worthwhile in choosing this method of anesthesia administration.

Sexing

Rabbits can be sexed when held on their backs. Gentle pressure is applied around the genital orifice with the thumb to evert the genitalia. In females, the vulva only protrudes cranially and is slit at the caudal end. In males, the penis protrudes in a complete circular tube shape. Bucks are usually smaller than does. Bucks lack an os penis and have hairless scrotal sacs.

Nutrition

Rabbits require a diet high in fiber for normal digestive function. Pellets that contain 20% to 27% fiber along with quality grass hay are recommended. Other pellets may be too high in calories because they were originally designed to feed rabbits that were produced for meat and did not live long lives. If pellets are used, vitamin supplements are unnecessary. A general rule is ¼ cup of pellets per five pounds body weight per day with ad libitum grass hay for mature nonbreeding rabbits.

High-fiber hay may be offered to pet rabbits. Supplementing the diet of rabbits with high fiber helps prevent some gastrointestinal problems and is important in maintaining a healthy gastrointestinal tract. Hairball prophylaxis is recommended via feeding a high-fiber diet and, if necessary, giving 10 milliliters of fresh pineapple juice or papaya juice daily for three to five days per month. Timothy hay is a good example of a high-fiber hay for pet rabbits. Because most pellets contain alfalfa, alfalfa hay is not recommended as a supplemental hay source because alfalfa is high in calcium. Too much calcium in the diet may result in the passage of white urine and may predispose rabbits to the development of urinary crystals.

Fresh vegetables and fruits can be offered in small amounts, and fresh water should be available at all times. A general rule for feeding is five grams of food per 100 grams of body weight per day and 100 milliliters of water per kilogram of body weight per day.

■

Bibliography

Carmen RJ: Clostridial enteropathies of rabbits. *Proc North Am Vet Conf*:795, 1993.

Fowler ME: *Restraint and Handling of Wild and Domestic Animals*, ed 6. Ames, IA, Iowa State University Press, 1987, pp 161–165.

Fraser CM (ed): *The Merck Veterinary Manual*, ed 6. Merck and Company Inc, 1986, pp 988–999.

Harkness JE: Rabbit husbandry and medicine. *Vet Clin North Am Exotic Pet Med* 9:1019–1044, 1987.

Harkness JE, Wagner JE: *The Biology and Medicine of Rabbits and Rodents*, ed 2. Philadelphia, Lea & Febiger, 1983, pp 7–16.

Hawkey CM, Dennett TB: *Color Atlas of Comparative Veterinary Hematology*. Ames, IA, Iowa State University Press, 1989.

Hillyer EV: Pet rabbits. *Vet Clin North Am Small Anim Pract* 24(1):25–67, 1994.

Weisbroth SH, Flatt RE, Kraus AL (eds): *The Biology of the Laboratory Rabbit*. San Diego, Academic Press, 1974.

Husbandry of the Rabbit—Part II

Janet Amundson Romich, DVM, MS
Madison Area Technical College
Madison, Wisconsin

Laura Ayers, CVT
National Wildlife Health Laboratory
Madison, Wisconsin

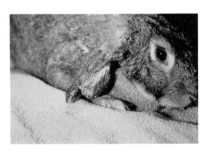

In the first part of this two-part series, the anatomy and physiology, general care, restraint techniques, injections, medicating, blood collection, anesthesia, sexing, and nutrition of the rabbit were discussed. Part II presents various diseases that affect rabbits, including bacterial, enteric, and parasitic diseases. Other disorders commonly encountered in rabbits, such as sore hocks, malocclusion, posterior paralysis, uterine adenocarcinoma, and urinary problems are also discussed. Where appropriate, treatment regimens and therapy are included.

Viral Diseases

Rabbits can contract a variety of viral diseases, such as infectious myxomatosis (Figure 1), rotavirus, and coronavirus. Viral diseases are rarely diagnosed in pet rabbits in the United States. Infectious myxomatosis is discussed in this review, however, because it is a well documented viral disease in rabbits.

Infectious myxomatosis, a fatal disease of domesticated rabbits, is a poxvirus. The disease is transmitted to rabbits by mosquitoes, biting flies, fleas, or through direct contact with an infected rabbit. Clinical signs generally begin with conjunctivitis, which rapidly becomes more marked and is accompanied by a milky discharge from the inflamed eyes. Animals may demonstrate mild lethargy and have an elevated body temperature. Death occurs within 48 hours in a large percentage of animals. Rabbits that survive become progressively depressed, with an edematous face, rough haircoat, and potential cutaneous hemorrhages. At this stage, animals are anorectic and dehydrated. Lesions can either regress during a one- to three-month period or develop into skin tumors that may rupture and suppurate. In chronic cases, the disease can be complicated by pasteurellosis.

No known treatment for patients with infectious myxomatosis is available in the United States. The virus is not zoonotic. The disease can be prevented by insect control and by screening outdoor hutches. Infectious myxomatosis is primarily found on the West Coast of the United States and is not a common problem in pet rabbits.

Bacterial Diseases
Pasteurella multocida (Snuffles)

Pasteurella multocida (snuffles) (Figure 2) is a common, enzootic, contagious disease commonly found in domesticated rabbits. Several serotypes of this bacteria, with varying virulence, have been found in rabbits. The bacteria tends to live in the nares or sinuses but may be found in any organ of the body. Asymptomatic carriers of *Pasteurella* are common in rabbit colonies. Any of

Figure 1—Infectious myxomatosis in a rabbit. The rabbit shown is demonstrating severe cutaneous involvement with multiple skin tumor growth. (Courtesy of the School of Veterinary Medicine, University of California, Davis, California)

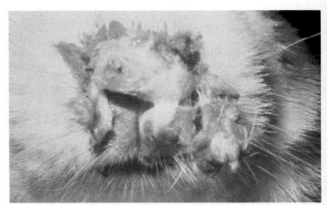

Figure 2—*Pasteurella multocida* (snuffles) in a pet rabbit. The rabbit shown is demonstrating severe signs of *Pasteurella* infection (i.e., severe crusting around the nares). Less severe signs include conjunctivitis, nasal discharge, and genital infections. (Courtesy of the School of Veterinary Medicine, University of California, Davis, California)

the following signs can be exhibited clinically: nasal discharge, pneumonia, otitis media (or wry neck caused by *Pasteurella* or *Staphylococcus* infection), conjunctivitis, abscesses, genital infection, or septicemia. Environmental stressors (e.g., high concentrations of ammonia in the air, poor sanitation, and high-protein diets) contribute to the development of clinical pasteurellosis. Some rabbits (usually old animals) may develop immunity after being infected and become asymptomatic carriers.

Transmission between rabbits occurs via direct contact, fomites, and airborne spread. Animals can be tested by taking a deep nasal swab and growing the organism on culture. Most laboratories only perform cultures for *Pasteurella* species; however, serologic testing is also available. An ELISA test designed to detect antibodies to *Pasteurella* is available for whole blood analysis through the Oregon State University Rabbit Research Center. A microagglutination test that requires one milliliter of serum is also available through the Texas Veterinary Medical Laboratory in Amarillo, Texas. Currently, most veterinarians only perform culture for diagnosis of pasteurellosis.

Antibiotics may provide temporary remission of clinical signs, but the next period of stress may cause a relapse. Some patients that are treated may not have another recurrence of the disease; however, they can never be completely cured and subsequently become carriers. Antibiotics used to treat rabbits with *Pasteurella* infection include trimethoprim-sulfa or enrofloxacin; drug therapy should be conducted for a minimum of three weeks. Tilmicosin phosphate, an antibiotic used to treat *Pasteurella* in cattle, has recently been used in rabbits. The agent, however, is not approved for use in rabbits

and fatal consequences may occur if the drug is overdosed. If tilmicosin phosphate is used, all other medication should be discontinued for one week before treatment, the rabbit should be hospitalized for 15 minutes after the injection, owners should not be permitted to give the drug, and a release form should be signed by the owner.

A follow-up culture after antibiotic treatment is important, and any abscess should be drained and cleaned. Isolation of the affected animal is also important. No effective preventive vaccine or treatment is available; therefore, purchasing animals from breeding stock that is free of *Pasteurella* and culling infected animals are the best methods of control. Although transmission to humans is extremely unlikely, *Pasteurella* can cause skin infections, arthritis, meningitis, peritonitis, pneumonia, and septicemia in susceptible individuals.

Staphylococcus Infections

Staphylococcus aureus is a common organism found in suppurative lesions in rabbits. Young rabbits affected with the septicemic form of *S. aureus* generally die. Clinical signs in cases of acute septicemia usually include fever, depression, and anorexia. Rabbits with this form of infection usually succumb within one week of the onset of clinical signs.

Rabbits may be infected with *S. aureus* but show little or no signs of clinical disease. Conjunctivitis may be the only evident clinical sign. In older rabbits, infection may involve almost any organ or tissue. Abscesses commonly contain *Staphylococcus* organisms. Mastitis has also been linked to *Staphylococcus* infections. In some cases, the infection may develop to septicemia and rapid death. Kits should not be fostered to another mother because the organism can be spread by the kits to the foster mother. Skin lesions are also evident with *Staphylococcus* infection. Diagnosis of the organism is by culture, and treatment of patients is similar to treatment of animals infected with *Pasteurella*, pending sensitivity testing.

Treponematosis

Treponematosis, or rabbit syphilis, is a venereal disease of domesticated rabbits. The disease clinically appears as scabbed external genitalia and genital ulcers and occurs in both sexes. Lesions may also be evident near the ears, nose, eyes, and lips. The disease is transmitted by coitus as well as from mother to offspring. Treponematosis is caused by the spirochete *Treponema cuniculi*, which can be observed using dark-field microscopy. Treatment of patients is attempted with subcutaneous penicillin injections, which may eradicate the organism in individuals, but all rabbits in the herd must be treated to eliminate the disease entirely.

Tyzzer's Disease

Tyzzer's disease is characterized by profuse diarrhea, anorexia, dehydration, lassitude, and death within one to three days. Tyzzer's disease was once believed to be caused by the enteric bacteria *Bacillus piliformis* but has been reclassified as an infection caused by *Clostridium piliforme*. The disease generally affects rabbits 6 to 12 weeks of age. Tyzzer's disease is uncommon in pet rabbits and is usually diagnosed at necropsy.

Bordetella bronchiseptica

Rabbits can be asymptomatic carriers of *Bordetella* bacteria. Transmission of *Bordetella bronchiseptica* occurs via direct contact or aerosolization; incubation of the organism is five to seven days. Clinical signs of the disease may include rapid death, nasal and ocular discharge, dyspnea, abortion, and stillbirth. Treatment of infected patients is accomplished by injectable trimethoprim-sulfa and supportive care. Isolation of affected animals is important. The disease is rapidly fatal in guinea pigs; therefore, guinea pigs and rabbits should not be housed together.

Enteric Diseases

Enteric complex is a general term used to describe gastrointestinal problems in rabbits. Many diseases (e.g., infectious, iatrogenic, and environmental) have clinical signs that include diarrhea. Infectious diseases, such as rotavirus, coccidiosis, and bacterial diseases (e.g., *Clostridium* species and *Escherichia coli*) are evident in young, stressed animals. Iatrogenic causes of diarrhea secondary to antibiotic treatment may be seen with such agents as penicillin, ampicillin, erythromycin, clindamycin, and lincomycin. Environmental alterations (pertaining to changes in diet and temperature stresses) may also affect fecal consistency. These factors, usually in the presence of stress, can predispose rabbits to the development of enteric complex.

Acute enteropathies generally affect very young or weanling rabbits. Lassitude, rough haircoat, a perineal area covered with a greenish brown fecal material, a watery feel when the animal is palpated, and death within 48 hours is evident clinically. As discussed in Part I, rabbits pass soft stools (cecotrophs) at night; cecotrophs should not be confused with signs associated with acute enteropathy. Also, soft stools passed at certain times of the day, mixed with normal stools, may be caused by a diet that is too low in fiber. Enteropathies are evident less often in animals that are fed a high-fiber diet.

Treatment varies with the presentation of the disease and age of the animal. Treatment of patients may include maintaining food intake with an increase in the fiber content of the food, fluid therapy, and a repopulation of normal gastrointestinal flora by feeding fecal material from a healthy rabbit. (Night stools from a healthy individual are best.)

Trichobezoar (Figure 3) or hair accumulation in the stomach of mature rabbits can also cause gastrointestinal problems. The reason rabbits ingest hair can range from a nutritional deficiency to boredom. Clinical signs often include anorexia, oligodipsia, bloat, hypothermia, weight loss, agalactia, depression, and absence of feces or diarrhea. Death from starvation and metabolic abnormalities may occur in three to four weeks. Diagnosis, which may be difficult, is generally based on clinical signs and radiographic examination. Treating patients with fresh pineapple juice or papaya enzyme tablets (if the rabbit is still eating) may be helpful. Pineapple juice contains the enzyme bromelin, which seems to help break up the hair ball. In terminal cases, gastrotomy and hair ball removal can be attempted but is associated with high mortality. Prevention of trichobezoar is accomplished by providing rabbits with quality grass hay and changing the diet to high-fiber feed.

Parasitic Diseases
Mite Infestation

Ear mites (*Psoroptes cuniculi*) (Figure 4) are seen in domesticated rabbits. Signs of infestation are head shak-

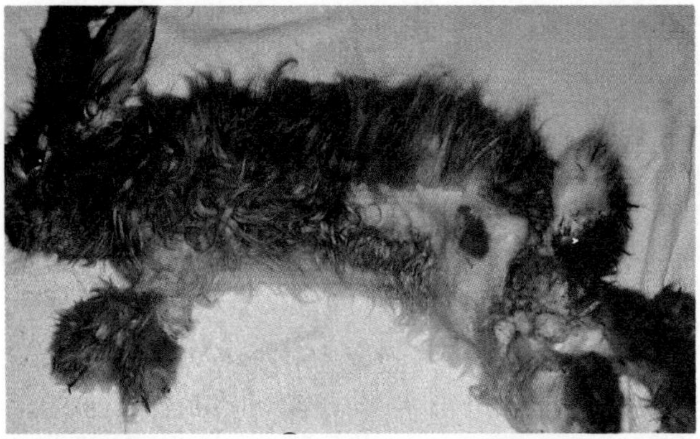

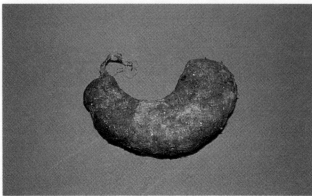

Figure 3A

Figure 3B

Figure 3—(A) Rabbit with trichobezoar. Clinically, the rabbit was emaciated, depressed, and hypothermic. (B) Trichobezoar after surgical removal. (Courtesy of the School of Veterinary Medicine, University of California, Davis, California)

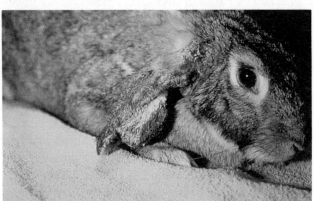

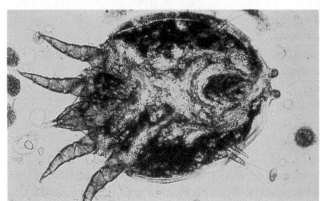

Figure 4A

Figure 4B

Figure 4—Ear mites in a pet rabbit. (A) The rabbit shown has a bilateral ear infection caused by *Psoroptes cuniculi*. (Courtesy of the School of Veterinary Medicine, University of California, Davis, California) (B) Photomicrograph of *Psoroptes cuniculi*. (Courtesy of Linda Sullivan, DVM, School of Veterinary Medicine, University of Wisconsin, Madison, Wisconsin)

ing; ear flapping; crusting around and in the external ear; scratching at the ears with the hind feet; or a loss of hair at the base of the ears, eyes, and head. If rabbits are infested, an examination of the ears will reveal a brown, crusty exudate. Normal ear exudate in rabbits should be minimal and can vary from white to yellow in color. Treatment of patients with subcutaneous ivermectin injections is the best choice; however, topical miticides have also been used. Ear cleaning is not needed before treatment and may cause unnecessary irritation in the ear. When rabbits are being treated, owners should be told that the mites can live outside the ear; therefore, the miticide should also be applied around the external ear and down the side of the neck. Rabbits that are being treated for infestation should be isolated and bathed, and the environment should be cleaned.

Pinworms

Pinworms may be seen as live worms in feces (usually found by an upset owner) or the eggs may be present in the feces and observed on fecal examination. The rabbit pinworm (*Passalurus ambiguus*) is transmitted via contaminated food or water. The adult parasite lives in the cecum or anterior colon. Eggs may be evident during a routine parasitologic examination. The adhesive tape test alone is not reliable for pinworm detection, and a complete fecal examination is recommended for diagnosis. The preferred treatment for rabbits with pinworms is piperazine or fenbendazole. More than one treatment, however, may be necessary to eliminate the worms.

Cheyletiella parasitovorax

Cheyletiella parasitovorax (Figure 5) is a fur mite of rabbits. This parasite may cause no clinical signs or result in loose hair that is easily pulled out in clumps. The exposed skin may appear reddened, oily, and hairless; scaly patches may be evident on the back and head of the rabbit. An increase in dandruff may be seen in infected animals. Diagnosis of the parasite is via skin

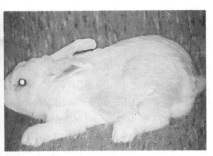

Figure 5A

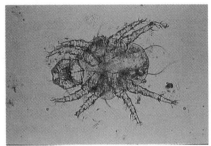

Figure 5B

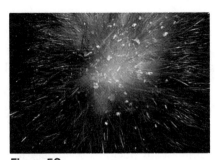

Figure 5C

Figure 5—Fur mites in a pet rabbit. (**A**) The rabbit shown has multiple areas of alopecia secondary to mite infestation caused by *Cheyletiella parasitovorax*. (Courtesy of the School of Veterinary Medicine, University of California, Davis, California) (**B**) Photomicrograph of *Cheyletiella parasitovorax*. (Courtesy of Linda Sullivan, DVM, School of Veterinary Medicine, University of Wisconsin, Madison, Wisconsin) (**C**) *Cheyletiella* organisms on the fur of a rabbit. (Courtesy of the School of Veterinary Medicine, University of California, Davis, California)

scraping. Injectable ivermectin given every two weeks for three doses or lime sulfur dip and/or shampoos and insecticidal dusting powders have been used to treat patients with *Cheyletiella* infestation. When rabbits are dipped in lime sulfur, technicians should remember to remove all jewelry. Isolation of rabbits affected by the parasite is important. *Cheyletiella parasitovorax* can cause dermatitis in humans and other animals.

Other Problems
Sore Hocks

Sore hocks is an ulcerative dermatitis that may occur on the plantar surface of the metatarsus in rabbits housed in cages with wire or solid floors. The incidence of disease may increase with an animal that is older and/or overweight or may be a genetic component of some rabbits that have a thin layer of fur over the feet and hock areas. In addition, lack of movement by the rabbit, which usually can be associated with being housed in a small, wet, unkempt cage, may also contribute to the development of the disease.

Topical antiseptics are generally used to treat patients with the condition; however, systemic treatment may be required. Protective dressings may also be helpful. The housing environment must be corrected in order to eliminate the problem. A soft, dry bedding material that provides a solid flooring in part of the cage can be used.

Malocclusion

Malocclusion is commonly seen in rabbits and small rodents. Chewing usually keeps the teeth at the proper length. If the teeth do not occlude properly, they can overgrow. The factors involved in tooth overgrowth can be nutritional, infectious, traumatic, or genetic. Patients with clinical signs of malocclusion may be presented because of salivation, anorexia, weight loss, starvation,

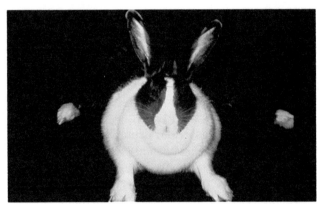

Figure 6—Posterior paralysis in a pet rabbit. The rabbit has a lumbosacral fracture secondary to improper handling. Posterior paralysis in rabbits has a poor prognosis for return to normal function. (Courtesy of the School of Veterinary Medicine, University of California, Davis, California)

and eventual death. Incisors should be routinely examined by pulling up on the lips; the molars and premolars should be examined by using an otoscope. Gauze that surrounds the upper and lower incisors may be helpful to open the mouth so that the back teeth can be examined. Isoflurane gas via a mask (used by an experienced examiner) or injectable anesthesia may be necessary to perform a thorough oral examination of the rabbit. Food, pus, oral ulcers, and excessive saliva in the mouth is abnormal and may indicate a malocclusion problem. Sedation and radiographs may be indicated to diagnose root infections.

Treatment of rabbits with dental malocclusion involves trimming of the teeth. This should be done with a Dremel drill or other similar grinding instruments. Bone rongeurs may be used to trim premolars and molars. Incisors can also be surgically removed; however, when rabbit teeth are extracted, the extensive curve of the tooth should be kept in mind. Teeth should not be clipped with a guillotine-style clipper because it may cause splitting, shattering, or growth of teeth in an abnormal fashion due to the stress placed on the teeth when they are clipped.

Posterior Paralysis

Posterior paralysis (Figure 6) is usually caused by lumbosacral fractures secondary to improper handling. Return to normal function in these animals is rare depending on the degree of neurologic damage; therefore, proper handling should be emphasized with owners (refer to Part I).

Uterine Adenocarcinoma

Uterine adenocarcinoma is a slow-growing tumor that is common in older rabbits. Unspayed female rabbits can develop a bloody vaginal discharge secondary to uterine adenocarcinoma. The color of rabbit urine can vary from clear to brown; therefore, a thorough examination should be performed to rule out disease of the urinary system. Other signs of urinary adenocarcinoma include infertility, anorexia, depression, dyspnea secondary to metastasis, and death. Prevention of the disease is best accomplished via ovariohysterectomy of rabbits; therefore, technicians should recommend this procedure (which is best performed in rabbits younger than two years of age) to all rabbit owners.

Urinary Problems

The color of urine in rabbits can vary from clear to brown. White, gritty urine can result from feeding a diet too high in calcium. High-calcium or high-protein diets may predispose rabbits to the development of uroliths. Urolithiasis can be a common problem in rabbits; ammonium magnesium phosphate and calcium carbonate are the most common uroliths found in the urine of rabbits. Urinalysis of abnormal urine is an important diagnostic test that should be performed on all sick rabbits. Performing urinalysis on urine from a healthy rabbit may help in dietary and disease management as well. Abdominal radiographs are an important diagnostic test in diagnosing urolithiasis; most uroliths in rabbits contain calcium and are therefore radiodense. Surgical removal, calculus analysis, and bladder culture are the optimum methods of treating rabbits with urolithiasis.

Conclusion

The diseases discussed in this article represent some of the more common diseases found in the pet rabbit population. Understanding such conditions in rabbits will enable technicians to aid veterinarians and rabbit owners in the care of this species. A more thorough description of other diseases may be found in the sources listed in the bibliography.

■

Bibliography

Carmen RJ: Clostridial enteropathies of rabbits. *Proc North Am Vet Conf*:795, 1993.

Fowler ME: *Restraint and Handling of Wild and Domestic Animals,* ed 6. Ames, IA, Iowa State University Press, 1987, pp 161–165.

Fraser CM (ed): *The Merck Veterinary Manual,* ed 6. Merck and Company Inc, 1986, pp 988–999.

Harkness JE: Rabbit husbandry and medicine, in *Vet Clin North Am Exotic Pet Med* 9:1019–1044, 1987.

Harkness JE, Wagner JE: *The Biology and Medicine of Rabbits and Rodents,* ed 2. Philadelphia, Lea & Febiger, 1983, pp 7–16.

Hawkey CM, Dennett TB: *Color Atlas of Comparative Veterinary Hematology.* Ames, IA, Iowa State University Press, 1989.

Hillyer EV: Pet rabbits. *Vet Clin North Am Small Anim Pract* 24(1):25–67, 1994.

Weisbroth SH, Flatt RE, Kraus AL (eds): *The Biology of the Laboratory Rabbit.* San Diego, Academic Press, 1974.

Anesthetic Management of Vietnamese Potbellied Pigs

Jeff C. H. Ko, DVM, MS
John C. Thurmon, DVM, MS
    Diplomate, ACVA
William J. Tranquilli, DVM, MS
    Diplomate, ACVA
G. John Benson, DVM, MS
    Diplomate, ACVA
Department of Veterinary Clinical Medicine
College of Veterinary Medicine
University of Illinois
Urbana, Illinois

Vietnamese potbellied pigs (Figure 1) have become increasingly popular pets during the past few years. Because many potbellied pigs are owned by urban and suburban families, small animal practitioners are frequently responsible for examining and treating these pigs and veterinary technicians are expected to be able to handle these pets and assist veterinarians during the examination and treatment procedures. Such procedures frequently require sedation and/or general anesthesia. This article discusses the anesthetic management of potbellied pigs with emphasis on special anatomic features, preanesthesia management, induction of anesthesia, anesthesia monitoring, and the recovery period.

ANATOMIC FEATURES

Potbellied pigs have several unusual anatomic features that significantly affect anesthetic management. Small ears, dark skin, and small ear veins make intravenous injection or catheterization difficult. Thick necks and lumpy jaws nearly preclude puncture of the anterior vena cava for intravenous injection. Direct visualization of the laryngeal opening

Originally published in Volume 13, Number 6, July 1992

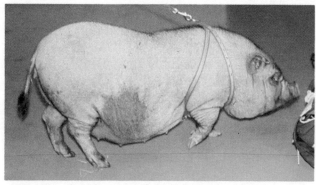

Figure 1—Vietnamese potbellied pigs have become increasingly popular pets. Note the thick neck and lumpy jaw.

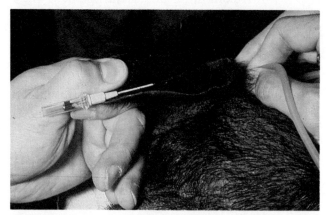

Figure 2—The ear veins can best be visualized when a rubber tourniquet is applied at the base of the ear. A 22-gauge 3.8-cm (1¹/₂-inch) catheter has been used to catheterize the vein.

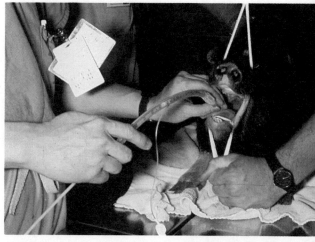

Figure 3—A plastic stylet is passed through the larynx into the trachea to serve as a guide for positioning the endotracheal tube.

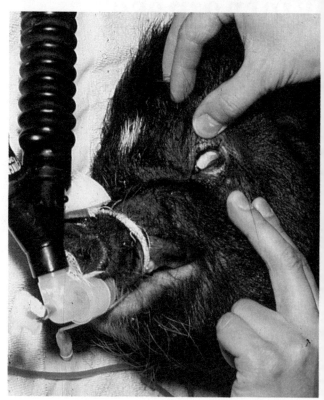

Figure 4—A surgical plane of anesthesia is characterized by ventral rotation of the eyeball and loss of the palpebral reflex.

(i.e., for tracheal intubation) is difficult because of a small oral orifice, prominent dorsal protrusion of the base of the tongue, and ventral sloping of the larynx. Thick subcutaneous fat over most of the body surface prevents intramuscular injection unless a long-enough needle is used.

PREANESTHESIA MANAGEMENT

Food must be withheld from potbellied pigs for at least 12 hours and water withheld for four to six hours before anesthesia. If the animal has not fasted, tracheal intubation is essential. We have found that potbellied pigs are more sensitive to anesthetics than are swine of most other breeds. Accurate weighing is essential because all doses of anesthetics are determined by body weight. Administering anesthetics on the basis of estimated body weight is unreliable and dangerous. Physical examination, including determination of heart rate and respiration rate, should be completed before induction of anesthesia. Because potbellied pigs are easily stressed, physical examination should be done in a fashion that minimizes excitement and therefore reduces stress and cardiopulmonary stimulation.

Because of their unusual anatomic features and temperament, potbellied pigs are difficult to restrain for intra-

venous injection. Consequently, it is prudent to tranquilize potbellied pigs with intramuscularly injected tranquilizers to allow subsequent induction of anesthesia without excessive excitement.

When properly used, a combination of tiletamine and zolazepam is an effective anesthetic for swine. The package insert for one product (Telazol®—Fort Dodge Laboratories) recommends reconstitution with 5 ml of sterile water. At the University of Illinois Veterinary Teaching Hospital, we mix Telazol® with ketamine hydrochloride and xylazine hydrochloride. When preparing this mixture for potbellied pigs, 2.5 ml of ketamine hydrochloride (100 mg/ml; 250 mg) combined with 2.5 ml of 10% xylazine hydrochloride (100 mg/ml; 250 mg) is used as the diluent. The intramuscular dose of the mixture required to sedate and immobilize potbellied pigs is 0.006 to 0.013 ml/kg.

Intramuscular injections are best made in the semimembranosus and semitendinosus muscles, which are located just above the hock, or in the caudal portion of the biceps femoris muscle. The area over these muscles has less fat, and the muscles can be more easily reached with a 3.8-cm (1½-inch) 20-gauge needle. Pigs usually assume lateral recumbency within three to five minutes after administration of the tranquilizer mixture into the semitendinosus muscle. Sedation and immobilization after the injection usually range from 35 to 40 minutes.

Once the pig is sedated, catheterization of an ear vein can be achieved. Ear veins are catheterized because they are the only readily visualized superficial veins on the external surface of pigs. Other veins are less visible and less accessible. An intravenous ear-vein catheter provides a route for administration of drugs or fluids and helps prevent inadvertent perivascular injection, which commonly results when only a needle is used.

The following material is required for catheterization of an ear vein:

- Rubber tourniquet
- 3.8-cm (1½-inch) 22-gauge intravenous catheter (Figure 2)
- Injection cap
- Small roll of gauze
- Suture material
- Adhesive tape.

The ear vein can best be visualized when a rubber tourniquet is applied at the base of the ear (Figure 2). Alcohol sprayed on the surface of the ear increases the visibility of the vein. Once the ear vein is catheterized, the catheter should be secured with skin sutures and taped in place over a gauze roll. Tape should not be placed over the ear proximal to the tip of the catheter. If this occurs, the vein will probably collapse, thus impeding blood flow and drug injection.

INDUCTION

Once the pig is tranquilized, anesthesia can be induced with injectable anesthetics or by mask with an inhalation anesthetic. When a mixture of Telazol®, ketamine hydrochloride, and xylazine hydrochloride is used, half of the calculated sedative and immobilization anesthetic dose is given intravenously for tracheal intubation. When mask induction is used, we routinely preoxygenate the pig (3 to 4 L/min for three to five minutes) and then introduce 3% to

5% isoflurane or halothane in oxygen. Within three to four minutes of administration of inhalant anesthetic, tracheal intubation is readily accomplished.

For tracheal intubation, the following materials are required: laryngoscope with a large (205-mm Miller) human blade, plastic stylet, 2% lidocaine, endotracheal tube, and gauze. After a surgical plane of anesthesia has been achieved, the mouth is opened and the tongue withdrawn (Figure 3). The tip of the laryngoscope blade is used to depress the base of the tongue. This maneuver displaces both the tongue and the epiglottis ventrally, thus exposing the laryngeal opening.

After it is visualized with a laryngoscope, the laryngeal opening is sprayed with 2% lidocaine to decrease the sensitivity of the larynx to intubation. A plastic stylet is placed in the trachea and serves as a guide for passing the endotracheal tube through the larynx (Figure 3). The plastic stylet should be held stationary while the endotracheal tube is positioned in the trachea (Figure 3). The stylet is then withdrawn and the cuff of the endotracheal tube inflated. During the course of intubation, failing to hold the plastic stylet stationary and permitting it to be advanced too far into the airway can result in injury to lung tissue. The endotracheal tube can be tied to either the upper or lower jaw; a gauze strip is used to secure the endotracheal tube (Figure 3).

MAINTENANCE AND MONITORING

Intravenous fluid, such as lactated Ringer's solution, should be administered at a rate of 11 to 22 ml/kg/hr during the maintenance of anesthesia. If surgery is prolonged, a heating pad should be provided. Mucous membrane color and capillary refill time should be monitored during anesthesia. Palpebral and corneal reflexes, eyeball position, anal tone, respiration rate, and heart rate are important indicators for monitoring the depth of anesthesia.

Surgical anesthesia is characterized by ventral rotation of the eyeball, with the cornea being partially or completely hidden by the lower eyelid (Figure 4) and loss of palpebral reflex and anal tone. As anesthesia deepens, the eyeball becomes centered and the pupils dilate. Palpebral and corneal reflexes are lost. Respiration and heart rates decrease. If anesthesia is too light, the eyeball is also centered but strong corneal and palpebral reflexes are present. Nystagmus (horizontal movement of the eyeball) may also be seen. Heart and respiration rates will increase, and anal tone will return.

RECOVERY

Potbellied pigs should not be extubated until the swallowing reflex is present and a chewing motion has begun.

The cuff of the endotracheal tube should be deflated and the tube carefully withdrawn from the mouth to prevent damage to the cuff and tube. After extubation, the pig should be observed until the tongue is withdrawn into the mouth. Heart and respiration rates and rectal temperature should be monitored. If body temperature is lower than 37°C (98°F), a heating pad should be provided. Breathing noise after extubation indicates possible airway obstruction. Mucous membrane color should be inspected and reintubation performed if necessary.

Compared with dogs and cats, potbellied pigs have unique anatomic features and unusual physiologic responses to anesthesia; the pigs present a challenge to small animal practitioners and veterinary technical staff. Thorough understanding of anatomic and physiologic peculiarities helps ensure safe anesthesic procedures for these unusual swine.

UPDATE

Jeff C. H. Ko, DVM, MS
Luisito S. Pablo, DVM, MS, Dip. ACVA
Anesthesiology Section
Department of Large Animal Clinical Sciences
College of Veterinary Medicine
University of Florida
PO Box 100136
Gainesville, FL 32610-0136

Injectable Anesthesia

There are two additional useful injectable combinations that can be used for potbellied pig anesthesia. The first combination is Telazol®-xylazine (TX) which is very similar to the Telazol-ketamine-xylazine (TKX) combination as we described in the original article. For preparation of TX, 5 ml of xylazine (10%) is added into a bottle of Telazol® powder. The preparation of the TX is summarized in Table I. We evaluated TX and TKX combinations in potbellied pigs in the clinical setting. We found that TX is the drug of choice. TX produced better analgesia (approximately 30 minutes), longer duration of endotracheal intubation, and smoother recovery than TKX in potbellied pigs.

The second combination is ketamine and xylazine (KX). This combination when compared to either TKX or TX combination has the following advantages and disadvantages: 1) Telazol® is a controlled substance under Drug Enforcement Agency regulations. Ketamine and xylazine are not controlled substances and may be more suitable for the practitioner who does not want to deal with regulations governing the use of controlled substances such as Telazol®; 2) TKX, TX, and KX are all suitable for tranquil-

TABLE I
Summary of Anesthetic Combinations and Their Preparation in Potbellied Pigs

Group	Diluent Volume (total 5 ml)	Drug Concentration (mg/ml)	Sedation IM Dosage (mg/lb)	Anesthesia IM Dosage (mg/lb)
TKX				
Tiletamine	—	50	0.5	1.0
Zolazepam	—	50	0.5	1.0
Ketamine	2.5	50	0.5	1.0
Xylazine	2.5	50	0.5	1.0
TX				
Tiletamine	—	50	0.5	1.0
Zolazepam	—	50	0.5	1.0
Ketamine	—	—	—	—
Xylazine	5	100	1.0	2.0
KX				
Ketamine	—	100	2.0	4.0
Xylazine	—	100	1.0	2.0

ization of potbellied pigs; 3) KX is not as potent as either TKX or TX in terms of analgesia and sedation in potbellied pigs. The analgesic property of the KX combination can be improved by simultaneous administration (IM with KX in the same syringe) of butorphanol, an opioid agonist-antagonist, 0.2 mg/lb.

The sedative and anesthetic doses of TX for potbellied pigs are similar to TKX. For sedation the TX is 0.01 ml/lb intramuscularly. For injectable anesthesia, the dose of TX is 0.02 ml/lb. Potbellied pigs receiving this dose can be intubated approximately 5 minutes after injection. A summary of TX and KX for sedation and anesthesia dosages is listed in Table I.

Inhalational Anesthesia

Malignant hyperthermia (MH) is a life-threatening syndrome and usually fatal in pigs. Malignant hyperthermia can be triggered by halothane and isoflurane. Suspected MH has been reported in a miniature potbellied pig undergoing isoflurane anesthesia.[1] This suggests that potbellied pigs may be as susceptible as other domestic pigs to MH. The clinical signs of MH include tachycardia, tachypnea, muscle rigidity, and hyperthermia. To date, there has not been a confirmed case of MH in potbellied pigs. However, it is important to closely monitor potbellied pigs under inhalational anesthesia for development of signs suggestive of MH. For further detailed information regarding MH in pigs, please refer to reference 1.

REFERENCES
1. Claxton-Gill MS, Cornick-Seahorn JL, Gamboa JC, Boatright BS: Suspected malignant hyperthermia syndrome in a miniature pot-bellied pig anesthetized with isoflurane. *JAVMA* 203(10):1434–1436, 1993.
2. Ko JCH, Thurmon JC, Benson GJ, Tranquilli WJ, Olson WA: Problems encountered when anesthetizing potbellied pigs. *Vet Med*, May 435–440, 1993.

MINIATURE PIGS
A VETERINARY PERSPECTIVE

George H. D'Andrea, DVM, MS, Dipl. ACVP
Charles S. Roberts Veterinary Diagnostic Laboratory
Auburn, Alabama

Jim Floyd, DVM, PhD, Dipl. ACT
Auburn University, Auburn, Alabama

Miniature pigs are exotic pets that have attained a degree of popularity in the last decade. While market values have dropped precipitously in recent years, they still enjoy widespread distribution. The August 16, 1993 issue of *Time* magazine featured a picture of a "miniature pig" at a placement shelter. The Vietnamese potbellied pig was described in this same article as one of the three animals most commonly abandoned by their owners.

Miniature pigs kept as pets in this country predominantly stem from three lines of Vietnamese potbellied pigs, the African pygmy and the Yucatan miniature pig. The Yucatan miniature pig has been used in research but the most popular pet pig is the Vietnamese potbellied pig. Various lines of these pigs have different physical characteristics and it is beyond the scope of this article to elaborate on them. However, buyer beware since "miniature pigs" tend to become "big pigs" and care should be exercised in purchasing these animals. Several associations now exist in this country to provide information and these should be consulted. An abridged list is given at the end of this article.

Miniature pigs fall under the regulatory auspices of USDA. Health certificates are needed for transport and when in doubt the appropriate officials in the state of destination should be contacted. Pseudorabies and *Brucella* are highly visible diseases that require a current test.

A pet assumes a different monetary value than the animal kept for production. Urban practitioners should remember that they are dealing with a farm animal and the swine production specialist must develop a companion animal attitude toward the miniature pig owner. Some basic clinical parameters are available for some miniature pigs, including the Yucatan and Vietnamese potbellied pigs. It is presumed that as a population of geriatric pigs evolves, more cases of neoplasia will be found. At this juncture hemangiomas, melanomas and probably embryonal nephromas have been recognized in Vietnamese potbellied pigs.

Commercial diets are available for miniature pigs. These and other commercial swine feeds require an added source of fiber to comprise about 20% of the diet. Vietnamese potbellied pigs have a large stomach capacity and supplementation with alfalfa is beneficial. Miniature pigs can have weight problems and careful attention should be paid to energy intake. Feeding of table scraps should be discouraged.

Miniature pigs require exercise time of at least one hour per day to help maintain their weight and conditioning. These animals will entertain themselves given appropriate toys and they can be trained to a leash.

Miniature pigs are probably susceptible to the same diseases noted in commercial swine operations. However, the potential for exposure varies due to the nature of the confinement. In one retrospective study of pigs submitted for necropsy, slightly fewer than half of the animals had enteric disease and about one third had respiratory disease. *Escherichia coli* was the most common enteric pathogen followed by *Clostridium perfringens*, rotavirus, and coronavirus(TGE). *Pasteurella multocida*, *Mycoplasma* sp. and swine influenza were implicated in the respiratory disease. These disease conditions were similar to those noted in necropsies of swine from commercial operations processed during a similar period. *Streptococcus suis* arthritis, meningitis, and septicemia are not uncommon in Vietnamese potbellied pigs.

Vaccines against *Erysipelas*, atrophic rhinitis, *Mycoplasma hyopneumoniae* and *Leptospira* are recommended. Vaccination programs can begin at 4 to 6 months and repeated semiannually thereafter. Breeding stock should be vaccinated against parvovirus twice a year. In regions where tetanus is common, toxoid should be used.

Pigs kept in modern production facilities have a very low incidence of rabies. However, when kept as pets concern should be exercised as to the appropriate protection from this disease. Because the incidence of rabies in pigs is low compared to other species we have not broached the needs for vaccines. In the pet environment where pet pigs can be exposed to our vaccinated pets or wild caught pets such as the raccoon, the need for vaccination should be considered. At this writing there is no approved vaccine for pet pigs and the incubation time has not been defined.

In some climates the skin may become dry and require applications of moisturizers. Sarcoptic mange, stress alopecia, and sunburn are common medical conditions. Sarcoptes may be treated with Ivermectin (1%) at 1 ml/75 pounds twice at 10 day intervals. Hypoallergenic sun screens may be used if animals are exposed for prolonged periods to summer sun.

Congenital conditions have included aplasia of the radius, fused lumbar vertebrae, hydrocephalus, cryptorchism, and shaker pigs syndrome. A condition described as epilepsy has been noted. Congenital entropion may require intervention.

The examination of the miniature pig requires either physical or chemical restraint. The spine of the potbellied pig is subject to physical stress and grasping or elevating the rear limbs can result in injury. The forelimbs should be elevated with the animal's back resting against the legs of the holder and the hams resting on the floor. Since these pigs can develop aggressiveness toward strangers, care should be exercised in physical handling, particularly boars. Some pigs will fight the snare rather than backing away and caution is needed to avoid injury to oneself and the pig.

Various forms of chemical restraint have been used to include xylazine/ketamine, telazol/ketamine and azaperone. Acepromazine and ketamine alone give inconsistent results. Only azaperone is approved for use in the pig. Azaperone is given at 0.5 mg/kg IM for relaxation, 2 mg/kg IM for preanesthesia, and 8 mg/kg IM for anesthesia. The Vietnamese potbellied pig has a thick subcutaneous fat pad and a 2.5 inch needle may be needed for IM injections. Both halothane and isoflurane are suitable anesthetic gases although malignant hyperthermia may occur with the use of halothane.

The Vietnamese potbellied pig has increased body fat and a poor thermoregulatory capacity. The small heart, lung and circulatory capacity of this animal requires attention to handling techniques and close monitoring when restrained.

Since many of the miniature pigs are kept in a home environment, certain surgical procedures may become commonplace. Castration, ovariohysterectomy and tusk cutting are commonly performed. Castration is best performed in younger animals and follows procedures given for domesticated production swine. Ovariohysterectomy requires some caution since the ovarian ligaments are short and friable. Care should be exercised in exteriorizing them. Tusk of adult males should be cut, preferably with Gigli's wire, every 6 to 12 months while the animal is under sedation/anesthesia. Electroejaculation and artificial insemination in Vietnamese potbellied pigs has been successfully performed.

In summary, most of the literature concerning the miniature pig is directed to the most common of the pets, the Vietnamese potbellied pig. Protocols for disease prevention and treatment frequently are extrapolated from those used for production swine operations. Philosophical and physical difference exist when attending pets compared to commercial pigs. Much is still to be learned about disease processes in the miniature pig and no one reference source is complete.

Other Sources of Information:

Pot-bellied Pet Pigs: Mini-Pig Care and Training
Kayla Mull and Lorrie Blackburn.
All Publishing, 10958 Meads Avenue, Orange, CA 92669
(Client Information Source) $9.95 + $2.00 Handling

Guidelines for the Care and Management of Miniature Pigs.
David Reeves, Editor
Veterinary Practice Publishing Company
P.O. Box 4457, Santa Barbara, CA 93140-4457
(805) 965-1028
(Veterinary Reference Source) $40.00

Potbellied Pigs
Sarman Publications, Box 853, Ooltewah, TN 37363
(Published Bimonthly)

Potbellied Pig Registry Service, Inc.
American Miniature Pig Association
22819 Stanton Road
Lakeville, IN 46536 (219) 784-2989

North American Potbellied Pig Association
Box 784
Columbia, MO 65205

References

1. Care and Management of Miniature Pet Pigs, Guidelines for the Veterinary Practitioner. Ed D. E. Reeves, Veterinary Practice Publishing Company, Santa Barbara, AL, 1993.
2. Bradford, JR. Caring for potbellied pigs. Vet Med 86:1173-1181, 1991.
3. Duran O, Walton J. Treatment and care of pet pigs. Vet Rec 1992;131:572-573.
4. Evans LE, Ko JCH. Electroejaculation and artificial insemination in Vietnamese potbellied miniature pigs. J Am Vet Med Assoc 1990;197:1366-1367.
5. Gleed R. Anesthesia for parlor pigs (Vietnamese potbellied pigs). Proc of The North Am Vet Assoc 1993;7:582-583.
6. Hall, RF. The Vietnamese potbellied pig: a porcine companion animal. Proc Am Assoc Swine Pract 1991:285-289, 1991.
7. Lawhorn, Bruce. Exotic Pet Medicine Seminar, Texas Veterinary Medical Center.
8. Pace LW, Kreeger JM, Miller, MA, et al. Necropsy findings from Vietnamese potbellied pigs, 33 cases. J Vet Diagn Invest 1992;4:351-352.
9. Sawatsky JD. Vietnamese potbelly pigs. Proc of The North Am Vet Assoc 1992;6:582-583.
10. Swindle MM. Minipigs as pets. Proc of The North Am Vet Assoc 1993;7:648-649.

Introducing the Ostrich

To successfully manage, diagnose, and treat ostriches, veterinary professionals need to understand various aspects of the species.

Kathleen M. Kimminau, CVT
Pitts Veterinary Hospital
Lincoln, Nebraska

Ostrich farming, although seemingly new to the United States, is in fact an old, established industry. Ostrich farming began in 1857 in South Africa.[1] It flourished and rapidly spread to other countries, including Germany, France, and Australia. The industry crashed, however, with the onset of World War I in 1914 as the demand for ostrich plumes declined. After World War II, the demand for ostrich products increased and ostrich farming revived.[1]

The current demand for ostrich meat (in Europe), leather, and feathers far exceeds supply, and future international demand is optimistic. Ostrich meat may be the meat of the future because it contains less cholesterol, fat, and calories than beef, pork, lamb, turkey, or chicken. Ostrich leather is one of the most valuable exotic skins. In the United States, ostrich leather is used mainly in the manufacturing of cowboy boots, which represent $9,000,000 in tanned ostrich hides annually. Prime ostrich plumes sell for as much as $150 per pound and are marketed worldwide.[1] New ostrich farms are being established throughout the United

Originally published in Volume 14, Number 8, August 1993

States to share in this profitable market.

The revival of the ostrich farming industry and the subsequent increase in ostrich patients has prompted the need for educating veterinary professionals about these birds. To successfully manage, diagnose, and treat ostriches, veterinary professionals need to understand various aspects of the species.

This article presents a general introduction to the ostrich. Readers are encouraged to seek information beyond the scope of this article.

GENERAL INFORMATION

The ostrich, *Struthio camelus*, is a native bird of the African plains and belongs to the avian division of flightless birds called *ratites*. Ostriches are the largest of all living birds, standing six to nine feet tall and weighing between 300 and 400 pounds. The male feathercoat is solid black, whereas the female feathercoat is brownish gray; both have white wings and tail plumes. Skin color varies (i.e., pink, blue, red, or yellow) depending on the subspecies.[2] Males and females reach maturity between two and four years of age. Hens begin laying at two to three years of age and can lay 40 to 50 eggs per year for 40 years. Ostriches can live from 30 to 70 years.[2,3]

The eyes of ostriches are proportionally the largest of all land animals. Ostriches have excellent eyesight and hearing. Their strong muscular thighs are well adapted to swimming and running. They can run up to 30 to 50 miles per hour for periods of 15 to 30 minutes.[2-5] In nature, ostriches are found in breeding pairs or in large groups of mixed flocks and individuals. Their social system is the most complex of the animal world.[3]

BEHAVIOR
Social

Ostriches generally are not aggressive and show no social order of feeding. These characteristics stem from their natural alertness and constant scanning of the landscape for predators. The duty of scanning is rotated among the members of the group; those not involved in scanning eat and drink. In their native habitat, ostriches enjoy communal sandbathing or feather dusting.[3]

Daily

In addition to eating, walking, and sandbathing, ostriches spend their time pecking and sleeping. Their constant pecking (2000 to 4000 times daily) permits not only food consumption but also examination of the environment. Pecking can be a problem with young chicks because they are likely to pick up foreign objects that may obstruct the gastrointestinal system. Pecking is a behavior that young chicks must learn by mimicking others, or it must be taught by the producer. Sleeping habits involve sitting with the eyes closed and the head and neck erect; the head and neck eventually become prone as deep sleep is reached. Ostriches produce various sounds—pleasant calls, guttural sounds, hisses, and snorts. They are particularly vocal with the onset of breeding season.[3]

Sexual

Behavior becomes aggressive as summer, with its long days and short nights, approaches (long-day breeders).[6] The jumps and forward kicks of ostriches can deliver fatal blows of up to 500 pounds per square inch.[2] Depending on mate availability, ostriches may be polygamous and/or monogamous. To attract a prospective male, the female ostrich stands erect, urinates, and defecates. It may drive away unwanted females and males by kicking, hissing, and pecking.[3] To signal receptivity, the hen lowers its head and extends and flutters her wings. This behavior is commonly referred to as fluttering.

Sexual behavior of the cock increases along with the red pigmentation on its face, feet, and shins. Courtship is a series of displays, dances, vocalizations (announcing territory), and synchronized behavior. Males signify their readiness to breed by a characteristic precopulatory behavior known as kantel, in which the wings alternately sweep the ground and the head rhythmically sways from side to side. After the eggs are fertilized, the male shares in the rearing of the offspring by building and guarding the nest. Cocks, camouflaged in black, incubate the eggs at night; the female, camouflaged in brown, sits on the eggs during the day.[3]

HUSBANDRY
Chicks

In breeding farms, 24 to 48 hours after hatching, chicks are moved to a brooder box (temperature ranges between 88°F and 92°F [31°C to 33°C]) and are fed commercial ratite starter (at least 18% protein).[2] The water should contain an electrolyte and vitamin mix for added nutrition. After two to three weeks, chicks can be slowly introduced to brooder pens by frequent, short visits, which allow them to familiarize themselves with the new surroundings and to distinguish food. Close observation of chicks is necessary to prevent impactions of the proventriculus caused by ingestion of inappropriate material. Environmental temperature should be maintained between 70°F and 80°F (21°C to 27°C).[2,3]

Juveniles and Adults

Juvenile and adult ostriches should be carefully examined for signs of illness or injury. Ratite grower, grit, and succulent plants (e.g., alfalfa, wheat, and rye) are usually fed. After one year of age, ostriches can adapt well to various climatic conditions.

Transportation

Adult ostriches should be transported in a closed trailer because the darkness inside provides a calming effect. Rubber mats should be used to cover the trailer floor; these provide traction. The use of hay or straw, which, if consumed, can cause stomach impactions, should be avoided. Small chicks may be transported in a pet caddie. Movement should be done slowly to avoid exciting the birds, which may result in injury to the birds themselves or to the handler. Hooding birds (see the section on restraint) on entrance to and exit from the trailer is helpful.[3]

Housing

Ostriches should be kept in a one- to three-acre, wedge-shaped pen for easy corralling. Fences should be six to seven feet high and constructed of wood, welded oil-field pipe, chain link, or any dull fence material. Lots may be sand, dirt, gravel, or ideally short grass. When switching substrates, a gradual change to the new substrate is necessary to decrease the risk of stomach impaction. Shelter, such as a three-sided shed, is recommended in regions with inclement weather.[3]

Sanitation

Proper hygiene is essential in controlling bacterial, viral, and fungal diseases. All areas should be kept clean and free of foreign material. Routine group fecal examination is recommended to control intestinal parasites. Commonly used disinfectants are quaternary ammonium compounds, a 5% bleach and water solution, and phenolic cleaners. Any of these compounds can be used to clean hatcheries, brooder boxes and pens, and breeding areas.[3]

NUTRITION

Little research has been done on the proper nutritional requirements of ostriches. In general, the staple of the diet comprises commercial ratite pellets. Approximate adequate ostrich nutrient levels are 16% to 20% protein, ≤10% fat, ≤10% fiber, 2.5% calcium, and 1.5% phosphorus. Many dog, rabbit, and horse chows have similar nutrient concentrations.[3] Free-choice feeding adult ostriches approximately 1 pound of feed per 40 pounds of body weight is recommended. Ostriches will also consume insects and succulent plants. Water should be available at all times.

Diet is particularly important in sick or debilitated birds and may be supplemented with fresh fruits (e.g., apples and prunes) and vegetables (e.g., peas, lettuce, and carrots). Administration of protein boluses to anorectic ostriches may be necessary. During cold weather, cracked corn may be added to the diet to provide extra calories.

RESTRAINT

Restraint methods vary with the size of the animal. Chicks that weigh less than 30 pounds can be easily herded and restrained by holding their abdomens and leaving the legs free. Gentle restraint is imperative to avoid bruises or fractures.[6] When a chick is released, it must be momentarily stabilized to prevent uncoordinated takeoffs.

Adults are more difficult to handle. The main concern for the handler is the threat of the ostriches' forward kick by their strong legs. *Handlers should not stand in front of adult birds.* To restrain the ostrich for a procedure, the base of the neck must be grasped and the head lowered to just above ground level. An opaque hood (a stockinette, shirt sleeves, or a sock) should be placed over the head and neck (Figure 1). *The nostrils should never be covered.* This method quiets the bird for manipulation. To move the ostrich, two people should each grasp the base of a wing and a third person should control the rump. Adult birds can be herded with visual barriers or arms.[6,7] Portable ostrich chutes are also available to allow safe manipulation of the birds.

Darkness aids in restraint. It disorients the ostriches, causing them to assume their nighttime sitting position. The reluctance to move facilitates examination.

COMPARATIVE ANATOMY

Understanding ostrich anatomy is important in clinical medicine and in management of these birds.

Skin. The ostrich feathercoat resembles hair because the feathers have no barbules. The thighs of ostriches are devoid of feathers. Like other birds, ratites have no sweat glands. To protect their bony prominences from trauma when sitting, ostriches have thick skin pads characterized by calluses, which cover such pressure points as the plantar digits, hock, sternum, and pelvic bones.[8]

Muscle. The inability of ostriches to fly is in part the result of the lack of breast muscles. Their strong, muscular upper legs, however, provide an alternate method of escape.

Bone. The absence of the keel bone for flight muscle attachment also contributes to the inability of ostriches to fly.

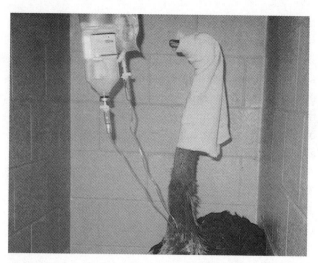

Figure 1—Juvenile ostrich hooded for manipulation.

TABLE I
Mean Hematologic Values for Adult Ostriches[3]

Parameter	Mean Value
Packed cell volume	32%
Total red blood cell count	$1.7 \times 10^6/\mu l$
Hemoglobin	12.2 g/dl
Mean corpuscular volume	174 fl
Mean corpuscular hemoglobin concentration	33.0%
Total white blood cell count	$5.5 \times 10^3/\mu l$
Lymphocytes	1705
Heterophils	3443
Monocytes	154
Eosinophils	16.5
Basophils	11

An ostrich has no patella, although an unfused tarsal bone may radiographically resemble one. The femur is the only air-filled bone. The ostrich is unique among the ratites in that it has only two toes instead of three; each toe has four phalanges. In an adult, the scapula, coracoid, and clavicle are fused and attached to the sternum. The pelvic girdle consists of fused ischial and pubic bones, which form a pubic symphysis.[3,4,8]

Circulation. The significance of the renal portal system in ostriches is controversial. Ostriches are reported to have a renal portal system that directs venous blood flow from the lower body through the kidneys before it reaches general circulation; therefore, nephrotoxic drugs (e.g., aminoglycosides) administered in the leg muscles may reach the kidneys in high concentrations. Conversely, drugs excreted by the kidneys may be removed before they reach appropriate circulatory levels.[4,8] According to Jensen, however, there was no discrepancy in blood concentration or clearance rates when an aminoglycoside (amikacin sulfate) was investigated. Amikacin sulfate was administered intramuscularly in cranial and caudal regions of the body. The results indicate that the renal portal system is not physiologically or pharmacologically significant in ratites.[3]

Digestion. In most birds, the entire inner surface of the proventriculus secretes digestive enzymes and acid; however, the proventriculus of an ostrich has only a single enzyme and acid secretory patch. Ostriches have no crop or gallbladder. Their paired ceca function in fermentative digestion.[3,4,8]

Reproduction. Male ratites have a phallus (analogous to the penis), but it does not contain a urethra.[3,4]

Respiration. Ostriches breathe laterally, not ventrally like other species of birds.[3]

PHYSIOLOGIC PARAMETERS

Normal body temperature and heart and respiratory rates in ostriches are greatly influenced by such stress factors as handling, trauma, or surgery. With isoflurane anesthesia, body temperature decreases; heart rate may increase to 120 beats/min; and respiratory rate may increase to 40 breaths/min.[7] Normal temperature for ostriches is 99°F to 104°F (37.2°C to 40°C), and normal respiratory rate is 6 to 12 breaths/min.

Hematologic assessments are important tools in diagnosing disease. Mean values for adult ostriches are summarized in Table I. White blood cell counts must be performed manually using a hemocytometer because avian red blood cells are nucleated. Automated machines cannot distinguish between leukocytes and erythrocytes. Natt and Herrick's solution is the recommended stain and diluent for the white blood cell count.[3] The packed cell volume (32%) in ostriches is lower than that of other birds (35% to 55%). Juvenile ostriches exhibit lower packed cell volumes than do adults.[3,5] The total red blood cell count ($1.7 \times 10^6/\mu l$) and white blood cell count ($5.5 \times 10^3/\mu l$) are also slightly below the normal avian range of 2 to $4 \times 10^6/\mu l$ and 4 to $15 \times 10^3/\mu l$, respectively. Adult ostriches have higher hemoglobin and mean corpuscular hemoglobin concentrations than do juveniles.[3,5]

Normal serum chemistry values for ostriches vary according to the laboratory testing method and the environmental factors affecting the bird. Average values listed in Table II are from the Animal Reference Laboratory of Houston, Texas. Serum chemistry values differ because of variation in blood collection technique, stress, and diet.

Young ostriches have lower total serum protein levels (3.7 g/dl) than do adults (4.5 g/dl).[3,5] Serum glucose levels are much higher than those of mammals. Serum values for

TABLE II
Normal Serum Chemistry Values for Ostriches

Parameter	Mean Value
Albumin	1.8–3.2 g/dl
Alkaline phosphatase	46–242 IU/L
Alanine transaminase	1–16 IU/L
Aspartate transaminase	250–469 IU/L
Bilirubin	0.1–0.3 mg/dl
Blood urea nitrogen	1–8 mg/dl
Cholesterol	32–177 mg/dl
Creatinine	0.1–0.6 mg/dl
Creatine kinase	1465–8310 IU/L
γ-Glutamyl transferase	0–10 IU/L
Glucose	168–289 mg/dl
Lactate dehydrogenase	412–1700 IU/L
Phosphorus	1.9–7.0 mg/dl
Calcium	10.2–15.2 mg/dl
Total protein	3.7–5.6 g/dl
Uric acid	4.7–15.8 mg/dl

TABLE III
Average Plasma Electrolyte Levels for Ostriches[3]

Electrolyte	mEq/L
Sodium	147
Potassium	3.0
Chloride	100
Calcium	2.3

the primary avian nitrogen by-product uric acid are higher in young ostriches (9.4 mg/dl) than in adults (6.3 mg/dl).[3] Further research on normal blood chemistry values is needed. Plasma electrolyte levels for ostriches are given in Table III.

VENIPUNCTURE

Knowledge of the location of the superficial veins is essential for blood collection and catheter placement. The jugular, brachial, and medial metatarsal veins are all suitable sites. The left jugular vein is significantly smaller than the right. The brachial and medial metatarsal sites (Figure 2) are recommended for catheter placement and for sedative administration.[4,8] Catheters must be secured with skin adhesive and bandaging to minimize the risk of the catheter being pecked and ingested.[3,4,6,8]

Blood for a complete blood count is collected with lithium heparin. The blood smear must be prepared before being mixed with heparin (the anticoagulant) because heparin destroys the membranes of the blood cells. Sodium citrate and EDTA may be used in other hematologic tests.[3]

Blood collection for chemical evaluation requires special consideration. Ratite blood clots quickly and forms gelatinous clots. The serum therefore may not be separated from the clots. For best results, the blood tubes should be warmed slightly in a water bath before centrifugation.[3]

THERAPEUTICS
Oral

The simplest route and method of administration is self-treatment, which uses the ostriches natural pecking behavior for consumption of pills. Coating the pills with molasses encourages eating. Soluble medication also may be placed in water troughs. Oral liquid medication may be delivered directly via a lubricated stomach tube. The distance from the beak to the sternum must be measured to ensure proper tube placement. An esophagostomy tube can be surgically placed for long-term administration of nutrients, fluids, or oral medications.[3,6]

Parenteral

Subcutaneous administration of medication (excluding ivermectin) is not recommended. Medication is poorly absorbed because of insufficient subcutaneous tissue and vasculature. If subcutaneous administration is warranted, the medication must be given in the loose skin cranial to the thigh.

Because ostriches do not have breast muscles, intramuscular injections should be given in the lumbar muscles on either side of the spine. The thigh muscles should not be used as injection sites because of potential bruising of this prime meat cut.

Intravenous sites are usually brachial or medial metatarsal veins. Standard isotonic electrolyte solutions (e.g., lactated Ringer's solution or 0.9% sodium chloride) can be used for fluid therapy at doses of 300 ml/hr. The abdominal skin cranial to the thigh is an acceptable site for the evaluation of hydration status.[3]

Antibiotics

The dosages of antibiotics used for dogs and cats are not appropriate for ostriches. Some research has been done on antibiotics for ostriches, but more research is needed. Subjective dosages for commonly used antibiotics are given in Table IV.

ANESTHESIA

Anesthesia is required for ostriches undergoing simple procedures, such as laceration repair, or complicated procedures, such as bone plating (see Anesthetic Agents). If the

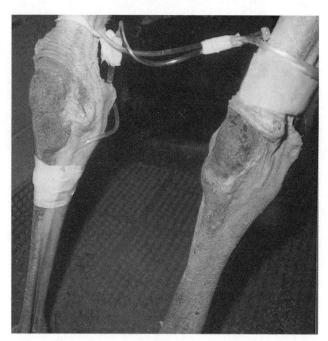

Figure 2—Intravenous catheter in the medial metatarsal vein of an ostrich.

ostrich is intubated, the neck should be kept straight to prevent kinking of the endotracheal tube. For all types of anesthesia, supplemental heat to reduce hypothermia and ample ventral padding to prevent ischemia and nerve injury should be provided. Recovery should take place in a dark, padded room, with the patient under constant observation.

INFECTIOUS DISEASE AGENTS
Parasites

Because of the long history of ostrich farming, much information on parasites is available (see Common Nematodes, Cestodes, and Trematodes of Ostriches). Internal parasites in hand-raised ostriches are infrequently seen in comparison with those in pasture-raised or free-roaming birds. Because most eggs are artificially incubated and chicks are hand-raised, offspring are isolated from potentially infested adult birds. This separation interrupts the parasitic life cycle.[3]

Nematodes are primarily a problem in range-raised birds. The ostrich wire worm (*Libyostrongylus douglassii*) is the most problematic in the African ostrich industry. It inhabits the proventriculus and causes severe pathologic changes in the organ. In the past, the wire worm was treated with levamisole hydrochloride, but resistance to this anthelmintic has developed; therefore, fenbendazole or ivermectin is the preferred drug.[3]

Ostriches may also be host to a tapeworm, *Houttuynia struthionis*, which typically is diagnosed by the presence of

Anesthetic Agents

Sedatives
Xylazine hydrochloride[3]
- Immobilization: 1 to 2.2 mg/kg intramuscularly
- Tranquilization: 0.2 to 1.0 mg/kg intramuscularly
- Xylazine may be partially reversed with yohimbine (0.125 mg/kg intravenously)
- May be used in combination with ketamine hydrochloride

Acepromazine maleate[3]
- 0.1 to 0.2 mg/kg intravenously or 0.25 to 0.5 mg/kg intramuscularly
- Produces good muscle relaxation

Diazepam[5,9]
- 0.1 to 0.3 mg/kg intravenously
- Minimizes thrashing during anesthetic recovery

Injectable Anesthetics
Ketamine hydrochloride[3,9]
- 50 mg/kg intramuscularly
- Ketamine does not produce acceptable analgesia in ratites
- Intramuscular injection may cause convulsive behavior during anesthetic recovery

Ketamine hydrochloride and xylazine hydrochloride[3]
- Xylazine: 2.2 mg/kg intramuscularly
- Ketamine: 2.2 to 3.3 mg/kg intravenously 15 minutes after the xylazine injection

Tiletamine hydrochloride-zolazepam hydrochloride[3]
- 2 to 5 mg/kg intramuscularly
- May cause excitement stage during induction
- Recovery is difficult

Fentanyl citrate-droperidol[3,9]
- 1 ml/9 kg intramuscularly
- Antagonist: naloxone hydrochloride 0.4 mg/9 kg

Inhalant Anesthetics
(oxygen flow rate: 2 to 4 L/min)
Isoflurane[3,7,9]
- Induction: 4% to 5%
- Maintenance: 2% to 3%
- Heart rate: 60 to 120 beats/min
- Respiration rate: 25 to 40 breaths/min

Halothane[3,7,9]
- Induction: 4%
- Maintenance: 2% to 3%
- Heart rate: 30 to 50 beats/min
- Respiration rate: 5 to 15 breaths/min

TABLE IV
Subjective Antibiotic Dosages for Ostriches[7]

Antibiotic	Dose	Frequency
Amikacin sulfate[a]	7 mg/kg	Three times daily
Amoxicillin	11–22 mg/kg	Two to three times daily
Enrofloxacin	4.4 mg/kg	Two to three times daily
Amoxicillin clavulonate	22 mg/kg	Two times daily
Gentamicin	2.2–6.6 mg/kg	Three times daily
Clindamycin	5.5 mg/kg	Three times daily
Lincomycin	22 mg/kg	Three times daily
Tylosin	17.6 mg/kg	Two to three times daily
Erythromycin	22 mg/kg	Three times daily
Trimethoprim-sulfadiazine	33 mg/kg	Two times daily
Ketoconazole	5–20 mg/kg	One to two times daily

[a]No kidney damage resulted from this nephrotoxic drug at stated dosage.[3]

proglottids. This tapeworm is treated with fenbendazole.[7]

The ostrich eye fluke (*Philophthalmus gralli*), like the tapeworm, requires an intermediate host—in this case, certain freshwater snails. The worms irritate the conjunctival sac and are treated with 5% carbamate powder.[3]

Ostrich lice (*Struthiolipeurus struthionis*) cause economic loss to the producer via feather damage to the ostrich. Quill mites (*Pterolichidae* species) damage quills during their life cycle and cause itching, which leads to further irritation. Quill mites are treated with ivermectin at 200 µg/kg every four weeks for three treatments.[3] Because they are also hosts to several species of ticks, ostriches are vectors of tick-borne diseases, such as Rocky Mountain spotted fever.[3]

Bacteria

In ostriches, the digestive tract is the most common site of infection by disease-causing bacteria. The tendency of ostrich chicks to consume feces of penmates contributes to the high rate of enteritis. Intestinal infections that do not result in death may affect growth and development of the bird.[3]

Gram-negative bacteria constitute the normal flora of the lower intestinal tract. Pathogenic intestinal bacteria in ostriches include *Escherichia coli* as well as *Salmonella*, *Klebsiella*, *Clostridium*, *Pseudomonas*, *Proteus*, and *Campylobacter* species. Treatment of bacterial enteritis involves keeping the bird warm and administering fluids and antibiotics.[3]

Bacterial infection of the yolk sac (yolk sacculitis) is one of the major causes of neonatal illness and death in ostriches. During the hatching process, the yolk sac is drawn through the umbilical area and into the abdomen of the chick. This process can take hours and may result in expo-

Common Nematodes, Cestodes, and Trematodes of Ostriches[3]

Ascaridia struthionis (the ostrich roundworm)
Dicheilonema rheae
Dicheilonema spicutarum
Libyostrongylus douglassii (the ostrich wire worm)
Paronchocerca struthionis (the ostrich lungworm)
Houttuynia struthionis (the ostrich tapeworm)
Philophthalmus gralli (the ostrich eye fluke)

sure of the umbilicus to bacteria from the environment (e.g., contaminated incubators or egg surfaces). The infection results in sudden death or retarded growth. Treatment of the ostrich entails administering a broad-spectrum antibiotic, restoring the energy deficit, and rehydrating fluid reserves.[3]

Inflammation of the respiratory system (rhinitis) is highly contagious and is caused by a bacteria, *Haemophilus gallinarum*. The condition is characterized by clear to purulent nasal discharge, inflamed infraorbital sinuses, and lacrimation of the eyes. It is spread by contact and is particularly common in ostriches less than one year of age that are subject to stress (e.g., cold, a new environment, or overcrowding). Isolation and treatment with trimethoprim-sulfadiazine are recommended.[10]

Candida albicans, a yeast, is a fungus that commonly affects ostriches and is characterized by a yellowish pseudomembrane on the oral mucosa. It infects the digestive tract and is treated with ketoconazole at a dose of 5 to 20 mg/kg.[10]

NONINFECTIOUS DISEASE AGENTS
Foreign Bodies

Ground-fed birds have an increased chance of consuming foreign objects. Ostriches are prone to impaction of the stomach with indigestible materials. The following factors contribute to the ingestion of foreign material: brightly colored or shiny objects that attract attention; relocation, which encourages oral sampling of the new environment; poor social training by older adult birds with regard to food intake; and the lack of continuously available food. Stomach impactions (complete or partial) result in scant or no passage of pelleted feces, dehydration, simulated eating or pecking, and decreased urine output. Proventriculotomy may be necessary to correct the impaction. Various objects retrieved from the proventriculus include sand, rocks, hay stems, leaves, nails, wood, plastic, and rubber products.[3,10]

Fractures

Fractures of long bones of the legs are almost always associated with extensive soft tissue trauma. Because of the excitable nature and powerful legs of the ostrich, fractures are usually severe and compound and result in exposure of bone. External fixation (bone plating) or internal fixation (Kirschner-Ehmer apparatus) may be attempted to repair the fracture.[3,10]

SUMMARY

Ostriches, the largest of all birds, lack the ability to fly but have exceptional running ability. These birds are strong and potentially dangerous with their forward kicks. Adult ostriches should be transported in closed trailers and kept in seven-foot-high, wedge-shaped pens. Proper sanitation of ostrich facilities is crucial in maintaining healthy birds. Nutritional requirements of ostriches are subjective because precise nutrient values have not been established. Many anatomic features of ostriches are different from those of other avian species and mammals. Hematologic parameters vary with the blood collection technique and diet of the ostrich as well as the testing laboratory. The jugular, brachial, and medial metatarsal veins are used for venipuncture and intravenous injections. Oral administration of therapeutic agents is easy because of the ostrich's tendency to peck. Intramuscular injections should be given only in the lumbar muscles along the spine to preserve the thigh meat cut. Antibiotic dosages are still in the experimental stage, although accepted extrapolated dosages are available. Many of the anesthetics commonly used in other species also are used in ostriches; however, ostriches require special anesthetic considerations. Ostriches are vulnerable to various diseases, as are all living things. The ostrich is a unique bird that will be seen more often in veterinary clinics and hospitals in years to come.

ACKNOWLEDGMENTS

The author thanks James J. Higgins for his assistance and Fran Savage, DVM, Pitts Veterinary Hospital, for her inspirational interest in ostriches.

■

REFERENCES

1. Stewart J: Overview of ratite industry: Past, present, and future. *1992 Proc Assoc Avian Vet*:304–305, 1992.
2. Cooperative Extension Service of Kansas State University, *Ostrich Production*. Manhattan, KS, Cooperative Extension Service, 1989.
3. Jensen J, Johnson JH, Weiner S: *Husbandry and Medical Management of Ostriches, Emus, and Rheas*. Texas, Wildlife & Exotic Animal Teleconsultants, 1992, pp 1–114.
4. Fowler M: Clinical anatomy of ratites. *1992 Proc Assoc Avian Vet*: 307–309, 1992.
5. Palomeque J, Pinto D, Viscor G: Hematologic & blood chemistry values of the Masai ostrich (*Struthio camelus*). *J Wildl Dis* 27(1):34–37, 1991.
6. Blue-McLendon A: Clinical examination of ratites. *1992 Proc Assoc Avian Vet*:313–315, 1992.
7. Gilsleider E: *Ratite Medicine and Surgery* (Meeting handout). Nebraska Veterinary Medical Association, Ogallala, NE, 1991.
8. Fowler M: Comparative clinical anatomy of ratites. *J Zoo Wildl Med* 22(2):204–221, 1991.
9. Ramsay E: Ratite restraint, immobilization and anesthesia. *Avian/Exotic Anim Med Symp*:176–178, 1991.
10. Dolensek E, Bruning D: Ratites, in Fowler M (ed): *Zoo and Wild Animal Medicine*. Philadelphia, WB Saunders Co, 1978, pp 167–180.

An Introduction to Llamas

Penny Miller

North Fork Veterinary Clinic

Wheeling, West Virginia

Llamas are domesticated, even-toed, modified ruminants that belong to the family Camelidae. The relatives of llamas are Bactrian camels, dromedaries, guanacos, vicunas, and alpacas.

Native to the Andes Mountains of South

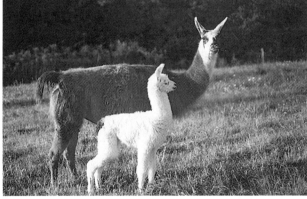

America, llamas were probably domesticated from wild guanacos approximately 7000

Originally published in Volume 12, Number 1, January/February 1991 years ago by the Incas.[1] The Incas relied on llamas as a source of meat, fuel, and fiber and used the animals in religious practices and as pack animals.[2]

North America did not become home to llamas until late in the 19th century. Imported pairs began to appear in zoos along the East Coast in the 1870s.[3] In the early 1970s, horse breeders Dick and Kay Patterson purchased their first llamas from the Catskill Game Farm and developed one of the largest herds (500 head) in the United States.[4]

During the 1980s, llamas skyrocketed in popularity. Pet owners and livestock producers are attracted to the animals because of their gentle and inquisitive nature, regal stature, diverse color patterns, and simple husbandry requirements. The intelligence and curiosity of llamas allow easy training and handling; people without livestock experience are thus apt to join the ranks of llama owners.

Biology

Adult llamas weigh 250 to 450 pounds (Figure 1), and newborns weigh 18 to 40 pounds. Normal rectal temperatures are 99.0° to 101.8° F for adults and 100.0° to 102.2° F for babies. The normal resting heart rate is 60 to 90 beats/min, and the normal resting respiratory rate is 10 to 30 breaths/min. The average life span is 15 to 20 years.[5]

The upper lip is split by a labial cleft, which permits flexibility and discrimination in selecting food materials.[2] Llamas are considered to be grazers and browsers. The tongue is rarely extended from the mouth. The animals do not lick themselves or their newborns and seldom use salt blocks.

Llamas have six lower incisors, a hard upper palate with no incisors, upper and lower molars, and fighting teeth (or fangs). The fighting teeth of males are well developed, curved, sharp, and capable of inflicting severe lacerations during fights with other males. There are three sets of fangs (two upper and one lower). Eruption begins when llamas are two years of age. It is recommended that the fighting teeth be removed or blunted by one of several methods.[2]

Llamas differ from true ruminants in that the stomach of a llama comprises three compartments rather than four. The first and second compartments are the sites of mixing and fermentation.[6] Motility in the first compartment is the reverse of that in true ruminants; the contraction wave moves in a caudal-to-cranial direction.[2]

Normal llama feces consist of small, firm pellets or a mass of pellets. Feces are deposited in a pile that is used by the entire herd for defecation and urination.

Llamas are natural pacers. A llama moves both legs on one side then both legs on the other side. The unique foot comprises two digits. The bottom (weight-bearing) surface is a tough but pliable pad, and the top of each toe is covered by a toenail. The soft feet damage ground vegetation less than the feet of burros and horses do; llamas are thus permitted on some National Park Service trails that are off-limits to other pack animals.

Feeding and Nutrition

Well adapted to the harsh climate and sparse vegetation of the high plains of the Andes, llamas are efficient users of poor-quality forage. Although most species require a dry-matter intake of 2.5% to 3% of body weight, llamas require only 1.8% to 2%.[6] In studies at Colorado State University, llamas fed a 10% protein diet performed as well as or better than llamas on a 16% protein diet. For most llamas, an adequate maintenance diet is 8% to 10% protein; growing, pregnant, or lactating llamas require 12% to 14% protein diets.[6]

An adequate diet is at least 25% fiber[6]; most llama owners feed mixed grass hays or oat hay to supplement pasture feed. If there are higher energy requirements, such concentrates as sweet feed or pelleted rations (e.g., Llama Chow®—Ralston Purina) should be fed.

There is concern about the growing number of obese llamas.[2,5,6] Such animals are at increased risk of hyperthermia, decreased libido and fertility, and (if pregnant) dystocia and poor milk production.[6]

Salt and trace minerals should be provided in loose form rather than in blocks. There is circumstantial evidence that some llamas are deficient in selenium; in regions that are known to be deficient in this mineral, owners should supplement the ration and monitor selenium blood levels. Normal selenium values have not been established for llamas, but comparison with other ruminants is helpful. A level of 0.1 to 0.3 µg/ml of whole blood is desirable.[7]

Restraint and Handling

Llamas do not naturally enjoy being touched. Although their curiosity makes them easy to approach, they tend to stay at arm's length. The animals are easily halter-broken and trained to lead. Most breeders desensitize llamas by routinely touching them, beginning with the least sensitive areas (the neck and shoulders) and progressing to the tail area, legs, and feet. Well-trained llamas may tolerate routine examination and minor procedures while cross-tied. Less cooperative animals may require additional restraint

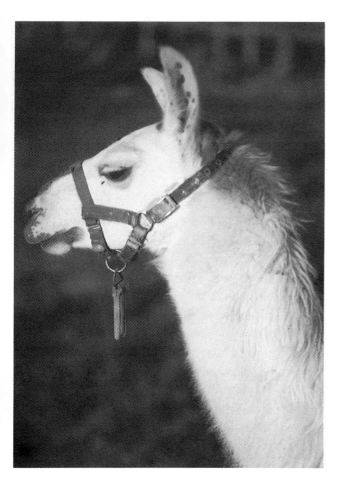

Figure 1—An adult llama.

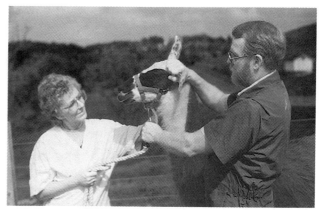

Figure 2—Grasping a llama at the base of the ears to stabilize the head.

by being grasped at the base of the ears (Figure 2).

A llama may attempt to defend itself by spitting, kicking, rearing, or slamming its neck or chest into the handler. Llamas rarely bite people; hand-reared males are the exception to this rule. Spitting can be controlled by placing a cloth under the noseband of the halter and over the nose and mouth or by draping a towel over the head.

The hindlegs are used for kicking defense; the leg is usually swung out to the side but also can kick to the rear. Owners of large herds use homemade or commercial restraint chutes to prevent llamas from swinging the hindquarters or rearing up. To avoid injury to the animals, chutes must be used judiciously.

Some llamas fall into a submissive, sternally recumbent position during restraint. Minor procedures may be better tolerated in this position.

To prevent injury to llamas and handlers, fractious animals are sedated for safe treatment. Xylazine hydrochloride at 0.10 to 0.15 mg/kg provides light sedation for minor procedures[2]; 0.44 to 0.66 mg/kg is adequate for immobilization.[8] Atropine (0.04 mg/kg) can be given to control salivation.[2] The effects of xylazine can be reversed with yohimbine (0.25 mg/kg).[2] Compared with intramuscular injection, administering xylazine subcutaneously permits smoother sedation and less pain and stimulation.[8]

Housing

Llamas are easy to house and to maintain. Although adapted to a wide range of temperatures, llamas are more tolerant of cold than heat and humidity. Three-sided sheds are usually adequate for healthy adults. Most owners have enclosed barns for sick, aged, or stressed animals and for bouts of severe weather. Many owners in hot climates provide air conditioning, sprinkler systems, or wading pools to prevent hyperthermia; some producers recommend at least partial shearing of body wool, particularly in pregnant females.

Various types of fencing are used in the llama industry. If wild and domesticated predators are not a concern, a three-rail fence works well. Other options include woven-wire, board, high-tensile, and chain-link fences. Barbed wire is unnecessary and seldom used.

Fence heights vary. Although llamas are capable of jumping 4.5 feet high, many are kept behind 40-inch fences. Farms that house studs require sturdy, high fences and often use buffer zones between fields of intact males.

Because many llamas have been killed or maimed by canids, farms in regions that are frequented by coyotes or dogs must have predator-proof fences. Electric or chain-link fences are used, and some producers keep livestock guard dogs with llama herds.

Hematology

Blood collection from the jugular vein is complicated by thick skin, the lack of a jugular groove, and the proximity of the carotid artery.[2] To avoid accidental cannulation of

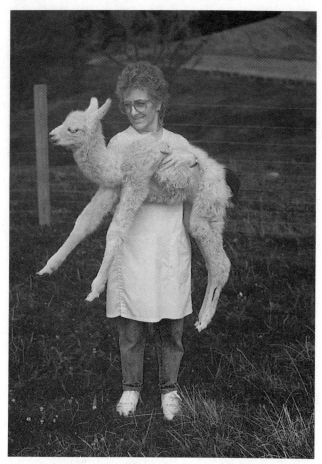

Figure 3—A two-day-old cria.

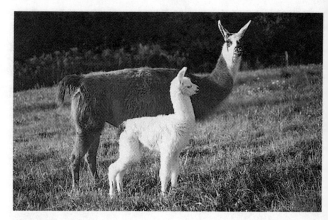

Figure 4—A female with a one-week-old cria.

the artery, a line is imagined from the ventral border of the mandible to the neck. With the head in a slightly flexed position, the tendon of the sternomandibular muscle is palpated; the site of penetration is just dorsal to the intersection of the imaginary line and the tendon.[2] Venipuncture can also be accomplished in the coccygeal vein (under the tail), the vein on the caudal border of the ear, or (in a recumbent patient) the saphenous vein (on the medial aspect of the stifle).[2]

Hematologic values are comparable to those in horses and cattle, with some notable exceptions. The leukocyte count is higher (7.2 to 22.2 $\times$ 10^3/μl) in llamas than in other domesticated species.[2] Llama erythrocytes are small and elliptic; normal values range from 9.9 to 17.7 $\times$ 10^6/μl.[2]

Reproduction

Males are routinely put into breeding service at two and one-half or three years of age; some are capable of breeding younger. A male that is put into service too early may be rebuffed by aggressive females and thus lose the confidence to mount. Females are bred at 18 months to two years of age or sooner if they are near adult size. Fertile matings can occur in any month.

The testicles of the adult male are relatively small compared with those of other livestock. Several testicles have been measured at 2 to 3 inches long and 1 to 1.5 inches wide.[2] In an unaroused male, the prepuce points backward; this fact explains the backward urination between the hindlegs. In an aroused male, the prepuce is pulled forward by the preputial muscle.[9] The adult llama has a long penis with a tapered tip that ends with a curved cartilaginous process; the process is believed to help the penis through the spiral cervical rings and into the uterine horn.[2]

Llamas are induced ovulators but differ from other induced ovulators (e.g., rabbits, cats, ferrets, and otters). Recent studies confirm that mature female llamas continuously have numerous small follicles on both ovaries; mature follicles are produced during a 10- to 12-day period in repeated, overlapping waves. If copulation occurs when a mature follicle is present, ovulation will take place in 24 to 30 hours.[10]

The llama uterus is bicornate. The left horn may be slightly larger; more than 95% of successful pregnancies occur in this horn.[2]

Female llamas do not exhibit an estrous period, and sexual receptivity is apparently not based on ovarian follicular status.[2,9] Llamas breed in a prone position. If the female is receptive, she becomes sternally recumbent when mounted. Intromission occurs after the female is down. Copulation lasts 5 to 50 minutes; 20 to 30 minutes is average.[2] During breeding, the male continuously vocalizes with a loud guttural sound that is referred to as orgling.

Because several breedings may be necessary to stimulate ovulation, most breeders continue to present the serviced female to the male for a few days. After ovulation, the female is no longer receptive and rejects the male by refusing to lie down or by spitting at him.

Although nonreceptivity usually indicates pregnancy, several methods can be used for confirmation. Progesterone assay of blood 21 days after breeding should indicate a serum value of at least 1 ng/ml; some laboratories use analytic techniques that require at least 2 ng/ml to confirm pregnancy.[2,9] A retained corpus luteum or pyometra can cause elevated progesterone levels that mimic pregnancy.[9]

At 40 to 45 days, greater reliance is placed on rectal palpation to determine pregnancy. After 90 days, the uterus is below the pelvic brim and palpation is difficult.[2] With ultrasound techniques, pregnancy has been observed as early as 15 days; the greatest accuracy begins at 28 days.[9]

Among domesticated animals, llamas have the highest incidence of early embryonic death; 30% to 50% of pregnancies terminate before 90 days of gestation.[11] Most breeders thus routinely recheck females at 60 to 90 days.

Gestation usually ranges from 335 to 350 days but exceeds one year in some llamas.[12] Udder development can occur one to three weeks before birth or after birth.

Parturition takes place during daylight, usually in the morning. Most births occur with the dam standing. The head and front feet of the newborn appear first. Assistance may be needed if birth is not completed in 30 minutes.[13] Dystocia is reported in 2% to 5% of births.[12]

Newborn llamas are referred to as crias (Figure 3). At birth, a cria is covered with an epidermal membrane that does not cover the mouth or nostrils; suffocation is thus unlikely.[2] The placenta should be expelled in four to six hours.

Healthy crias stand in two hours and nurse in six hours (Figure 4). Crias may sample foodstuffs at three weeks of age but are not weaned until four to six months of age.

Dams can be rebred at 10 to 15 days postpartum. The average period between births is 13 to 14 months.[9]

Herd Health Programs

Routine vaccinations should include *Clostridium perfringens* types C and D. Many veterinarians use seven-way clostridial vaccines.[14] Leptospirosis vaccinations may be indicated in endemic areas. The first reported case of rabies in a llama in the United States occurred in Oklahoma on November 28, 1989.[15] Although there is no licensed rabies vaccine for llamas, the use of a killed vaccine in endemic areas is prudent.[14]

Conclusion

Llamas are hardy, versatile, unique creatures that have won the hearts of owners throughout the United States. The International Lama Registry currently lists 70,400 llamas.[a]

Llamas are used as pets, wool producers, and pack animals. Because of their gentle nature, llamas are suitable for pet therapy programs, nursing home visitation, petting zoos, and 4-H programs.

Although most large animal diagnostic and treatment regimens apply to llamas, llama medicine is still in its infancy. Veterinarians and veterinary staff will find that working with llamas is challenging and rewarding.

---

[a]Utley M: Personal communication, International Lama Registry, Rochester, MN, 1994.

■

REFERENCES

1. Fowler ME: Conformation and soundness. *Vet Clin North Am [Food Anim Pract]* 5(1):21, 1989.
2. Fowler ME: *Medicine and Surgery of South American Camelids.* Ames, IA, Iowa State University Press, 1989.
3. Hoffman E: History of llamas in U.S. *Llama Life* 5:12, 1988.
4. Ebel S: The llama industry in the United States. *Vet Clin North Am [Food Anim Pract]* 5(1):4, 1989.
5. Hoffman C, Asmus I: *Caring for Llamas: A Health and Management Guide.* Livermore, CO, Rocky Mountain Llama Association, 1989, p 130.
6. Johnson L: Nutrition. *Vet Clin North Am [Food Anim Pract]* 5(1):38–48, 1989.
7. Smith JA: Noninfectious diseases, metabolic diseases, toxicities, and neoplastic diseases of South American camelids. *Vet Clin North Am [Food Anim Pract]* 5(1):125, 1989.
8. Heath RB: Llama anesthetic programs. *Vet Clin North Am [Food Anim Pract]* 5(1):76, 1989.
9. Johnson L: Llama reproduction. *Vet Clin North Am [Food Anim Pract]* 5(1):160–165, 1989.
10. Bravo W, Fowler ME: Basic physiology of reproduction in female llamas. *Llamas* 4(3):37, 1990.
11. Fowler ME: Early embryonic death in llamas and alpacas. *Llamas* 3(4):81, 1989.
12. Paul-Murphy J: Obstetrics, neonatal care, and congenital conditions. *Vet Clin North Am [Food Anim Pract]* 5(1):183–184, 1989.
13. Smith B, Reed P, Long P: Llama neonatal care. *Llamas* 3(7):36, 1989.
14. Long P: Llama herd health. *Vet Clin North Am [Food Anim Pract]* 5(1):230–231, 1989.
15. Centers for Disease Control: Rabies in a llama in Oklahoma. *Morbid Mortal Weekly Report* 39(12):203, 1990.

Llamas: An Overview

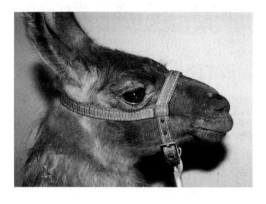

Kriss A. Hoffman, RVT, MS
Department of Veterinary Clinical Medicine and Surgery
Washington State University
Pullman, Washington

Llama is a general term used to describe the four species within the genus *Lama.* All llamas are members of the South American Camelidae family. *Lama glama,* the focus of this article, is the species most often reated by veterinarians and technicians. Excluding the general description section, the information presented in this article pertains to the *Lama glama* (which will be referred to as the llama).

Unique features of the anatomy and physiology of the musculoskeletal, digestive, and reproductive systems of the llama are followed by a discussion of behavior characteristics and defense mechanisms, restraint procedures, reasons for ownership, and major medical disorders.

GENERAL DESCRIPTION

The four species within the genus *Lama* are the llama (*Lama glama*), the alpaca (*Lama pacos*), the vicuna (*Lama vicugna,* syn. *Vicugna vicugna*), and the guanaco (*Lama huanacos,* syn. *L. guanicoe*). Of the four species, only two (the llama and alpaca) have been domesticated. All species have a common body

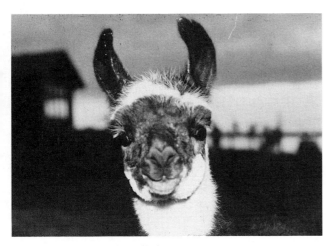

Figure 1—Inquisitive juvenile llama.

shape but vary in size and color.

The llama (Figure 1) is the largest of the four species. It has been domesticated for more than 5000 years.[1] The male weighs between 162 and 243 kilograms, and the female weighs between 108 and 189 kilograms. Llamas have a characteristic angular face that is crowned with long, erect ears. Wool and guard hair cover much of the neck and body. The flank and brisket areas usually are not covered by wool. The absence of wool provides a *thermal window*, which enables the animal to regulate body temperature by finding cover for this area when it is cold or by lying on cool surfaces when it is warm. Hair rather than wool covers the lower extremities. Markings range from solid to multicolored in various shades of brown, gray, black, and white.

The second domesticated species, the alpaca, is smaller than the llama and is known for its high-quality fleece. Male alpacas range in weight from 60 to 80 kilograms, and females have an average weight of 55 kilograms. Characteristics that typically differentiate the alpaca from the llama are a forelock of wool, smaller ears, and the continuation of long staple wool to the lower extremities and throughout the belly and flank areas. Alpacas vary in color from solid white, brown, or black to any multicolored combination.

The vicuna is the smallest of the four species of llamas. The vicuna is undomesticated and is protected in the wilds of South America. The average male weighs between 40 and 65 kilograms, and the average female weighs between 30 and 40 kilograms.

The guanaco is also undomesticated. Males typically weigh between 100 and 150 kilograms, and females weigh between 100 and 120 kilograms. The soft brown color on the upper body and white underbelly as well as the slightly smaller body size and unpredictable disposition distinguish the guanaco from the other species of llamas.

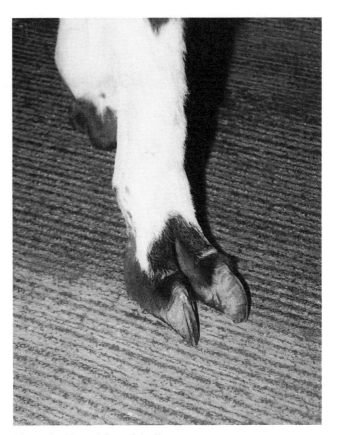

Figure 2—Normal foot of the llama.

Males of all four species are called bulls, females are called cows, and castrated males are called geldings. The birthing process is called calving, and offspring are called cria. As the young grow, they are referred to as juveniles and weanlings.

Basic temperature, pulse, and respiration values in llamas are similar to those of other ruminants. Normal body temperature is between 37.2°C and 38.6°C (99°F to 102°F), heart rate ranges from 60 to 90 beats per minute, and respiration ranges from 10 to 30 breaths per minute. The normal life span of llamas is between 15 and 20 years.

Hematologic and serum biochemical values for llamas[2,3] are similar to those of cattle and horses. Erythrocytes are more numerous (10.1 to 12.3 x 10^6/μl), but values for packed cell volume are lower (25 to 45) because the cells are smaller in size and are packed more tightly together.

Venipuncture in llamas, as compared with other domestic species, is not a simple task.[1,4,5] This is because of the thickness of the skin on the upper third of the neck, which does not allow good visualization or palpation of the veins. The technician should remember that the hemoglobin molecule in the blood of llamas has a high affinity for oxygen; thus, a venous sample is much brighter red in llamas than it is in most domestic animals. Care must be taken when injecting solutions to ensure that needle placement is intravenous and not intraarterial.

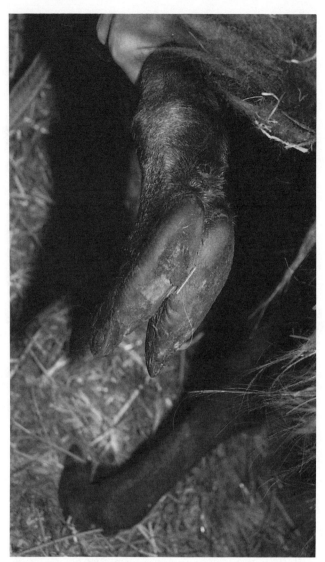

Figure 3—Palmar surface of the foot of a llama. Note the small nail on the distal end.

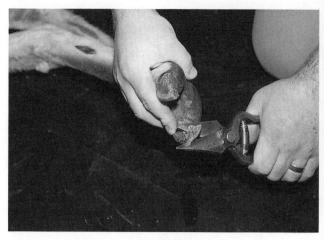

Figure 4—Trimming a nail on the foot of a llama.

UNIQUE ANATOMY AND PHYSIOLOGY OF THE LLAMA

The musculoskeletal, digestive, and reproductive systems of the llama have several unique features. Beginning with the musculoskeletal system, there are two digits on each foot of the llama (Figure 2). Phalanx-3 (P-3) and phalanx-2 (P-2) are positioned in a nonweight-bearing, horizontal plane, and phalanx-1 (P-1) is positioned in an upright position at approximately a 45-degree angle.[6] A small nail is located at the extremity of each digit, and the remainder of each foot is supported by a digital cushion and a soft pad on the palmar surface (Figure 3). The nail is the only portion that must be trimmed periodically to prevent overgrowth (Figure 4).

The digestive system of the llama is also unique and is characterized by the dentition, prehensile lip, and modified digestive system. Because of the sensitive split lip, llamas have selective grazing habits and therefore do not often experience penetration of the stomach by foreign bodies (traumatic reticulitis). The tongue of the llama is not as freely movable as it is in ruminants and thus is rarely seen. Llamas do chew a cud and often alternate from one side of the mouth to the other with each mastication.

Llamas, primarily males, have canine (fighting) teeth, which are often cut (pulpotomy) when the animal is two years old. This procedure is done to protect other llamas and may be required every two to three years. The age of a llama can be determined by examining the lower three pairs of incisors. The first set erupts at 2.2 years of age, the second at 3.1 years, and the third at 4.0 years of age. Llamas have an upper dental pad with no incisors.

The llama is classified as a modified ruminant because of its digestive system. The stomach is divided into three sections called compartments one, two, and three.[7] Compartment one (approximately 83% of the entire stomach) consists of a dorsal and ventral sac in which most fermentation occurs. Compartment one is similar to the rumen in cattle and sheep. The ventral sac contains saccules, which evert during digestion and secrete buffering sodium bicarbonate into the digestive system. Compartment two (approximately 6% of the stomach) has been compared with the reticulum of cattle. It contains absorptive cells and some mucous cells. Compartment three (approximately 11% of the stomach) is similar to the abomasum in ruminants. The proximal four fifths of this compartment contain mucous glands, and the distal fifth contains gastric glands for acid production.

In the neonatal llama, compartment three is used primarily for the digestion of milk. Neonates begin to browse as early as one week of age, and some juveniles have partial physiologic function by one month of age. The nature of compartmental development changes with age, similar to that observed in bovine calves. In South America, poor nutrition is believed to be a problem in llamas, whereas in the United States, obesity is a problem.

Stomach motility in the mature llama can be variable and irregular. Compartmental contractions range from 0 to 4 per minute; in ruminants, 1 or 2 per minute is expected. Digestion is very efficient, with good absorption of volative fatty acid. Gastric and duodenal ulcers, conditions seen in foals, may also be seen in neonatal llamas. Llamas do not have gallbladders, but they do have multilobulated livers with fringed (serrated) edges. The normal stool is elongated and pelleted.

Some aspects of reproduction also are unique in llamas. Puberty in the male occurs between 18 and 36 months (average, 30 months) of age. The scrotum is located in the perineal region, similar to swine, and has a horizontal axis. Accessory sex glands include a prostate and bulbourethral glands but no seminal vesicles.[1] The penis is fibroelastic and has a prescrotal sigmoid flexure and urethral process. The penis may remain adhered to the prepuce until the animal reaches puberty. When in a relaxed position, the penis is in a caudal direction, and when erect, the penis is in a cranial direction. Copulation occurs in a recumbent position and takes 10 to 20 minutes.

In the female, puberty is associated more with weight than with age. At puberty, the female llama weighs 60% of its adult weight; this figure can be compared with sheep (which weigh 40% to 55% of their adult weight at puberty), dairy cattle (which weigh 40% of their adult weight at puberty), and beef cattle (which weigh 45% to 55% of their adult weight at puberty).

Llamas are nonseasonal, induced ovulators. Ovulation can be induced through rectal palpation and hormonal injections. The uterus is bicornate and is Y- or T-shaped. The left horn, where nearly 100% of pregnancies occur, is often larger than the right horn.[8] The presence of a corpus luteum seems to be required throughout the entire pregnancy, although the site of the corpus luteum—on the ipsilateral ovary (same side as the gravid horn) or contralateral (opposite side, i.e., right side)—is insignificant.[9] Estrus continues for 30 to 40 days after intromission and is characterized by periods of nonacceptance (lasting approximately 48 hours). Ovulation occurs from either ovary 24 to 26 hours after copulation. Multiple ovulations take place in 10% of cycling llamas, although twinning is rare.[10]

Pregnancy can be determined by various methods. Rectal palpation is restricted by the arm size of the person performing the procedure and by the body size of the llama. An accurate determination of pregnancy can be made via rectal palpation after 45 days of gestation. Ultra-sonography (used in conjunction with rectal palpation) allows visualization of the embryo as early as 15 days. An additional method, the use of progesterone assays, is fairly accurate at 21 days of gestation. The results of all three methods should be reconfirmed after an additional 30 days.

Placentation is simple, diffuse (similar to the mare), and epitheliochorial (six layers). More specifically, six layers of tissue are found in the placenta of a llama. There are three maternal layers (endothelium, connective tissue, and epithelium) and three fetal layers (trophoblast, connective tissue, and epithelium). Parturition usually takes place during daylight hours. The time frame of the three stages of labor is similar to that of the mare. Dystocia is rare. The length of gestation is 335 to 360 days. Llamas do not lick their young when they are born and do not chew the umbilical cord.[1] Estrus usually occurs within two to three days postpartum (similar to foal heat in mares) and is followed by normal uterine involution in approximately 20 days. All four species of llamas have 37 pairs of chromosomes and, therefore, can intermix and produce viable offspring.[6]

BEHAVIOR

The body language of llamas can indicate temperament. Ear set is a primary indication of attitude.[1] When llamas are comfortable with the environment, the ears are erect and slightly forward (Figure 5A). As changes take place in the environment, the ears will point toward the back of the head (Figure 5B). This is not a sign of anger but rather of change. If llamas are extremely upset, the ears will be flat against the back of the head and neck. The nose will be elevated and the animal will begin to vocalize (orgle), immediately after which it will spit and continue vocalizing. Spitting of ingesta is often one of the first lines of defense. To handle a spitting animal comfortably, a cloth can be placed over the muzzle (Figure 6).

Llamas, primarily males, can inflict damage by biting one another. Llamas rarely bite humans. Males possess four canine teeth, which are used for fighting and establishing dominance. The primary targets of fighting males are the neck and genitals. As natural protection, the skin on the upper third of the neck can be up to one centimeter thick and the genitals are held close to the body wall.[5,11]

An additional defense mechanism is kicking. Most llamas kick in rapid, sideswiping motions, similar to the kick of a cow. Although the foot of the llama is primarily a soft pad and not a hard hoof or claw, there is considerable force to the blow. Llamas also can charge or butt as methods of obtaining domination. The long neck of the llama allows

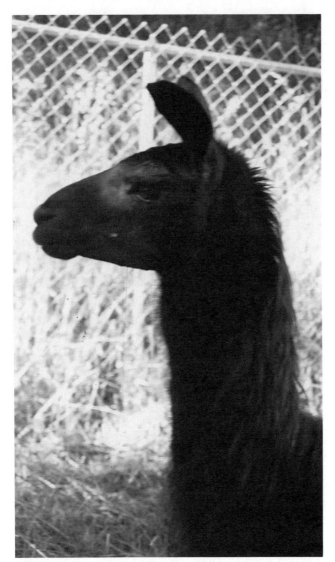

Figure 5A

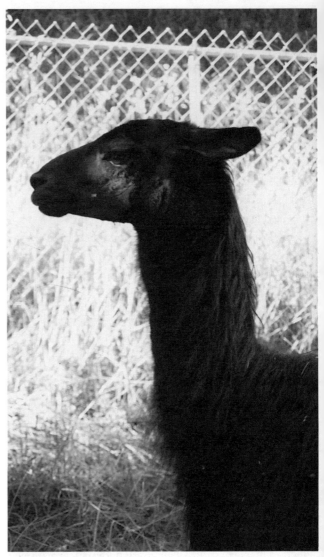

Figure 5B

Figure 5—(**A**) The ear set of a llama that is comfortable with its environment. (**B**) The ear set of a llama after a change has taken place in its environment.

considerable leverage when striking an opponent with its head. For these reasons, it is safer to stand very close to llamas (as with all large animals) when an examination or treatment is required.

Few behavioral problems have been noted in llamas. The so-called berserk male syndrome,[1,12] or aberrant male syndrome, has been observed in a small percentage of male llamas that are either hand-raised (bottle-fed) or interfered with considerably as neonates. Affected males imprint on humans and essentially treat humans as other male llamas. Signs become apparent at puberty, at which time the llama becomes very aggressive toward humans and other animals. The llama orgles, butts humans and animals, bites, and becomes extremely dangerous. The most advocated method of prevention of the berserk male syndrome is castration between one to six months of age or, at the latest, before weaning. After the syndrome has manifested itself,

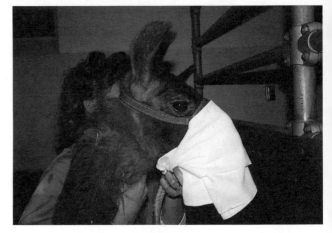

Figure 6—Cloth wrap that can be used on a spitting llama.

many experts believe that castration (and/or behavior modification) is not effective, and the llama must be euthanatized.

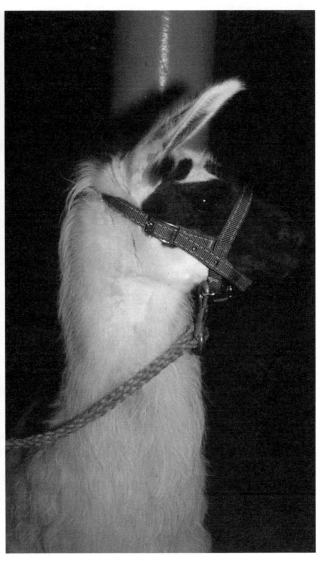

Figure 7—Llama halter and lead.

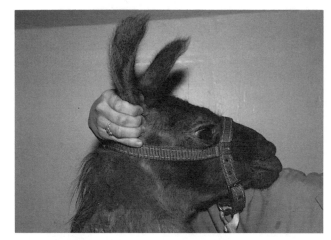

Figure 8—Ear twitch.

RESTRAINT

Physical restraint of llamas requires minimal specialized equipment. A halter and lead rope are standard equipment (Figure 7). Catching a llama in a pen or pasture can be performed easily with only two people. Stretching a rope between two people at a height of 90 to 100 centimeters (approximately one meter) creates the illusion of a fence, which llamas usually will not challenge.[1] Another method is to drive the llama toward the corner of a small pen. The corner of the pen closes off two sides to the llama and a rope held between two people closes off the third side.

A llama should be approached from its left side. A hand is placed on the withers or around the neck. Most domesticated llamas will stop moving when the neck is encircled. It must always be remembered that llamas have considerable leverage with their necks. By holding the neck close to the body of the handler, serious injury can usually be avoided. Llamas in the wild or those that are rarely handled can be roped and will usually stand still after the rope is tightened.

Llama halters are commercially available, but most rope halters will work on a temporary basis. Because llamas are obligate nasal breathers, special care must be taken to ensure that the nose piece of the halter does not cover the cartilaginous nares.[1] A small llama or juvenile can be handled by placing one hand around the front of the neck and grasping around the rump or base of the tail with the second hand.

Large llamas and llamas that are head shy can be restrained for brief periods by using an ear twitch (Figure 8). The base of an ear is encircled in the palm of the hand between the thumb and forefinger and squeezed. The ear should not be twisted.

Many llamas are very sensitive to handling of the ears, legs, and feet. Producers can help to desensitize these areas by stroking the head and legs. A llama that is nervous or very reactive to handling can be difficult to examine because the animal often will act head shy or lie down (in a sternal recumbent position termed *cush*) to cover its legs and feet. A handler can attempt to force the llama to rise by pulling the rear legs out behind the llama, which will make the animal so uncomfortable that it will stand up.

For additional restraint, modified large animal working chutes (Figure 9) or stocks can be used as well as commercially available llama chutes. Chemical restraint is also common for llamas. The same anesthetics and tranquilizers that are used for ruminants and horses can be used for llamas.[13,14] Intubation is possible in llamas, although it should be noted that some general inhalant anesthetics have produced hepatotoxicity in ruminants[14]; the same problem may occur in llamas.

REASONS FOR OWNERSHIP

Llamas are owned because they provide companionship, can be used for wilderness packing, and can be a source of

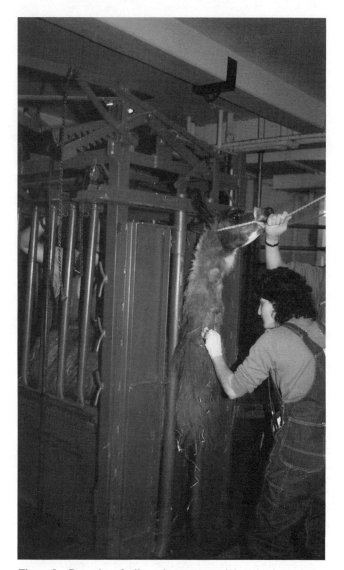

Figure 9—Restraint of a llama in a commercial cattle chute.

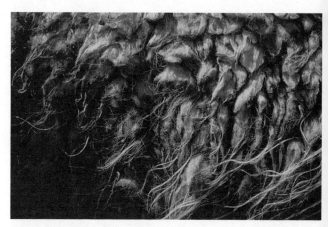

Figure 10—Llama wool. Note the long guard hair covering the wool undercoat.

income. Llamas are low maintenance, docile, hardy animals that are well suited to various environments.

A renewed interest in wilderness packing in North America has increased the popularity of llamas. These animals historically come from the high-altitude countries of South America, such as Peru and Chile, where they traditionally are used for packing. Llamas can pack approximately 30% of their body weight.[15]

An additional consideration for ownership is wool production. Llama fleece has dual purposes: the soft undercoat of wool provides thermal regulation and the covering of guard hair (approximately 20% of the fleece bulk) sheds moisture (Figure 10). Unlike sheep wool, llama wool does not contain lanolin. The weight of the fleece of an average llama ranges between 2.5 to 4.0 kilograms; some males have fleece that weighs more than 7.5 kilograms. Alpaca wool is more desirable than llama wool because alpacas have a lower percentage of guard hair than do llamas. In terms of micron diameter, the undercoat wool fibers of llamas are similar to the fibers of medium- and fine-wooled sheep, which makes this wool desirable to handspinners.

Some producers shear llamas; others prefer to groom the llamas using various types of brushes, most commonly slicker brushes, which are used on dogs. Combing gives a full, clean coat year-round and allows the producer to handle the llamas regularly, which has the added benefit of permitting early detection of possible abnormalities. Shearing is done every one to two years. Staple length of fiber ranges from 7 to 30 centimeters (3 to 12 inches).

Heat stress is an increasingly recognized syndrome in llamas. Fleece that is considerably long can exacerbate the syndrome.[16] Natural cooling mechanisms in the llama are the open-fleeced ventral body (thermal window), groin, and axillary areas, which allow dissipation of heat.

MAJOR MEDICAL DISORDERS

Because llamas are very stoic animals, observing them may give little indication of the type or severity of illness that may be present. Often, the practitioner must do a complete physical examination and diagnostic workup before even attempting a diagnosis.

Llamas have few if any reproductive diseases that are unique to the species and no known venereal diseases.[17] There have been reports of various reproductive tract deficiencies and anomalies in males and females (e.g., hypoplastic penis and vaginal segmental hypoplasia).

Congenital cardiovascular disorders in llamas are similar to those observed in other species and include atrial septal defects, patent ductus arteriosus, and ventricular septal defects. Additional congenital defects seen in llamas include angular limb deformity, arthrogryposis, choanal atresia, atresia ani, and cleft palate. The metabolic disorders common to most ruminants are also seen in llamas. Most of

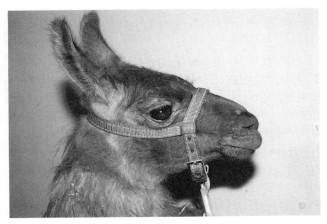

Figure 11—Zinc-deficient dermatitis on the face of a llama. Note the areas around the eyes and lips.

these disorders are caused by mineral deficiencies and imbalances and include zinc-deficient dermatitis (Figure 11), decreased immunoglobulin levels, and failure to thrive.

A basic understanding of medicine and surgical techniques serves as a solid foundation for the examination and treatment of llamas. Herd health programs should be established for llamas and they should include routine vaccinations, deworming, and nutritional programs.

SUMMARY

The number of llamas in North America is increasing, and these animals require appropriate health care. Llamas offer companionship, can be used as pack animals, and are an economic asset because of their valuable wool. Because llamas are mammals, the basic medical and surgical information that pertain to most mammals can be applied to llamas. The unique aspects of the musculoskeletal, digestive, and reproductive systems of llamas are easily mastered. Physical restraint techniques and behavior characteristics are also easily learned.

ACKNOWLEDGMENTS

The author thanks Dr. Steven Parish for numerous consultations regarding all aspects of llama medicine and surgery. Thanks is also given to Diane Odell, RVT, Shirley Sandoval, RVT, and Mary Shepard for their editing and technical assistance.

REFERENCES

1. Fowler ME: *Medicine and Surgery in South American Camelids.* Ames, IA, Iowa State University Press, 1989a, pp 7-279.
2. Lassen ED, Pearson EG, Long P, et al: Clinical biochemical values of llamas: Reference values. *Am J Vet Res* 47(10):2278-2280, 1986.
3. Fowler ME, Zinkl JG: Reference ranges for hematologic and serum biochemical values in llamas (*Lama glama*). *Am J Vet Res* 50(12):2049-2053, 1989.
4. Fowler ME: The jugular vein of the llama (*Lama pervana*): A clinical note. *J Zoo Anim Med* 14(2):77-78, 1983.
5. Amsel SI, Johnson LW: Choosing the best site to perform venipuncture in a llama. *Vet Med* 82(5):335-338, 1987.
6. Johnson LW: An orientation to llama medicine or what every veterinarian has always wanted to know about llamas but was afraid to ask. Handout #127, 1990 AVMA Meeting, San Antonio, TX.
7. Vallenazs A, Cummings JF, Munnell JF: A gross study of the compartmentalized stomach of two world camelids, the llama and the guanaco. *J Morphol* 134(1):399-424, 1971.
8. Weipz DW, Chapman RJ: Nonsurgical embryo transfer and live birth in a llama. *Theriogenology* 24(2):251-257, 1985.
9. Johnson LW: Llama reproduction. *Vet Clin North Am [Food Anim Pract]* 5(1):159-182, 1989.
10. Fowler ME: Twinning in llamas. *Llama* 4(7):35-38, 1990.
11. Fowler ME: Skin problems in llamas and alpacas. *Llama* 3(8):45-48, 82, 1989b.
12. Rolfing S, Herriges S: Berserk male syndrome: Not a pretty problem. *Llama* 1(9):70-73, 1987.
13. Heath RB: Llama anesthetic programs. *Vet Clin North Am [Food Anim Pract]* 5(1):71-80, 1989.
14. O'Brien TD, Raffe MR, Cox US, et al: Hepatic necrosis following halothane anesthesia in goats. *JAVMA* 189(12):1591-1595, 1986.
15. Ebel S: The llama industry in the United States. *Vet Clin North Am [Food Anim Pract]* 5(1):1-20, 1989.
16. Strain MG, Strain SS: Handling heat stress syndrome in llamas. *Vet Med* 83(5):494-498, 1988.
17. Johnson LW: Major causes of abnormal embryonic/fetal attrition in camelids. *Llama* 4(6):35-38, 1990.

Basic Avian Health Care and Nutrition for the New Bird Owner

Shelly L. Vogt, AHT
Las Vegas, Nevada

Veterinary clients frequently ask technicians to recommend an appropriate type of pet–either for the client or for a family member. One animal that is frequently overlooked but does make a good pet is a bird. Technicians

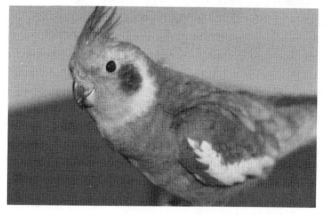

must be prepared to provide information on the choice of a type of bird and the preparation

Originally published in Volume 12, Number 6, July 1991

of the bird's new home as well as on the acquisition and care of a healthy bird.

Before-Purchase Considerations

Before purchasing a pet bird, clients should consider whether a bird fits their life-style. Birds need to have someone give them attention; owners must therefore have time to spend with the bird. Because birds do not demand such attention in the same manner as cats and dogs do, it is easy to get preoccupied with other activities and neglect the bird. A bird left alone too much can suffer from boredom and loneliness.[1]

Although most birds spend a considerable amount of time preening and grooming themselves, they are not the neatest of pets. They shed feathers and dust, leave behind droppings wherever they have been, and scatter their food around. The bird owner must be able to tolerate a certain amount of dirt.

The responsibility that pet care entails and the long life span of some birds must also be considered. It is inadvisable to surprise someone with a bird as a present; nor is it a good idea to purchase a bird for a small child. Many school-age children are responsible bird owners, but the parents must be willing and able to take over care of the bird if it becomes necessary. Birds need to have a proper-sized, safe cage with appropriate accessories; depending on the size of the bird, this purchase can also be expensive.

Other pets that may already be in the household must also be considered. Although a bird can live happily in a house with dogs and cats, the owner must keep a constant watchful eye on them. Because of the natural hunting instinct of cats and dogs, it can be very dangerous to leave the bird alone with these animals, especially if the bird is out of its cage.

If there are other birds in the household, adding a new bird usually causes no problems. Of course, the new bird will have to adjust to the new environment and should be confined to its cage until it has had a chance to get acquainted with the other birds.

Buying a Bird

Veterinary technicians are often asked to recommend the species of bird that makes the best pet. Technicians should therefore become familiar with the many varieties of avian pets, which range from small finches to large macaws. Books and magazines provide valuable information, and local pet shops and zoos permit technicians to observe many birds. Such research will make it easier to advise clients about various birds that might be enjoyable pets.

The appropriate species of bird is an important decision that depends largely on the client's life-style. The sex of a bird is rarely important unless the client wants to start breeding birds. Males and females adapt equally well to a new home and owner. In most species, neither sex is more intelligent or more likely to talk or whistle.[1] Cockatiels and budgerigars have distinctive secondary sexual characteristics, but it is impossible to sex birds of many other species just by looking at them. Some species can only be sexed surgically.

The most important consideration in purchasing a new bird may be selecting a healthy one. This point cannot be stressed to the client enough. Finding out that a newly purchased expensive bird is sick and requires a significant amount of costly veterinary care can be disheartening to the owner.

Veterinary technicians can perform an invaluable service by becoming familiar with pet stores and breeders that sell healthy birds and recommending these sources when asked about the purchase of a new bird. Also, technicians should recommend that the client bring the bird in for a veterinary examination soon after purchase. Most reputable pet stores and breeders offer a 48- or 72-hour guarantee that the bird is healthy. If the bird is found to have a health problem, it can be returned to the pet store or breeder within that time and exchanged for a different bird.

When a veterinary client expresses an interest in purchasing a pet bird, the technician should review with the client the following characteristics of a healthy bird:

- The bird should be active in its cage. A bird that sits quietly with fluffed-up feathers may be ill.
- A young, healthy bird should have shiny feathers that lie smoothly on its body with no bald spots (Figure 1).
- The eyes should be bright and alert and free of any discharge.
- The legs should be straight and the toes well shaped. The horny scales on the feet should be smooth and even with no overgrowth.
- The feathers around the cloaca should be clean. Feathers that are matted with fecal material may indicate illness[1] (Figure 1).

First Examination

The type of examination the bird receives on its first visit depends on the veterinarian's preferences; but it generally includes a physical examination, complete blood count, and one or more Gram stains. The bird's leg bands

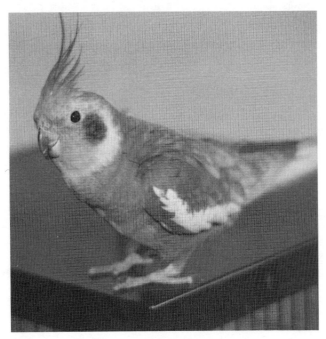

Figure 1—A healthy bird. Note the shiny feathers and bright eyes.

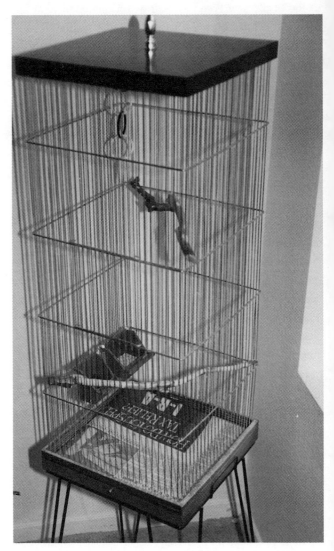

Figure 2—A cage with the proper accessories: natural branch perches, plastic food dishes, newspaper on the bottom, and a toy.

should be removed and the wings may be clipped to prevent escapes and flight injuries. Some birds require nail or beak trimming.

During the first checkup, it is also advisable to discuss nutrition and husbandry with the owner and to demonstrate to the owner how to use a towel to capture and restrain the bird. The client will need to be familiar with this technique in case the bird requires medication.

During the first examination, the technician should tell the client that most avian veterinarians recommend that a bird receive a checkup at least every six months or as soon as the client notices a problem with the bird. This way, any illness will be discovered early and treatment can be easier and more successful.

Husbandry
Cage

To allow the bird more freedom of movement, the owner should purchase the largest cage that is economically feasible. The cage should be big enough for the bird to move around without constantly running into perches and food dishes and to extend its wings fully sideways and upward without bumping into anything. The cage bars should be made from a rust-free metal that is strong enough to withstand chewing and pecking. Wooden cages are not recommended because most birds chew wood and thus ruin the

cage. The owner also should check how well the cage door locks. With a little practice, many birds can open the door and escape.

The perches that come with most cages are all of the same diameter; this design can be detrimental to the bird's leg and foot muscles. The perch should be thick enough so that the bird cannot reach all the way around it with its toes. A perch that varies in diameter provides proper exercise for the foot and leg muscles. Thus, the owner may want to replace some or all of the perches with natural branches. The owner must not, however, use a poisonous wood, such as yew (*Taxus* species), buckthorn (*Rhamnus* species), oleander (*Nerium oleander*), or horse chestnut (*Aesculus hippocastanum*). The owner must also make sure that fruit-tree branches have not been sprayed with insecticide.

Perches should be placed in the cage so as to avoid contamination of food and water with fecal matter. Also, any upper perches should be placed so that the bird cannot defecate onto a lower perch. Perches, food, and water must be kept free of fecal matter, which can cause serious health problems.[2]

Most cages come with two plastic dishes that are suitable for most birds and withstand continual use. Glazed ceramic dishes can also be used and are especially suitable for large birds because these dishes do not tip over easily.

Before the bird is placed in its new cage, it should be thoroughly cleaned and disinfected (including perches and dishes). All items should be washed in hot, soapy water (to remove dirt) and then rinsed with hot water. Items are then soaked in a disinfectant solution (e.g., benzalkonium chloride [2 to 4 teaspoons/gallon] or chlorine bleach [1 cup/gallon]) for at least 30 minutes to kill bacteria. Large cages can be sprayed with a generous amount of disinfectant solution to cover the bars and then thoroughly rinsed with water. Water from a garden hose should not be used because bacteria from inside the hose can contaminate the cage and accessories.[a]

This cleaning should be repeated daily for food and water dishes and weekly for cages and perches. Perches should be replaced twice a year. Following these steps helps prevent disease.

The bottom of the cage should not be covered with absorbent litter (e.g., sand, wood chips, or sawdust) because such material encourages bacterial growth and thus increases the chance that the bird will become ill. Lining the bottom of the cage with newspaper or paper towels works well. These papers should be changed daily or more often if necessary.

Many birds enjoy playing with toys, and owners can find a variety of toys at most pet stores. The main consideration in purchasing is that the toy is sturdy enough for the type of bird. A toy intended for a small bird can be easily destroyed by a large bird; resultant sharp edges can injure the bird.

Some old bird toys were made with lead parts and can be dangerous if ingested. It is wise to recommend that the client provide only new toys for the bird (Figure 2).

New Bird Care

Before bringing a bird home, the client should prepare for the bird's arrival. The cage should be ready for the bird (equipped with food and water) and in a permanent location. The cage should be placed in a quiet area of a room that is frequently used by the family. The cage must be away from drafts, which may stress the bird and make it less able to withstand disease. Most birds enjoy being by a window. If the sun shines into the cage, part of the cage must be shaded so that the bird is able to move away from the sun if the temperature gets too hot. The cage should be placed where the temperature never drops below 18 °C (65 °F).[2]

At night, the cage should be covered with a cloth to help the bird feel more secure in the dark and to facilitate sleep. The cloth will keep the bird somewhat warmer during the winter. The cloth should be removed early in the morning so that the bird can have 12 hours of daylight if possible.[1]

When the bird arrives at its new residence, the owner should encourage the bird to leave the transport box willingly. Many birds readily enter the cage. Others need to be gently slid from the transport box into the cage; this process frightens most birds. Attempting to catch the bird and place it in the cage increases fright.

For the next several days, it is advisable to keep a reasonable distance from the cage except to provide fresh food and water. During feeding, the owner should talk quietly to the bird and move slowly so that the bird does not become frightened.

The bird will become used to the owner gradually and will eventually let the owner stroke it without pecking or attempting to bite the owner's hand. The owner should set aside time each day to spend with the bird in this way. Soon, the bird will become hand tame and will perch on the owner's finger.

Removing Hazards

Because of the possibility of injury or escape, I do not recommend letting a bird fly free in the house. Some owners, however, insist on this practice. Several attendant problems must be addressed. First, the bird should be hand tame so that the owner does not have to chase the bird when it is time to return to the cage. Second, all items that could injure the bird (e.g., sharp objects and poisonous plants) should be removed from the room. Third, the doors and windows should be closed and the drapes or blinds pulled almost completely closed; otherwise, the bird may attempt to fly through a windowpane and may receive a serious injury.

Another hazard in many homes is the ceiling fan. Such fans must be turned off when the bird is released from the cage. Ceiling fans have caused severe injuries to birds (especially small birds) that have flown or been sucked up into them.

[a]Fudge AM: Personal communication, Avian Medical Center, Citrus Heights, CA, 1988.

Even birds with clipped wings enjoy being out of the cage. Birds love to climb on their cages or pieces of furniture. Birds also enjoy walking around on the floor or riding on the owner's shoulder. The owner should be sure to remove dangerous items from the room before the bird is removed from the cage.

Kitchens and bathrooms are filled with dangers for birds. A bird should not be allowed in these rooms even if its wings are clipped. At any time, the bird might flutter onto a hot stove or into the toilet.

Recognizing Illness

Veterinary technicians can help owners to recognize signs of illness in pet birds. Sick birds may show few signs of illness; disease often goes unnoticed until it is too late to help. The technician thus should recommend that the new owner spend as much time as possible watching the bird's behavior so that changes are noticed immediately.

The owner should examine the bird's droppings. A change in the amount or characteristics of the droppings is often the first sign of illness.

Owners should watch for the following signs of illness in birds:

- Sitting with the feathers fluffed out
- Sleeping during the day
- Eating less frequently or a small amount
- Talking or singing less
- Sitting weakly on the bottom of the cage (a sign of serious illness)
- Labored breathing (a sign that the bird is moribund)
- A change in the quality and quantity of the droppings (Normal droppings consist of green or brown formed stools, watery white urates, and a small amount urine.[1,a])

An owner who notices any of these signs should call the clinic promptly and make an appointment to have the bird examined. Few owners realize how fast a bird's condition deteriorates during illness. Waiting one day to see if the bird is any better might be waiting too long. Many owners try over-the-counter medications and treatments, which rarely help and in some cases add to the pet's problems. From the outset, the technician should teach the new bird owner that it is critical to call the clinic immediately if there seems to be a problem with the bird.

First-Aid Kit

As with other pets, some avian emergencies might necessitate immediate treatment by the owner. The technician should recommend that the client stock an avian first-aid kit with the following items:

- A towel for capture and restraint of the bird
- Ferric subsulfate to stop hemorrhage (e.g., from a broken toenail or feather)
- Blunt tweezers to remove a bleeding feather; needle-nose pliers may be necessary for large birds
- Gauze pads and gauze rolls to stabilize possibly broken wings and legs.

Nutrition

New owners of birds frequently ask veterinary technicians what type of food is best. Most owners are surprised to hear that an all-seed diet is not recommended and can be harmful. Seeds (especially sunflower seeds and peanuts) are high in fat and have slight nutritional value. Approximately 20% of a bird's diet should consist of seeds.[3] The rest should be made up of fruits, vegetables, and a high-quality source of protein (Table I).

Pelleted diets are generally easy to prepare. Manufacturers claim that pellets provide complete and balanced nutrition. It is nevertheless advisable to supplement pellets with other foods.[a]

Most birds prefer certain foods (e.g., sunflower seeds and peanuts) and may eat such items exclusively if given the chance. In such cases, it may be necessary to eliminate the items from the diet completely or give them as occasional treats.

If a bird maintained on an all-seed diet refuses to eat fresh foods or a pelleted diet, the owner can withhold seeds for as long as 12 hours while introducing new items.[a] Most birds eagerly eat a new food item once they have tried it. The owner can gradually reduce the amount of seed given each day until the bird is eating all fresh foods or a combination of fresh and pelleted foods.

Raw fruits and vegetables should be washed well to remove pesticide residues and then dried before being cut into bite-sized pieces. Cutting food into small pieces reduces waste and maximizes consumption. Fresh foods should be removed after 6 to 10 hours—sooner in hot weather, during which the rate of bacterial growth increases.[2]

Some owners may ask whether it is acceptable to give birds sprouted seeds. Birds generally eat sprouts readily, but special care is required in preparation because moist

TABLE I
Avian Diets

Type of Food	Large Parrots	Small Parrots	Canaries and Finches
Seeds	Sunflower seeds, safflower seeds, peanuts, Brazil nuts, almonds, walnuts, wheat, rice, corn, barley, and millet	Sunflower seeds, safflower seeds, oats, millet, canary seed, rapeseed, rice, and wheat	Millet, canary seed, rapeseed, and thistle seed
Fruits and vegetables (fresh or thawed frozen)	Yams, carrots, squash, cabbage, peas, beans (e.g., green, lima, or pinto), broccoli, parsley, bananas, peppers, berries, and sprouts	Yams, carrots, squash, cabbage, peas, beans (e.g., green, lima, or pinto), broccoli, parsley, bananas, peppers, berries, and sprouts	Yams, carrots, squash, cabbage, peas, beans (e.g., green, lima, or pinto), broccoli, parsley, bananas, peppers, berries, and sprouts
Fresh fruit and vegetable treats (slight nutritional value)	Apples, grapes, celery, lettuce, peaches, and pears	Apples, grapes, celery, lettuce, peaches, and pears	Apples, grapes, celery, lettuce, peaches, and pears
High-quality protein sources	Cheese, yogurt, cottage cheese, tofu, soy products, cooked lean red meats, chicken, fish, eggs (boiled or scrambled), and whole-wheat bread	Cheese, yogurt, cottage cheese, tofu, soy products, cooked lean red meats, chicken, fish, eggs (boiled or scrambled), and whole-wheat bread	Cheese, yogurt, cottage cheese, tofu, soy products, cooked lean red meats, chicken, fish, eggs (boiled or scrambled), and whole-wheat bread
Other protein sources	Commercial dog or cat food, monkey biscuits, and dog biscuits	Commercial dog or cat food	Protein powder put on moist food
Pelleted diets	Various brands available; selection depends on proper size of pellet for bird	Various brands available; selection depends on proper size of pellet for bird	Various brands available; selection depends on proper size of pellet for bird
Vitamins and minerals	Powdered forms that can be put in water or on moist food	Powdered forms that can be put in water or on moist food	Cuttlebone

sprouted seeds provide a fertile medium for bacterial and fungal growth. The sprouts must be rinsed and drained well just before feeding and must not be left in the cage for more than two hours.[2]

The technician and owner should discuss providing grit to the bird. Most avian veterinarians do not consider grit to be essential for a bird's digestion. Overingestion of grit can cause potentially fatal impaction.[2,a]

Fresh, clean water should be available at all times. Water should be changed daily or more often if it becomes contaminated with food or fecal matter. During hot weather, the water dish may need to be refilled several times a day because the bird's thirst increases with the temperature.

Vitamins and minerals are essential to the health of birds and should be supplemented daily. These nutrients are marketed in various forms. Some preparations can be added to the drinking water; other formulations can be sprinkled on soft foods. Supplements should not be added to seeds; powders do not adhere to seeds but fall to the bottom of the seed dish. Some small birds prefer a cuttlebone to supplements added to food or water. The cuttlebone should be available at all times.

Conclusion

Bird owners consult veterinary technicians concerning many aspects of avian care. In order to provide appropriate guidance to clients, technicians must be knowledgeable about such care.

REFERENCES
1. Wolter A: *Cockatiels*, ed 1. New York, Barron's Educational Series, 1984, pp 8–25.
2. Ring L: Aviary design and management. *Proc Assoc Avian Vet*:252–256, 1989.
3. Ableseth MK: Management husbandry and nutrition, in Frazer CN, Mays A (eds): *The Merck Veterinary Manual*, ed 6. Rahway, NJ, Merck & Co, 1986, pp 1157–1161.

Avian Anesthesia: Part I

Marlee A. Richter, LVT
Department of Small Animal Clinical Sciences
Michigan State University
East Lansing, Michigan

With the rise in popularity of birds as pets, technicians should be able to feel comfortable in performing avian anesthesia. The basic principles of anesthesia in mammals apply to birds, although birds have certain unique anatomical and physiological characteristics that influence the effects of anesthetic agents. With the information presented in this two-part article and some close attention to details, avian anesthesia cases can be an interesting challenge for animal health technicians.

Avian Respiratory Anatomy and Physiology

The respiratory system in birds is considerably different from that of mammals. The text by King and McLelland[1] provides an excellent introduction to avian anatomy and function and is the source of much of the information in this section.

The respiratory system begins at the nostrils, generally located at the base of the beak. Air is filtered, warmed and humidified in the nasal cavity; it then passes into the pharynx, and then into the larynx. The larynx contains the glottis which is the slit opening between the two arytenoid cartilages. An epiglottis is not present in birds. Air then passes down the trachea, which contains complete tracheal rings (not C-shaped as in mammals), and into the syrinx. The syrinx is located at the junction of the end of the trachea and the beginning of the right and left primary bronchi, and is responsible for the voice in birds. Each primary bronchus, after entering a lung, is termed a mesobronchus and courses to the caudal aspect of the lung, tapering as it goes and giving rise to secondary bronchi (Figure 1). The secondary bronchi give rise to the parabronchi (also called tertiary bronchi[2]) which anastomose freely with other parabronchi. The walls of the parabronchi contain the tissue and structures (air capillaries and blood capillaries) where gaseous exchange takes place.

The lungs are held closely to the dorsolateral chest wall by connective tissues. The pleura covers only the free surface of the lung.

Most birds have four paired air sacs and one unpaired air sac (Figure 2). In the budgerigar, the paired air sacs are the cervical, cranial thoracic, caudal thoracic and abdominal, and the unpaired air sac is called the interclavicular. Each air sac, except the abdominal sac, is connected to a secondary bronchus and most, except the cervical sac,[2] are also connected via recurrent bronchi (saccobronchi[2]) that branch and anastomose with the parabronchi. (The abdominal sac is connected directly to the end of the mesobronchi.) The air sacs also have connections with some of the pneumatic bones (Figure 2).

The function of the bird's respiratory system is unique. Unlike mammals, birds do not have a complete diaphragm; consequently, they rely heavily on the movements of the chest during breathing. During inhalation, the ribs move ventrally and cranially, expanding the chest and abdomen (this causes negative pressure in the air sacs[3]) and drawing air into the respiratory tract.[4] During expiration, this is reversed (ribs move dorsal and caudal), the structures are compressed, and air is forced out of the system.[4] The lungs themselves do not expand and contract as they do in mammals (they may undergo small changes in volume[1]); the air sacs act as a bellows, pulling air through the lungs during inspiration and pushing it out during expiration.[1,4] Therefore, it is easy to understand why it is so very important not to restrict movement of the chest during manual restraint and positioning—taping or tying down—for a surgical procedure.

The air flow through the lungs and air sacs is still controversial and not well understood.[1,3,5,6] It is thought, however, that during inspiration the caudal air sacs

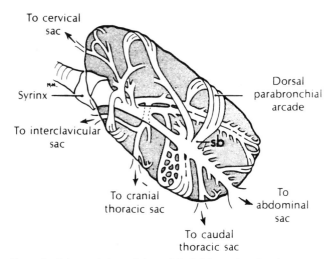

Figure 1—Schematic lateral view of the left lung showing the meso-bronchus and a secondary bronchus (*sb*) which gives rise to a dorsal parabronchial arcade. (Illustration and legend reprinted with permission. Evans HG: Anatomy of the budgerigar, in Petrak ML (ed): *Diseases of Cage and Aviary Birds.* Philadelphia, Lea & Febiger, 1969, p 83)

Figure 2—Schematic ventral view of the air sacs and their connections. 1, interclavicular sac; 2, lateral diverticulum of interclavicular sac; 3, subscapular diverticulum; 4, axillary diverticulum; 5, cervical sac. (Illustration and legend reprinted with permission. Evans HG: Anatomy of the budgerigar, in Petrak ML (ed): *Diseases of Cage and Aviary Birds.* Philadelphia, Lea & Febiger, 1969, p 86)

receive most of the air that is relatively fresh, i.e., some has already passed across the exchange tissues in the lung. During expiration, the anterior air sacs (interclavicular, cervical, and cranial thoracic) expel their gases into the primary bronchus and out the trachea. The caudal thoracic and abdominal air sacs expel their gases into the lung for passage through the parabronchi for gaseous exchange.[1] This *double passage* of gases through the lungs may account for the rapid induction and plane changes during the administration of inhalation anesthetic agents in birds. In mammals, anesthetic induction with inhalation anesthetics occurs more slowly.

Information on the tidal volumes of birds is limited. When compared to a mammal of the same size, a bird may have a tidal volume that is four times as large.[1]

Preanesthetic Considerations

The choice of anesthetic depends on the (1) age of the bird, (2) general condition of the bird, (3) anticipated duration of the procedure, (4) surgical disease, (5) coexisting diseases, and (6) equipment available.[7-10] Whenever anesthesia is contemplated, the benefits must be weighed against the possible risk involved.[8,11] In some cases, anesthesia should be avoided. For example, birds have very few pain receptors in the skin (except around the cere,[a] legs, and vent[b]), so a small wound or incision can be sutured without administering an anesthetic agent.[5,8,9] Very short procedures, such as amputating a toe or lancing an abscess, are other examples in which the risk of anesthesia may outweigh its benefits.[8,9] It should be remembered, however, that manual restraint is not without risk.[12] The stress of handling may cause the bird to go into shock or further injure itself by

struggling.[8,9,12-14] For these reasons, anesthesia may sometimes be necessary for diagnostic procedures such as radiology.

All patients should have a complete and accurate physical examination before any anesthetic is administered.[7-9,11,14,14a] Many of the signs of illness may be seen while simply observing the bird in its cage from a distance so as not to disturb it.[c] A normal bird is aware of its surroundings and is active, while the depressed or ill bird will sit in one spot on its perch or perhaps sit on the bottom of its cage, reluctant to move. The feathers of an ill bird will appear *puffed up* and the eyes may be closed or appear droopy. The eyes and nose should be examined for discharge. Respiratory rate and depth should also be noted. The vent area should be checked for *diarrhea*, indicated by pasted-looking feathers. Since the number of the bird's droppings is a good indicator of its appetite, owners should be counseled *not* to clean the bird's cage before transporting it to the veterinary hospital. Weight loss will be best indicated by a prominent keel (sternum). An accurate weight (using a gram scale) should be taken.[9,14] The average parakeet weighs

---

[a]*cere*—the tissue at the base of the beak that contains the nostrils.
[b]*vent*—the external opening of the cloaca.

[c]The author has attempted to briefly describe some of the signs a person may observe in a bird that is ill. This description should in no way be construed as being complete; nor should it be used in any way to circumvent the need for a thorough physical exam. All interested persons should consult the literature for further information.[23]

30 grams and the average canary only 20 grams,[9,11] so even a slight error in determining a bird's weight could lead to incorrect drug dosages, with potentially fatal results.[14]

Whenever possible, the patient should be acclimated to the hospital environment before proceeding with anesthesia.[9,14] Transporting the bird to the hospital and the handling required for examination can be very stressful. To immediately proceed to anesthetize the patient can be dangerous.[14] The bird should be kept in a quiet, warm, draft-free area of the hospital.[9,11] Before anesthesia, supportive care (i.e., tube feeding, fluids, warm environment, etc.) is indicated for those patients that are very weak, depressed, cold, emaciated or dehydrated.[9,11] Anesthetic dosages for sick or debilitated patients should be reduced.[11,14]

Birds have a rapid metabolism and, therefore, drugs (including anesthetics) are rapidly absorbed, detoxified and eliminated.[11,12] The bird's rapid metabolism also means that it cannot live very long without eating. A bird's liver cannot store large amounts of glycogen, so fasting prior to general anesthesia should be limited to two to three hours[5,11] or avoided altogether.[8,9]

Preanesthetic Agents

A tranquilizer or sedative is sometimes necessary for the extremely excitable or vicious animal prior to induction.[13] Because these drugs may have undesirable effects in birds, they are rarely used.[5] The dosage of an injectable anesthetic must be reduced if the bird is given a preoperative tranquilizer.

Atropine can be used to prevent bradycardia and to decrease respiratory secretions. The suggested dosage is 0.04 to 0.1 mg/kg.[8] Atropine should be diluted and accurately measured.[8] For example, the amount needed for a 30-gram patient is 0.0012 to 0.003 mg, or 0.024 to 0.06 ml of a 1:10 dilution of a 0.5 mg/ml solution.

General Anesthesia

General anesthetics can be broken down into two main categories: (1) injectable and (2) inhalation. These will be described in detail in Part II. The following discussion will focus on two important considerations relating to general anesthesia. The first is the prevention of hypothermia, which can be a serious problem in avian patients undergoing general anesthesia, and the second is the administration of oxygen, either alone or with inhalation agents, by way of an endotracheal tube or face mask.

Hypothermia

Hypothermia is a major consideration whenever a patient undergoes general anesthesia and, when the patient is a tiny bird, it becomes particularly important.[5,7,12,15] Anesthetics slow metabolism,[10] which reduces heat production, and eliminate the shivering reflex, thereby allowing the body to cool when the environmental temperature is less than the body temperature.[16] Birds also lose body heat when feathers are plucked and wet scrubs are applied to the skin in preparation for surgery.[5] This is especially true when a large area is plucked and the standard povidone-iodine[d]/alcohol scrub is applied. If inhalation anesthesia or oxygen therapy is used, the patient must warm and humidify the inhaled gases and this can result in additional heat (and fluid) loss.[5,7] Of course, the longer the patient remains anesthetized, the more severe and pronounced the hypothermia will be.[5]

Anesthesia time can be kept to a minimum by being certain that everything needed for the procedure is set up and ready to go, including personnel.[11] If inhalation anesthesia (or oxygen alone) is to be administered, the Bain Breathing Circuit[®e] should be used. It has many

[d]Betadine®, The Purdue Frederick Co., Norwalk, CT 06856.
[e]Bain Breathing Circuit®, Respiratory Care Inc., Arlington Heights, IL 60004.

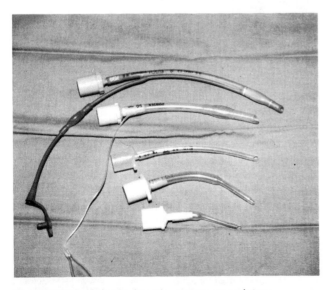

Figure 3—Endotracheal tubes of various types and sizes.

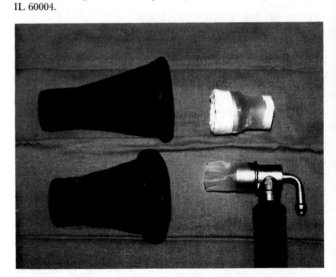

Figure 4—Anesthetic masks showing the commercially available types and two kinds of *homemade* masks—one made from the thumb of a rubber glove and the other made from a 20-ml syringe case.

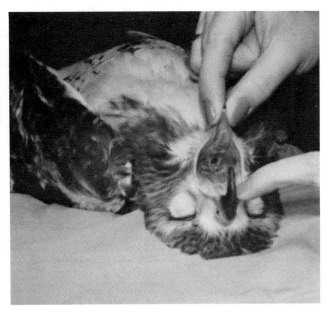

Figure 5—The location of the glottis in a red-tailed hawk.

advantages[7,17,18] including the fact that it warms and humidifies the gases, if they are used at recommended low flow rates. As few feathers as possible should be plucked from the surgical site. Prep the skin with povidone-iodine scrub[d] and avoid the excessive use of alcohol which has a cooling effect as it evaporates.[14a]

The patient should be placed on a circulating water blanket to protect against *cold* environmental temperatures.[7,15,19,20] A Vac Pack positioner® or sandbags can be placed under the water blanket to create a U-shaped area in which the patient lies, providing this does not interfere with the surgical site.[f] Alternatives to a water blanket include an electrical heating pad,[5,8] and a hot water bottle,[15] both of which have major disadvantages

---

[f]Olympic Vac Pac, 4400 7th South, Seattle, WA 98108.

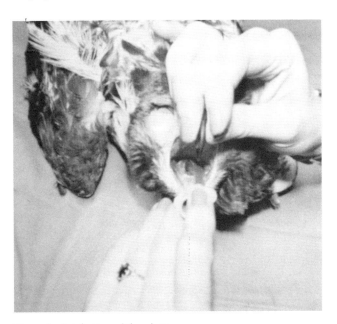

Figure 6—Intubation of the glottis.

and are not recommended. Serious burns have occurred with the use of electric heating pads.[21] A towel or blanket should be placed on top of the heating pad and the pad should be set at the lowest heat level to minimize the possibility of burns. The patient should be closely monitored. Hot water bottles are not recommended because it is difficult to get the water at the right temperature and the bottles tend to cool rapidly. Towels and blankets are used alone or in conjunction with any of the above methods.[15]

Oxygen Administration

Oxygen should be administered to all avian patients that receive a general anesthetic.[9] Both major types of general anesthesia, injectable and inhalation, will depress respiration.[16] Oxygen is administered in addition to inhalation agents, or alone if an injectable anesthetic is used. An endotracheal tube (Figure 3) or face mask (Figure 4) is used to deliver oxygen to the patient.[8,19] Most birds have a large fleshy tongue that can fall back into the mouth, obstructing the laryngeal opening,[8,19] and the masks themselves tend to be bulky and easily dislodged.[8] Intubating prevents these problems. Once the patient is connected to the oxygen delivery system, the anesthetist can readily visualize the rate, depth, and effort of breathing and can support ventilation as needed during anesthesia or apnea.[8]

Endotracheal Intubation

Intubation is easily accomplished in most birds due to the location of the glottis (Figures 5 and 6). Endotracheal tubes should not be lubricated with jelly-type materials. If the jelly gets into the lumen of the endotracheal tube, it hardens to form a solid plug that obstructs respiration. Water can be used instead. When the endotracheal tube has been inserted, the trachea should be gently palpated to check for proper tube length. The endotracheal tube should extend no farther than the thoracic inlet. To eliminate dead space, all tubes should

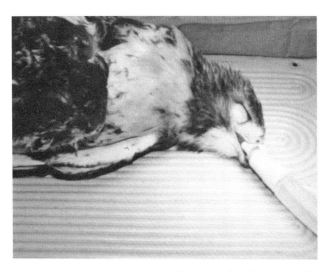

Figure 7—The endotracheal tube of the proper length is secured in place (to the upper beak) with a piece of adhesive tape.

be cut so that they do not extend beyond the beak.[8,19] This is crucial in small patients. The bird will rebreathe exhaled gases if the tube is not cut, and the results can include acidosis and/or insufficient depth of anesthesia if inhalation anesthesia is being used. The endotracheal tube is secured in place by taping the tube to the upper beak, being careful not to tape over the delicate cere tissue[5] (Figure 7).

The Cole-type of endotracheal tube[5,8] can be used in birds. Cole tubes do not have cuffs, but rather a narrow end that is placed into the trachea and a wider portion that rests against the glottis, preventing gas leakage around the tube.

The rubber and plastic types of endotracheal tubes with an inflatable cuff can also be used. When using this type of tube, it is important to avoid overinflating the cuff. Birds have continuous tracheal rings (360°) that cannot expand and may rupture with overinflation of the cuff.[8] Also, with the cuff overinflated, the tracheal epithelium may become damaged due to an insufficient blood supply, resulting in pressure necrosis.

If a commercial endotracheal tube suitable for the bird is not available, plastic or rubber tubing can be used to make one. The tubing is cut to length and sharp edges are filed; then, it is fitted with an adapter.

Oxygen Masks

If, due to patient size, intubation is not practical, a mask can be used.[22] With a mask, a paper clip can be bent and used to hold the tongue forward to prevent obstruction of the laryngeal opening.[8,9,19] A *mask* may not be necessary in a tiny bird as very often the head (beak) will fit inside the end of the nonrebreathing system or y-piece.[22] For slightly larger birds, a mask can be made by cutting the thumb from a rubber glove at the base and at the tip so that both ends are open. The narrow end is stretched on the end of the nonrebreathing (or semiopen) system and the patient's head is placed in the other end (Figure 4). Disposable cups, syringe barrels and syringe cases are other examples of materials that can be made into a mask (Figure 4). Commercial masks (Figure 4) can be used, if available,[19] but they are usually too bulky for the small bird. Appropriate size masks (as small as possible) will prevent problems that result from too much dead air space.

When using a mask, flow rates are variable and depend on the size of the patient and the equipment used. The flow rate should be high enough to compensate for the increased dead space of a mask.[8,19] Generally, a 3 liter total flow rate/minute should be adequate for most patients under 7 kg.[7] The patient should receive 100% oxygen until it has fully recovered from the anesthetic.

REFERENCES

1. King AS, McLelland J: *Outlines of Avian Anatomy*. New York, The Macmillan Publishing Co, Inc, 1975, pp 43-64.

2. Evans HG: Anatomy of the budgerigar, in Petrak ML (ed): *Diseases of Cage and Aviary Birds*. Philadelphia, Lea & Febiger, 1969, pp 82-88.

3. Farner DS: Some physiological attributes of small birds, in Petrak ML (ed): *Diseases of Cage and Aviary Birds*. Philadelphia, Lea & Febiger, 1969, pp 116-119.

4. Fowler ME: *Restraint and Handling of Wild and Domestic Animals*. Ames, Iowa State University Press, 1978, pp 262-264.

5. Sandford J: Avian anesthesia, in Soma LR (ed): *Textbook of Veterinary Anesthesia*. Baltimore, The Williams and Wilkins Co, 1971, pp 359-367.

6. Sturkie PD: *Avian Physiology*, ed 2. Ithaca, Cornell University Press, 1965, pp 152-174.

7. Sawyer DC, Evans AT, DeYoung DJ: *Anesthetic Principles and Techniques*. East Lansing, Department of Small Animal Surgery and Medicine, College of Veterinary Medicine, Michigan State University, 1973, pp 1-57.

8. Altman RB: Avian anesthesia. *Compend Contin Educ Pract Vet* 2(1):38-42, 1980.

9. Amand WB: Avian anesthesia, in Kirk R (ed): *Current Veterinary Therapy VI*. Philadelphia, WB Saunders Co, 1977, pp 705-710.

10. Booth NH: Introduction, in Jones LM, Booth NH, McDonald LE (eds): *Veterinary Pharmacology and Therapeutics*, ed 4. Ames, The Iowa State University Press, 1977, pp 191-207.

11. Friedburg KM: Anesthesia of parakeets and canaries. *JAVMA* 141(10):1157-1160, 1962.

12. Arnall R: Anesthesia and surgery in cage and aviary birds (I). *Vet Rec* 73(7):139-142, 1961.

13. Graham-Jones D: Restraint and anesthesia of small cage birds. *J Small Anim Pract* 6(1):31-39, 1965.

14. Gandal CP: Surgical techniques and anesthesia, in Petrak ML (ed): *Diseases of Cage and Aviary Birds*. Philadelphia, Lea & Febiger, 1969, pp 217-222.

14a. Harrison GJ, Harrison LR: *Clinical Avian Medicine and Surgery*. Philadelphia, WB Saunders Co, 1986, pp 543-548.

15. Amand WB: General techniques for avian surgery, in Kirk R (ed): *Current Veterinary Therapy VI*. Philadelphia, WB Saunders Co, 1977, pp 711-716.

16. Smith TC: Respiratory effects of general anesthesia, in Soma LR (ed): *Textbook of Veterinary Anesthesia*. Baltimore, Williams and Wilkins Co, 1971, pp 156-175.

17. Manley SV, McDonell WN: Clinical evaluation of the Bain breathing circuit in small animal anesthesia. *JAAHA* 15(1):67-72, 1979.

18. Manley SV, McDonell WN: A new circuit for small animal anesthesia: The Bain coaxial circuit. *JAAHA* 15(1):61-65, 1979.

19. Klide AM: Avian anesthesia. *Vet Clin North Am* 3(2):175-186, 1973.

20. Blair E. Hypothermia, in Soma LR (ed): *Textbook of Veterinary Anesthesia*. Baltimore, Williams and Wilkins Co, 1971, p 562.

21. Sumner-Smith G: Surgical nursing and anesthesiology, in Catcott EJ (ed): *Animal Health Technology*. Santa Barbara, American Veterinary Publications, Inc, 1977, p 195.

22. Soma LR: Systems and techniques for inhalation anesthesia, in Soma LR (ed): *Textbook of Veterinary Anesthesia*. Baltimore, Williams and Wilkins Co, 1971, pp 201-227.

23. Stone RM: Clinical examination and methods of treatment, in Petrak ML (ed): *Diseases of Cage and Aviary Birds*. Philadelphia, Lea & Febiger, 1969, pp 177-187.

Avian Anesthesia: Part II

Marlee A. Richter, LVT
Department of Small Animal Clinical Sciences
Michigan State University
East Lansing, Michigan

General anesthesia is necessary for many surgical and for some diagnostic procedures performed on avian patients. Part I of this series reviewed pertinent aspects of anatomy and physiology, preanesthetic considerations and agents, prevention of hypothermia, and oxygen administration in birds. This article will focus on anesthetic agents, equipment, and techniques used in performing general anesthesia on birds. Monitoring the bird during anesthesia and during the recovery period will also be discussed.

Anesthesia with Injectable Agents

Small doses of injectable anesthetic agents followed by inhalation agents are occasionally used for anesthesia induction[1] or to facilitate diagnostic procedures such as radiography in birds. Injectable agents are rarely used as the sole anesthetic, because the inhalation agents are safer and more reliable and with them recovery is much faster.

Injectable anesthetics must be used carefully, because the appropriate dosage varies according to the species and individual animal.[1,2] A small dosage error may result in death.[2-4] Administering the drug intravenously (IV) allows it to be more closely titrated *to effect*, but this is difficult in small birds.[1,2,4] Birds have small, thin-walled veins that contribute to poor hemostasis.[4,5] The veins that can be used are the jugular (right side only in the budgerigar[5]) and the brachial[a,6] veins; however they are not easily accessible.[2] IV injections are only practical in the larger species.[4]

Another disadvantage of injectable anesthetic drugs is the long recovery period associated with them.[2,3] Hypothermia and hypoglycemia are common problems. There is also the possibility of having to provide some type of restraint to prevent injury during the recovery period.

The intramuscular (IM) route is another method of administration that can be used in the bird. The amount of anesthetic injected should be proportionate to the bird's size, i.e., an injection of 0.3 ml in a 30-g parakeet is approximately equivalent to an injection of 500 ml in a 100-lb child.[2] IM injections are most commonly given in the pectoral muscles (breast), although the upper thigh can be used in bigger birds.[4] Birds have a large venous plexus in the pectoral muscles (associated with the extra venous drainage needed during flight), so deep injections should be avoided, and aspiration is essential before injection.[1,6]

Intraperitoneal (IP) injections are not recommended for birds, because there is a strong possibility of entering an air sac or other abdominal organ and causing severe damage.[1,4]

Injectable Anesthetic Agents
Barbiturates

The barbiturates are perhaps the least used group of the injectable drugs. Pentobarbital sodium, thiobarbiturates, and phenobarbital sodium have been used in birds. The dosages and responses are variable[1,7] and unreliable,[4] and therefore their safety and usefulness in birds is questionable.[1-3]

---

[a]The brachial vein crosses the ventral surface of the humerus.

Originally published in Volume 2, Number 4, July/August 1981

Cyclohexylamines

Ketamine[c,d,9,10] is probably the best-known cyclohexylamine. It is relatively safe for all species of birds;[3] it has a wide margin of safety and can be given IM.[3] It is frequently used as a restraining agent for diagnostic procedures and can be used as a preanesthetic or induction agent prior to inhalation anesthesia.[3,4] Ocular and oral reflexes and a high degree of muscle tone are present when it is used.[3,4] Analgesia is more somatic than visceral—therefore ketamine should not be used as the sole anesthetic agent during *deep* (abdominal or orthopedic) surgery. Ketamine can cause or stimulate fluttering, tremors, or convulsions.[3,4] Induction takes place in three to five minutes or less, and the duration of anesthesia is 10 to 30 minutes.[3] Complete recovery can take 30 minutes to five hours.[3] Ketamine should be used with caution in debilitated patients—especially in those that are dehydrated and/or have renal insufficiency—because it is excreted unchanged by the kidneys.[3,4] Dosages are variable. The dosage is 50 to 100 mg/kg for birds weighing up to 500 g,[e] and for birds weighing more than 500 g it is 25 to 50 mg/kg IM.[f]

Ketamine/Xylazine Combination

Xylazine[g] is commonly combined with ketamine because of its synergistic effects of sedation, analgesia, and muscle relaxation. This combination is considered generally safe and preferred over using either ketamine or xylazine alone in birds. It can be administered IV to effect for rapid induction and recovery or given IM. Recovery will be prolonged with IM administration. Violent recovery is seen in some birds probably due to the ketamine component. It has been reported that pigeons do not tolerate xylazine,[3] however it has been used successfully in combination with ketamine in that species.[24] Suggested IM dosage of ketamine is 10–30 mg/kg combined with an equal *volume* of xylazine (draw up xylazine into syringe first) and initially give one eighth to one quarter of dose, wait 5–10 minutes, and repeat if necessary for more depth or for longer procedures. Interested readers are referred to Harrison and Harrison for dosages for various avian species and further discussion.

Inhalation Anesthesia

Inhalation anesthesia is the method of choice for general anesthesia in birds. Although administering an inhalation anesthetic agent requires more equipment, technical knowledge, and skill than injections do, the benefits of this method are great.[4] Induction and recovery are smooth and rapid, and anesthetic depth can be precisely regulated.[3] The basic principles of inhalation anesthesia in mammals apply to birds, although

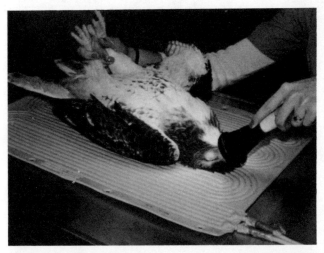

Figure 1—Mask induction.

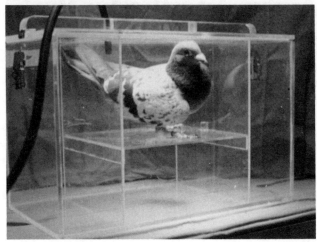

Figure 2—Chamber induction. Note the partitions that allow for size adjustments.

birds do have respiratory structural and physiological differences.[h,1,4,5]

Inhalation agents can be administered via a face mask (Figure 1) or an induction chamber.[1,6,12,13] Some anesthetic chambers[3] have partitions that allow them to be adjusted to the patient's size (Figure 2).[14] This not only conserves gases (Table I), but the bird is confined to a small enough area so that injuries during induction are not likely to occur. Other chambers that can be used are a clear plastic shoe storage box, a plastic freezer container, or a clear plastic bag placed around the bird's cage.[4] Freezer containers are usually opaque, but clear plastic wrap can be held or taped in place instead of the regular lid. Putting the bird's cage in a plastic bag works well for those patients not easily handled, but injuries can occur during the early stages of the induction. All perches, bowls, toys, etc. should be removed before the bird is anesthetized. There should be two holes in the induction chamber—one for the fresh gas inlet and one for escape of excess gases so that pressure does not build up inside the container.

The most commonly encountered pet birds are small (less than 7 kg); therefore, an anesthetic machine with a vaporizer outside the circle is the most easily adapted for

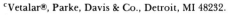

[c]Vetalar®, Parke, Davis & Co., Detroit, MI 48232.

[d]Ketaset®, Bristol Laboratories, Syracuse, NY 13201.

[e]1 to 3 mg/30 g (33 to 90 mg/kg)[23]; 1 mg/30 g, restraint dose; 2 mg/30 g, surgical dose (effects last 5 to 20 minutes); 3 mg/30 g, surgical dose (effects last longer).

[f]15 to 20 mg/kg for fowl and various raptors.[4]

[g]Rompun®, Haver-Lockhart, Shawnee, KS 66201.

TABLE I

Flow Rates for Various-Sized Anesthetic Chambers[14]

Size of Anesthetic Chamber (liters)	Total Flow Rate*,† (liters/minute)
18	5
14	4
10	3
7	2
3	0.75

*Flow rates must be adjusted for the various-sized anesthetic chambers so that induction time is kept constant.
†Oxygen alone or with nitrous oxide.

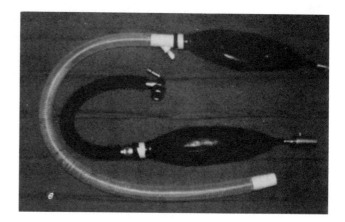

Figure 3—Commonly used nonrebreathing systems. Norman mask elbow, Bain breathing circuit.

use with a chamber and a nonrebreathing (semiopen) system.[12] Patients less than 7 kg should never be placed on a circle system.[3,12] A fairly large tidal volume is required to move the gases around the circle (and into the vaporizer on machines with the vaporizer located in the circle). There is some dead space in the y-piece, and the valves themselves offer some resistance to breathing. The combination of these factors is devastating to the small patient. Machines with vaporizers in the circle can be adapted for use with a nonrebreathing system with some modifications.[15]

The most commonly used nonrebreathing systems[13] are the Ayre's T-piece,[i] Norman mask elbow,[j] and the Bain Breathing Circuit®[k] (Figure 3). The total flow rate for the Norman mask elbow and the Ayre's T-piece is three times minute ventilation[l,m,2,12,15] (Table II). The recommended total flow rate for the Bain circuit is 100 to 140 ml/kg/minute.[n,12,16,17] Although these systems can be used at low flow rates, precision vaporizers may not be able to deliver accurate percentages of the anesthetic at these levels.[o,2,18] Oxygen and nitrous oxide flowmeters cannot always be precisely regulated at very low flow rates. Therefore a minimum flow rate of 0.5 liter/minute is recommended.

Inhalation Anesthetic Agents

Many of the volatile anesthetics, including ether, cy-clopropane, methoxyflurane, halothane, isoflurane and nitrous oxide, have been used in birds. Only the latter four agents will be discussed, since the others are fairly obsolete primarily because of their flammability and explosiveness.

Isoflurane

Isoflurane is the best inhalation agent to use in birds. It is nonflammable, has a greater molecular stability than halothane or methoxyflurane, and does not need a preservative. Metabolism accounts for only 0.17% of the uptake of isoflurane, compared to 50% with methoxyflurane and 20% for halothane.[25] This results in little or no effect on hepatic or renal function, an important feature for our patients as well as surgical personnel. Isoflurane has a lower blood:gas coefficient (1.4) than halothane (2.5) or methoxyflurane (1.5), which results in short induction and recovery periods, an important consideration for birds. The effects on cardiac function are minimal. Isoflurane provides a larger margin of safety than halothane or methoxy-flurane and is reported to have an extensive interval between apnea and cardiac arrest.[24] Isoflurane depresses respiration in a dose dependent fashion to a slightly greater extent than halothane. It may be necessary to

---

[i]Foregger Co., Smithtown, NY 11787.
[j]Dupaco Inc., San Marcos, CA 92069.
[k]Respiratory Care Inc., Arlington Heights, IL 60004.
[l]Minute ventilation-respiratory rate times tidal volume.
[m]i.e., oxygen alone or with nitrous oxide.

[n]Some rebreathing of exhaled gases occurs at this flow rate. A total flow rate of three times minute ventilation must be used to prevent rebreathing.
[o]Manufacturer's recommendations for the vaporizer should be checked.

TABLE II

Oxygen Consumption and Minute Volume in Various-Sized Birds*

Bird	Weight (grams)	O₂ Consumption (ml/g/hour)	O₂ Consumption (ml/minute)	Respiratory Minute Volume (ml)
Chicken	2400	0.3	20	770
Pigeon	300	0.9	45	250
Sparrow	24	3.0	1.2	25

*From Klide AM: Avian anesthesia. *Vet Clin North Am* 3(2):184,1973. Reprinted with permission.

TABLE III

PROGRESSION OF SIGNS OF SURGICAL ANESTHESIA*

	Stages of Anesthesia			
	Induction and Narcosis	*Light*	*Medium*	*Deep*
Signs	Eyelids closing, wings starting to droop, head lowered			
Voluntary movement	Can be aroused and is pain sensitive	Absent	Absent	Absent
Respirations	Deep, rapid, and regular without stimulation	Deep and rapid	Slow, deep and regular	Slow, regular and shallow
Corneal reflexes	Present	Present	Slow or intermittent	Absent
Pedal reflexes	Present	Present	Slow or intermittent	Absent
Palpebral reflexes	Present	Present	Absent	Absent
Cere reflexes	Present	Present	Absent	Absent

*From Altman RB: Avian anesthesia. *Compend Contin Educ Pract Vet* 2(1):41,1980. Reprinted with permission. Information classified and compiled by Arnall.[7]

assist ventilation especially in the unstimulated patient. The vapor pressure of isoflurane is 239.5 mm Hg at 20°C which is very close to that of 244.1 mm Hg for halothane and therefore both must be used in a precision vaporizer located outside the circle.[2] Precision vaporizers calibrated for halothane, but properly cleaned, and filled with isoflurane, will produce a concentration very close to that indicated on the dial.[25] In birds, isoflurane concentration is 5% for mask induction with oxygen flow rates of 2–3 liters/minute. Anesthesia is maintained with 2–3% isoflurane in an oxygen flow rate of 0.5–1 liters/minute. The cost of isoflurane may be of concern. Sixty minutes of anesthesia with an oxygen flow rate of 0.5 liters/minute and an isoflurane concentration of 2% would cost $2.10. The slightly higher cost seems well worth it in terms of benefit and safety to our avian patients.

Halothane

Halothane is noninflammable,[3] nonexplosive, and nonirritating,[2] and is less expensive than isoflurane. Because of its low blood solubility, halothane is easily used with mask and or chamber inductions and the depth can be controlled with greater precision than with methoxyflurane.[4] Inductions at concentrations of 2–4% are recommended.[3,4] Inductions are generally complete in one to five minutes.[3] A brief excitement stage is indicated by trembling or wing flapping in birds.[3,4] Following induction, the bird is maintained at 0.5 to 1.5% halothane.[1,3] Because halothane only provides a moderate level of muscle relaxation, nitrous oxide at a 1:1 ratio (nitrous oxide:oxygen) is sometimes used (refer to next section). If using nitrous oxide, the halothane concentration is generally reduced to 0.5–1%. Halothane increases the sensitivity of the

heart to exogenous or endogenous epinephrine which may result in arrhythmias. This may be especially problematic in excitable birds. As mentioned, halothane, and all inhaled anesthetics, depress ventilation in a dose-related manner. Since 20% of halothane is metabolized, consideration needs to be given for proper scavenging of waste anesthetic gases and the use in patients with liver disease. (The maintenance percentage of halothane required will vary somewhat depending on the species and general condition of the bird, use of preanesthetic sedation, etc.) Recovery is generally complete in 5 to 10 minutes.

Methoxyflurane

Methoxyflurane, like halothane, is nonexplosive,[3] nonirritating, and noninflammable. It has the highest solubility of the inhalation anesthetics discussed, which results in longer inductions and recovery times. It can be used in precision vaporizers out of the circle or with less expensive wick vaporizers in the circle. The advantage of the vaporizer out of the circle is that it can be used for mask and chamber induction and maintenance with a *nonrebreathing system*, because exact percentages can be delivered to these systems. The vaporizer in the circle can be adapted for use in these systems as previously mentioned, but this is not commonly done (or recommended for birds) because this type of vaporizer's output depends on many variable factors.[12] Induction with methoxyflurane by placing a measured amount of the liquid in a jar or chamber has also been described but not recommended.[1,5] Induction with methoxyflurane is done at 3%,[3] and anesthesia is generally maintained to effect at 0.5 to 2%.[3,4] Because of the potential for organ toxicity, this anesthetic is not recommended for use in debilitated or critical patients and careful attention should be given to scavenging waste gas.

Nitrous Oxide

Nitrous oxide is incapable of producing anesthesia alone; it is used as an adjunct to other anesthetics.[3,4,7,13] Nitrous oxide provides analgesia and muscle relaxation, so less primary anesthetic agent is required. Inductions are quicker because of the second gas effect.[12,19] Nitrous oxide should never be used in greater than 75% concentration with oxygen; if it is used at 75% concentration, it should be used only for a short time during the early phase of induction.[13] A 50 to 60% concentration[13] of nitrous oxide may be more appropriate for induction and maintenance of birds.[3] Nitrous oxide will diffuse into air pockets and cause their expansion; therefore it should not be used if intestinal obstruction is suspected. It is also not recommended in cases of respiratory and severe myocardial diseases.[12] Diffusion hypoxia will occur unless oxygen is administered following its use. In mammals, two to three minutes of oxygen is administered after nitrous oxide is discontinued, and this is necessary for birds as well. Because of the hazards of diffusion hypoxia, nitrous oxide is not as popular as it once was.

Monitoring Depth of Anesthesia

The stages and signs of anesthetic depth in birds with both inhalation and injectable anesthetics are listed in Table III.

The two main indicators in monitoring anesthetic depth in birds are respiratory variables (rate, depth, and effort) and reflex responses.[4] The respiratory variables are the most important indicators since reflex responses vary somewhat depending on the bird species[1] and the anesthetic agent.[4] It is therefore essential that the anesthetist be able to see the respiratory movements at all times; smaller-than-normal or clear plastic surgical drapes may be necessary.[3,20] Any change in respiration should alert the anesthetist to possible trouble and it should be investigated immediately.[4]

In the corneal reflex, the nictitating membrane flashes across the eye in response to corneal stimulation.[p] In the palpebral reflex, the eyelids close in response to a touch near the eye.[3] The cere reflex (a pain response) is tested by a pin prick.[p,3] The pedal reflex is withdrawal of the foot in response to pressure on the toes.[3]

Heart rate, sound, and strength can also be used to monitor the patient.[4] A stethoscope can be placed on the chest or, in larger patients, an esophageal stethoscope can be passed into the esophagus, although this may be difficult because of the bird's crop.[3] Since the heart rate in birds is so rapid, it is difficult to count; the anesthetist should instead listen for changes in rate, rhythm, or strength. An EKG is helpful in determining the heart rate and rhythm.[3]

Muscle tone is another variable that can be used to monitor the patient—especially during the induction period. The wings, legs, and toes can be moved to test for the amount of tone. When a round object (such as a pencil or pen) is placed on the ventral aspect of the foot, the lightly anesthetized patient will often attempt to grasp it. Slight movements of the wings are often one of the first signs that the bird is entering a lighter plane of anesthesia. An increase in respiratory rate before or at the same time as wing movements also signals lightening of anesthesia.

Recovery

The bird should be placed in a warm, quiet,[1,3,7] oxygen-enriched environment where it can be easily observed during the recovery period.[3,4] Patients recovering from inhalation anesthesia should receive oxygen via the endotracheal tube or mask.[3] Some birds will tolerate the endotracheal tube longer than mammals; they will often allow the tube to be left in place well into the recovery period. If the patient is awake (eyes open, but not yet able to stand) but still appears groggy, it can be placed in an oxygen chamber until fully recovered. The anesthesia induction chamber works well if an oxygen cage is not available. A bird will often appear alert when stimulated but will later become groggy; this may be because of the reservoir of gases in the air sacs. The recovery period generally takes approximately 10 to 30 minutes following inhalation anesthesia. Birds that received injectable anesthetics will often have long recovery periods which can lead to complications such as hypothermia and hypoglycemia.

Thrashing and disorientation may occur during the recovery period, especially following the use of injectable anesthetics, and restraint may be necessary to prevent injuries. Placing a stockinette, piece of tube gauze, or, for smaller birds, a cardboard cylinder (such as those found in paper towels or toilet tissue) over the bird will prevent it from trying to stand or fly too soon.[4,6,7]

Once the bird is recovered (this is indicated by the ability to perch), it can be placed back in its cage,[2,7,8] where it should be given food and water.[3,4] Birds that have had splints applied or their wings taped should be watched carefully to ascertain that they are able to maintain their balance well enough to eat and drink. Perches, food, and water can be placed near the bottom of the cage until the bird has completely regained its coordination.[4]

Other Considerations

Patients should be handled carefully while under anesthesia. Special care should be taken to avoid injury to the head and neck area when moving the patient and during surgical procedures (such as orthopedic) requir-

---

[p]This reflex is not routinely tested.

[q]A nonrebreathing system should never be flushed using the oxygen flush valve. On machines so equipped, this valve will deliver 30 liters/minute of oxygen directly to the system. Pressure will build rapidly, and it can rupture the bird's air sacs and/or lungs.

[r]Other methods of artificial ventilation have been described.[1,5]

ing manipulation.[2] Sudden cardiac arrest due to patient movement (especially when the head is lowered) during anesthesia has been known to occur.[2,21] This is probably because some anesthetic agents cause vasodilation and the body may not be able to compensate for sudden movements by normal mechanisms. Also, severe hypotension can result from a small amount of blood loss, and this may cause circulatory collapse.[1,4,7,8] "Small birds have a blood volume of 100 ml/kg . . . a canary of 20 grams has a blood volume of about 2 ml. If there are 20 drops per ml of blood, then 5 drops of blood is one-eighth of the canary's blood volume."[2] Hemostasis is very important;[5] fluids should be administered when necessary.[2,3,5,20] Fluids warmed to body temperature can be given IV (if possible) or subcutaneously (in the wing web or loose skin of the neck) in small patients.[3,4,20]

Emergencies (cardiac and respiratory arrest) can occur even with the best of efforts; they are most often associated with blood losses.[8] Early recognition is essential. The procedure to follow is the ABCs of emergency care:

A. The airway is checked for patency, anesthetics are turned off (if using inhalational agents), and oxygen is left on.[9]
B. The patient's ability to breathe is determined and, if necessary, the bird is ventilated with 100% oxygen via an endotracheal tube or close-fitting mask.[r,4]
C. If circulation is inadequate, cardiac massage is begun at a rate of two compressions/second.[4] With tiny birds, a finger can be used to gently compress the thorax.[1,5,8]
D. Drugs can be given at the veterinarian's discretion.

Local Anesthesia

Local anesthesia is indicated for conditions that require analgesia without loss of consciousness. The use of local anesthetics and their administration and precautions in birds are outlined here.

Local anesthetics produce analgesia and require less equipment than do general anesthetics. However, the use of local anesthetics in birds has been limited for many reasons. First, the bird may go into shock (especially wild and small pet birds) or be injured when manually restrained.[2-6] In addition, there is some controversy regarding the use of injectable local anesthetics in birds.[1-6] Birds, particularly parakeets,[2] have been reported to be sensitive or *allergic* to the drugs[e] commonly used as local anesthetics.[1,2,5,6,22] In one study, it was found that this may not be the problem; the apparent toxicity may have been simply attributable to overdosing the small patient on a milligram/kilogram basis.[2] It was suggested that the maximum total dosage in small birds not exceed 200 mg/kg of a 0.2% solution of procaine.[2,3] Epinephrine, used to slow the absorption of local anesthetics, should not be used in avian patients.[4,5] It is obvious, therefore, that when using injectable local anesthetics, one must be careful to weigh the bird accurately, calculate dosages carefully, use dilute solutions when necessary,[2,5] and measure the drug in a microliter or tuberculin syringe.[4] The needle size recommended for birds is 25- to 26-gauge, used with standard injection techniques.[4]

Topical local anesthetics are more widely used and accepted than injectable local anesthetics.[1,3,4] Examples are proparacaine HCl, which is used to anesthetize the eye, and lidocaine HCl ointment, which is used to control tenesmus and pain after a prolapsed cloaca.[3] Other topical anesthetics include Cetacaine®[s] and ethyl chloride,[1,5-8] in the spray form.

Conclusion

Careful evaluation and consideration should be given as to the type of anesthetic (if any) that is best suited for the bird. Intubation is easily accomplished in most birds and therefore should be done whenever practical. All avian patients should receive oxygen throughout the anesthetic period, whether injectable or inhalation anesthetics are used. Prevention of hypothermia, along with careful patient monitoring and handling, is of major importance. In general, mask induction and maintenance with isoflurane proves to be an effective and safe way of anesthetizing birds. The patient should be observed carefully during the recovery period for complications or the possible need for restraint to prevent injuries. The bird should be fed and given water as soon as it can perch.

Acknowledgment

The author is indebted to the following people (and many others) who have helped to make this article possible: Dr. Sally Oblas Walshaw and Dr. A. T. Evans for their editorial assistance.

---

[s]Cetylite Industries, Inc., Pennsauken, NJ 08110.

REFERENCES

1. Sandford J: Avian anesthesia, in Soma LR (ed): *Textbook of Veterinary Anesthesia.* Baltimore, The Williams and Wilkins Co, 1971, pp 359-367.
2. Klide AM: Avian anesthesia. *Vet Clin North Am* 3(2):175-186, 1973.
3. Altman RB: Avian anesthesia. *Compend Contin Educ Pract Vet* 2(1):38-42, 1980.
4. Amand WB: Avian anesthesia, in Kirk RW (ed): *Current Veterinary Therapy VI.* Philadelphia, WB Saunders Co, 1977, pp 705-710.
5. Gandal CP: Surgical techniques and anesthesia, in Petrak ML (ed): *Diseases of Cage and Aviary Birds.* Philadelphia, Lea & Febiger, 1969, pp 217-222.
6. Graham-Jones D: Restraint and anesthesia of small cage birds. *J Small Anim Pract* 6(1):31-39, 1965.
7. Arnall R: Anesthesia and surgery in cage and aviary birds (I). *Vet Rec* 73(7):139-142, 1961.
8. Friedburg KM: Anesthesia of parakeets and canaries. *JAVMA* 141(10):1157-1160, 1962.
9. Kittle EL: Ketamine HCl as an anesthetic for birds. *Mod Vet Pract* 52(11):40-41, 1971.
10. Mandelker L: Ketamine HCl as an anesthetic for parakeets. *VM SAC* 76(1):55-56, 1972.
11. Booth NH: Nonnarcotic analgesics, in Jones LM, Booth NH, McDonald LE (eds): *Veterinary Pharmacology and Therapeutics,* ed 4. Ames, The Iowa State University Press, 1977, p 367.

(continues on page 143)

Raptor Rehabilitation in the Private Veterinary Hospital

Terry W. Campbell, DVM, PhD
Sea World of Florida, Inc.
Orlando, Florida

Veterinarians in private practice are frequently presented with sick or injured wildlife, and many of these animals are raptors. Most veterinary hospitals involved in raptor rehabilitation provide intensive and short-term convalescent care, whereas long-term convalescent care is provided by licensed rehabilitators.

In general, birds considered to be raptors are the caracara, condor, eagle (Figure 1), falcon (Figure 2), harrier, hawk, kite, osprey (Figure 3), owl (Figures 4 and 5), and vulture. Many field guides that aid in identifying raptors are available to individuals who are not familiar with the various species of raptors.

Legal protection for raptors is provided by a number of federal statutes, specifically by the Migratory Bird Treaty Act of 1918, the Bald Eagle Protection Act of 1940, and the Endangered Species Act of 1973. Individual states may also have other laws and regulations that further protect birds of prey. Because of these laws, anyone involved in raptor rehabilitation must obtain the proper permits to satisfy legal requirements that support such activities. The appropriate state wildlife agency and the U.S. Fish and Wildlife Service's special agent in charge of the region should be contacted before any raptor rehabilitation activity is begun. It usually takes at least 90 days to obtain a permit. It may be possible for veterinarians and veterinary technicians to care for raptors under the permit of a licensed wildlife rehabilitator who presents the raptor patient for medical treatment.

General Considerations

With a few minor modifications and additions, most veterinary hospitals involved in the care of small domestic mammals are properly equipped to provide medical, surgical, and short-term convalescent care to raptors. Most veterinary facilities do not, however, have the proper facilities (i.e., flight cages) for long-term convalescence. Special considerations related to provision of medical and surgical care for raptors include proper housing, intensive care facilities, diet, and surgical equipment.

The standard stainless steel hospital cages used for dogs and cats can be used for critical and short-term convalescent care for raptors. Cages should be easy to clean. Bird droppings, especially the urate portion, can be difficult to clean from cages (especially cage bars). Therefore, constant attention to cage cleaning is required to prevent accumulation of feces. Newspapers are routinely used to line cage floors. Routine hospital disinfectants (e.g., quaternary ammonium compounds and phenols) can be used to clean cages as long as these chemicals are thoroughly rinsed from the cages before reintroduction of a bird.

Heavy tree branches are often used as perches for most raptors; however, flat perches are required for some species, such as falcons. It is recommended that perches be padded to reduce foot injury. Perches can be padded in several ways. One common method involves wrapping perches with a single layer of sisal rope. Perches should be kept

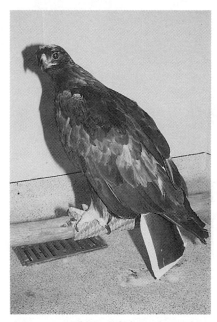

Figure 1—A golden eagle housed in a short-term convalescent facility that is easy to clean. The perch is wrapped with sisal rope to protect the feet, and the tail feathers are protected by a tail sheath.

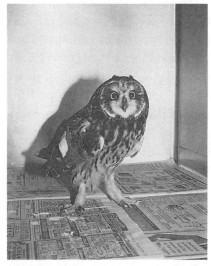

Figure 4—A short-eared owl is treated with a figure-of-eight bandage to support a radial and ulnar fracture. The ulna was repaired using intramedullary pinning.

clean at all times. The perch should be easily accessible to an injured bird but be high enough that the tail feathers do not touch the cage floor as the bird perches. The captive environment of a convalescing raptor should provide a photoperiod that closely matches that of the natural day length. Protected outdoor facili-

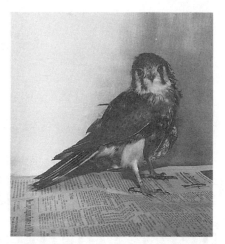

Figure 2—A kestrel with a coracoid fracture exhibits a drooping wing. No palpable fractures involving the bones in the wing were found. A radiograph confirmed the suspected coracoid fracture.

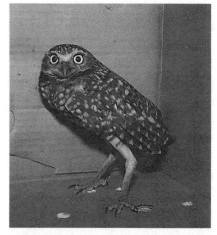

Figure 5—A burrowing owl is provided with a hiding place to ease the stress of captivity.

ties are ideal for birds that do not require intensive care. The captive environment should be as quiet as possible. It is advisable to keep raptors away from noise and activities of domestic animals and the hospital staff. Adequate ventilation also should be provided. Cages should ideally be placed in open areas or in rooms with 10 to 15 air changes per hour.

The size of an intensive care unit for raptors should be adequate for birds as small as screech owls and as large (if not larger) than bald eagles. The intensive care unit should be equipped to provide additional

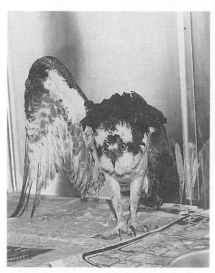

Figure 3—An osprey demonstrating the typical posture of raptors with luxations of the elbow. Luxations and fractures involving joints are associated with a poor prognosis for release of the raptor.

heat, humidity, and oxygen to critically ill raptors. Various intensive care units used in small animal medicine could also be used for raptors.

Equipment

Heavy gloves and netting are helpful in handling raptors. Gloves used by welders are commonly used to handle raptors.

Additional surgical equipment may be necessary because most raptor patients require surgical intervention. Small, delicate surgical instruments are recommended for use in raptors, especially the smaller species. Bipolar cautery is helpful in controlling hemorrhage from small vessels. For orthopedic surgery, Kirschner-Ehmer fixators, plastic rods for use as intramedullary pins, and material to create lightweight connecting bars for Kirschner-Ehmer fixators (i.e., cast material or epoxy) should be available.

Isoflurane is the anesthetic of choice for raptors. A nonrebreathing system should be used.

Small mammals and birds are the

TABLE I
Suggested Food Requirements for
Commonly Seen Raptors Fed a Diet of Mice

Species	Average Body Weight (kg)	Daily Food Intake (g/kg)
Bald eagles	4.0	68
Hawks (red-tailed, Swainson's, rough-legged)	1.0–1.5	42–55
Peregrine falcons	0.7	89
American kestrels	0.1	139
Owls (great horned, snowy, barred)	0.7–1.8	40–58
Small owls (short-eared, screech, saw-whet)	0.1–0.4	114–135

mainstay of the diet fed to most captive raptors. Natural whole food diets are best. Almost all food is stored frozen and thawed as needed. Accipiters are usually fed quail (coturnix or bobwhite) or mice. Eagles, hawks, harriers, and vultures are fed mice, rats, chickens, quail, and rabbits. Falcons can be fed quail or mice. Osprey are fed fish. Frozen fish diets require supplementation with thiamine. Table I lists the food requirements for maintaining commonly treated raptors.

Most raptors can be maintained in captivity without drinking water, as the oxidative water in the prey provides an adequate water supply. Fresh water is, however, usually provided to sick or injured birds during convalescence as well as to owls. Great horned owls require small amounts of water each day to compensate for evaporative water loss; the amount of water given depends primarily on environmental temperature.

Supportive Care

Supportive care considerations for raptors in short-term convalescence include proper attention to foot care, prevention of feather damage, and treatment for parasites.

Foot Care

Attention to foot care is directed toward preventing plantar pododermatitis (or bumblefoot). Padding perches, blunting the tips of talons, wrapping the feet, and providing an adequate diet and environment aid in preventing pododermatitis.

Feather Care

The goal of feather care during captivity is to prevent feather damage (especially to flight and tail feathers) that would delay the return of the raptor to the wild. Measures that help prevent feather damage include applying tail wraps, preventing excitable birds from clinging to cage bars, and proper handling of birds. Excitable birds should be placed in quiet areas where they are not likely to be disturbed by humans. Providing a hiding place in the cage or partially covering the cage may help calm excitable birds. Tail wraps are usually made from waterproof materials, such as used radiographic film. The film is folded into an envelope and slipped over the tail feathers to form a shield. The wrap is attached to the base of the feathers with tape that contains a small amount of adhesive (leaving adhesive on the tail feathers after the tape has been re-moved is undesirable).

Raptors often are presented with broken flight and tail feathers. Many damaged feathers result in the bird being unable to fly properly, and the convalescent period is greatly extended if the bird is forced to rely on molting to replace the broken feathers. A procedure known as imping can be used to repair broken feathers. In essence, the procedure involves replacing the missing section of feather with a portion of a molted feather or feather removed from a dead bird. The feather should be from the same or a related species. The feather is cut and fitted to repair the broken feather at the appropriate length. The broken end of the damaged feather and the replacement feather are trimmed to create a tight union. A lightweight wooden or plastic splinter tapered at both ends is inserted into the feather shafts of both the damaged feather and the replacement feather and glued in place to create a stable union, resulting in a feather with normal function.

Cyanoacrylate glue or epoxy work well for this procedure. If done properly, a repaired feather should be as strong and function as well as a normal feather. Sophisticated rehabilitators keep feather banks comprising feathers labeled according to feather type (i.e., flight or tail feather), feather position or number (e.g., left primary flight feather number one), species of bird, and age of bird (i.e., adult or juvenile). The number of birds requiring this procedure is generally small each year; thus, using feathers from other related species that closely match the damaged feathers works as well as matching the exact feather obtained from the same species.

Parasite Treatment

Raptors are often presented with various endoparasites and ectoparasites. Lice and mites are commonly found on raptors presented for medical treatment. Most of the ectoparasites are easily removed by dusting the birds with a 5% to 7% carbaryl powder.

Fecal examinations may reveal various parasite ova. It may be difficult to discern from the examination whether the parasite ova have originated from ingested prey or if the raptor is actually infested with parasites. Therefore, serial fecal examinations for detection of persistent parasite ova may suggest true parasitism, or the birds could be treated with antiparasitics as a routine procedure. Commonly used antiparasitics include fenbendazole, ivermectin, levamisole, mebendazole, niclosamide, and praziquantel.

Common Disorders

The common disorders of raptors presented for veterinary care include traumatic injury, aspergillosis, trichomoniasis, pododermatitis, pox, bacterial infection, and lead poisoning. Most birds presented to veterinary hospitals are victims of traumatic injury that has caused fractures of one or more bones. Humeral fractures are usually repaired with intramedullary pins and cerclage wires to hold fragments together. A figure-of-eight bandage applied to the wing is used to add further stability during the initial two weeks of convalescence.

Internal fixation is not usually required in fractures involving the antebrachium if only one of the bones (radius or ulna) is fractured. In such cases, the wing is stabilized with a figure-of-eight bandage and the unfractured bone acts as an internal splint for the fractured bone. If both bones are fractured, then fixation of the ulna and sometimes the radius is required. The ulna can be stabilized with a shuttle pin created from a sterile polypropylene plastic rod, a Kirschner-Ehmer fixator, or a bone plate (for large birds). Plastic shuttle pins are stabilized using small Kirschner wires with or without external stabilization or bone cement. A Kirschner-Ehmer apparatus is usually modified to provide a lighter weight appliance for small birds by replacing the heavy metal external clamps and screws with lighter casting material or tubes filled with epoxy. The affected wing should be stabilized by a figure-of-eight bandage with any fracture of the antebrachium for the initial two weeks of convalescence.

Fractures distal to the antebrachium usually require stabilization of the wing using a figure-of-eight bandage for at least two weeks. Use of a figure-of-eight bandage for longer than two weeks may, however, diminish the range of motion of the joints in the wing. Articular fractures and luxations or fractures near joints usually result in loss of normal function to the affected limb and are associated with a poor prognosis for complete rehabilitation.

Birds with fractures of the pectoral girdle usually present with clinical signs of wing drooping and no palpable fractures involving the bones of the wing. In such cases, radiographs often reveal a fracture of the coracoid, scapula, or furculum.

Coracoid fractures are the most common fracture in the pectoral girdle and usually do not require surgical management unless the fragments are greatly displaced. Most uncomplicated coracoid fractures are managed by immobilization of the affected pectoral girdle using a figure-of-eight bandage to the wing and taping the wing to the body.

Femoral fractures are usually repaired using intramedullary pins, Kirschner-Ehmer fixators, or bone plates. Fractures of the tibiotarsus are repaired using intramedullary pins or Kirschner-Ehmer fixators. A Schroeder-Thomas splint can provide additional support to the leg with a tibiotarsal fracture. Most fractures in raptors develop a solid fibrous callus within two weeks if there is effective stability and fixation.

Aspergillosis most commonly occurs in raptors held in captivity for an extended period and is rarely seen in newly acquired birds. Conditions that predispose raptors to this disease include immunosuppression, malnutrition, and unhygienic environmental conditions. Immunosuppression can result from stress, malnutrition, preexisting disease, or prolonged use of antibiotics or corticosteroids. Aspergillosis is primarily a disease of the lower respiratory tract, and an antemortem diagnosis can be difficult to obtain.

Clinical signs of aspergillosis vary; however, emaciation, lethargy, and dyspnea are common. The hemogram often reveals leukocytosis, heterophilia, monocytosis, and lymphopenia. Radiographic detection is often disappointing; however, serodiagnosis may provide a reliable diagnosis for this disease in some species. Golden eagles, goshawks, and gyrfalcons have temperaments that predispose them to the stress of captivity. Therefore, providing an environment that minimizes stress and oral administration of an antifungal medication, such as 5-fluorocytosine (50 mg/kg twice daily) are

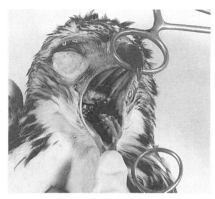

Figure 6—A red-tailed hawk shows multiple raised lesions and ulcerations in the oral cavity. The usual ruleouts include bacterial abscess formation, trichomoniasis, candidiasis, hypovitaminosis A, and possibly avian pox.

recommended during the initial two-week adaptation period for species known to be highly susceptible to aspergillosis. Successful treatment of chronic aspergillosis with antifungal medication can be difficult; therefore, emphasis should be placed on disease prevention.

The clinical signs of trichomoniasis include chronic weight loss, regurgitation, and oral ulceration (Figure 6). The diagnosis is made by visualization of piriform flagellate protozoa with anterior flagella and an undulating membrane in samples obtained from the upper alimentary tract. Treatment involves the use of parasiticides for flagellate protozoa, such as metronidazole and ipronidazole.

Plantar pododermatitis is a common disorder of captive raptors. Predisposing conditions for the disease include trauma to the plantar surface of the feet (usually puncture wounds made by the bird's own talons), malnutrition, and unhygienic environmental conditions. Treatment can be lengthy, depending on severity of the condition. Pododermatitis is generally treated using surgical debridement in addition to topical treatment with antimicrobial agents.

A ball bandage placed on the feet provides support for the foot and holds the medication in place. A window cut in the ball bandage allows easy access for daily treatment.

Raptors are occasionally presented with pox lesions, which appear as raised, crusty lesions on the head or feet. A definitive diagnosis can be made by the presence of pox inclusions on cytologic or histologic specimens. Cytologic confirmation of avian pox is provided by the presence of squamous epithelial cells that contain large cytoplasmic vacuoles. These vacuoles contain the pox viruses, which appear as small, pale eosinophilic inclusions in smears prepared with Wright's stain and an oil immersion objective. Treatment of avian pox is nonspecific and supportive and is designed to prevent secondary bacterial or mycotic infections.

Lead poisoning in raptors usually results from ingested lead obtained from prey containing lead particles, such as lead shot. The clinical signs vary, but raptors often present with generalized weakness, anorexia, or seizure disorders. Clinical suspicion of lead poisoning can be supported radiographically by the appearance of metallic densities in the ventriculus. The hemogram may show an inappropriate release of immature erythrocytes in a bird that is not anemic. Stippled basophilia may occur but is extremely rare. Levels of lead in the blood provide a definitive diagnosis; values greater than 60 µg/dl are considered significantly elevated. Treatment for lead poisoning may require surgical removal of lead particles from the gastrointestinal tract and chelation therapy. Intramuscular injections of calcium ethylenediaminetetraacetic acid (EDTA) should be given until clinical signs no longer recur after therapy is stopped.

Conclusion

Raptor rehabilitation can be a gratifying activity for the veterinary staff in private practice. Although there is often no financial compensation for practices that participate in wildlife rehabilitation, it has a positive effect on hospital public relations. The rewards obtained by helping animals that have no primary care giver to pay their medical bills often surpass the relatively small financial losses of the veterinary hospital.

BIBLIOGRAPHY

Campbell TW: Mycotic diseases, in Harrison GJ, Harrison LR (eds): *Clinical Avian Medicine and Surgery.* Philadelphia, WB Saunders Co, 1986, pp 464–471.

Campbell TW, Campbell LV: Physical restraint of exotic patients. *Vet Tech* 12(1):56–63, 1991.

Duke GE: Raptor physiology, in Fowler ME (ed): *Zoo and Wild Animal Medicine,* ed 2. Philadelphia, WB Saunders Co, 1986, pp 370–376.

Harrison GJ: Disorders of the integument, in Harrison GJ, Harrison LR (eds): *Clinical Avian Medicine and Surgery.* Philadelphia, WB Saunders Co, 1986, pp 509–524.

Knopf AA: *The Audubon Society Field Guide to North American Birds: Eastern Region.* New York, Chanticleer Press, 1977.

Peterson RT: *A Field Guide to the Birds.* Boston, Houghton Mifflin Co, 1980.

Redig PT: A clinical review of orthopedic techniques used in the rehabilitation of raptors, in Fowler ME (ed): *Zoo and Wild Animal Medicine,* ed 2. Philadelphia, WB Saunders Co, 1986, pp 388–401.

Redig PT: Mycotic infections of birds of prey, in Fowler ME (ed): *Zoo and Wild Animal Medicine,* ed 2. Philadelphia, WB Saunders Co, 1986, pp 420–425.

Redig PT: Basic orthopedic surgical techniques, in Harrison GJ, Harrison LR (eds): *Clinical Avian Medicine and Surgery.* Philadelphia, WB Saunders Co, 1986, pp 596–598.

Udvardy MDF: *The Audubon Society Field Guide to North American Birds: Western Region.* New York, Chanticleer Press, 1977.

Basic Avian Hematology: Techniques of Collection, Preparation, and Identification

Jennifer L. Jenkins, LVT
Sedgwick County Zoo and
Botanical Garden
Wichita, Kansas

Differential evaluation in avian hematology is becoming a necessary diagnostic procedure in exotic practices. The ability of a technician to evaluate these parameters properly benefits both the practice and the veterinarian. This article

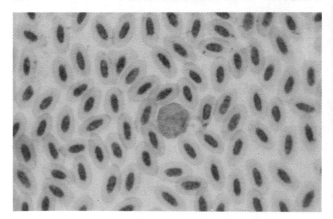

presents the basics of avian hematology so that technicians can assist practitioners in

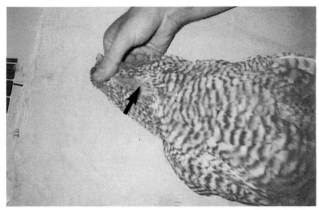

Figure 1—The jugular vein (*arrow*) is useful to collect large volumes of blood.

the differential diagnosis of avian patients.

Methods of Blood Collection

The medial metatarsal, the jugular vein, and the cutaneous ulnar are the three major sites of avian blood collection. The technician's decision of the site to use often depends on the amount of blood needed for evaluation and the amount of restraint necessary for successful collection.

The jugular vein (Figure 1) is a vein from which large samples of blood can be collected. This vein is located next to the cervical vertebra in a featherless furrow. One person can collect blood from this site without requiring assistance in restraining the patient. The jugular vein is an effective collection site in smaller birds. The disadvantages of using the jugular vein is that the right vein is often larger than the left and in some species the left jugular vein is often absent[1]; therefore, if the vein is lacerated and a hematoma forms, it is difficult to make another attempt at collection. Another disadvantage is that the vessel is very difficult to stabilize.

The cutaneous ulnar (Figure 2), or wing vein, is located over the ventral surface of the humeral or radial ulnar joint (i.e., the elbow). This vein is located transversely to the joint[1]; the cutaneous ulnar is very accessible, and collecting blood from this site is uncomplicated. In preparation, some feathers may need to be plucked and alcohol is applied to make the vein more visible. This site also has disadvantages. Hematomas form easily because the wing is difficult to stabilize in this position. Because this posture is abnormal for the patient, it requires firm restraint. For larger birds, two people may be necessary to restrain the bird in addition to the technician collecting the blood. If the wing moves, the vein is easily lacerated, thus forming a hematoma. To prevent this occurrence, a dry cotton ball should be placed on the site immediately after the needle

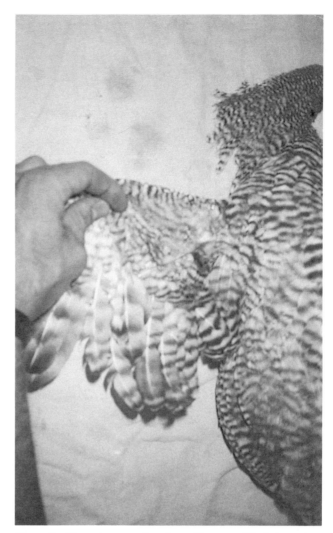

Figure 2—The cutaneous ulnar is readily accessible but requires firm restraint during blood collection.

has been removed. Pressure should be applied until the bleeding stops.

The medial metatarsal vein (Figure 3) is the preferred site for blood collection in larger birds. In most cases, the vein is visible unless the skin has dark pigmentation. Because the vein is surrounded by a muscle mass, hematomas do not readily occur. The leg is also easy to stabilize.[2] One disadvantage is that it is difficult to obtain blood from this site in small birds.

Other methods of blood collection exist, but they are only used to obtain small amounts of blood. One such method is by toenail clipping. Although the vessel in the toes is easily accessible, there are many disadvantages to this method. The blood does not flow freely, and the toe must be milked to obtain an adequate sample. The milking process often results in contamination of the blood.[3] Poor circulation, resulting in small samples, is another disad-

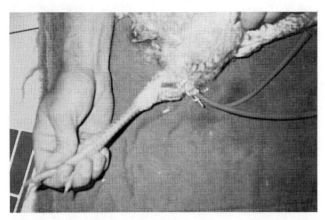

Figure 3—The medial metatarsal cannot be used in small birds but is a useful collection site in large birds because the chance of hematoma is minimized.

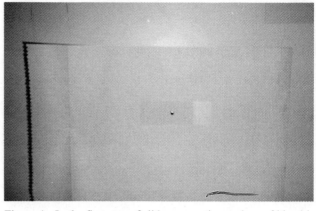

Figure 4—In the first step of slide preparation, a drop of blood is placed in the center of a slide.

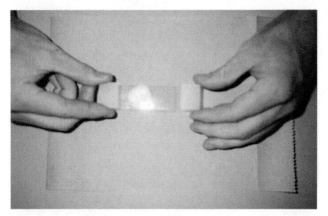

Figure 5—In the second step, another slide or large coverslip is placed directly on the blood and drawn away from the slide using an even motion.

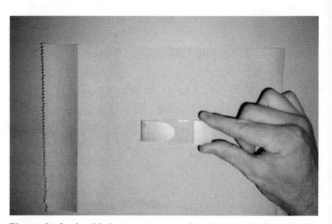

Figure 6—In the third step, a tongue-shaped smear is formed; the cells in the center of the smear are evaluated.

vantage. This procedure is also very painful to the patient and may not please the client.

Another method is skin pricking. The skin must be very clean for this procedure, and it can only be used for small amounts of blood. As a result, this method, which is used commonly during Pullorum testing in chicken, is not used often clinically.[4]

Cardiac puncture is the least desirable collection technique. Although large amounts of blood can be obtained very quickly, cardiac puncture is undesirable because it is very dangerous to the patient.[6]

Techniques of Blood Collection

A very steady hand is essential for blood collection. A 25-gauge or larger needle should be used because the blood cells are hemolyzed through smaller needles.[5] The syringe may need to be heparinized before collection because an inadequate blood flow may result in clotting before the entire sample is obtained. The heparin may inter-

fere with staining and cause the cells to pool on the slide; however, heparin remains the anticoagulant of choice. Ethylenediaminetetraacetic acid (EDTA) is not considered to be an ideal anticoagulant because it may cause the cells of some species to stain unusually dark.[5]

Slide Preparation

Preparing a slide of avian blood for evaluation is different from preparing a slide of mammalian blood. A 30° angle smearing technique is often used to prepare mammalian blood; however, in birds, this technique often distorts the blood cells. When the cells are smudged, the different types cannot be distinguished and the results of the testing may be altered.

The recommended procedure is a slide-to-slide or slide-to-coverslip method. To begin, a drop of blood is placed in the center of the slide (Figure 4). Either a long coverslip or another slide is placed on top of the drop of blood (Figure 5). The coverslip or slide that is on the top is then pulled away from the bottom slide using an even motion. The technician must be careful not to lift up on the coverslip or slide. The cells in the center of the slide are then evaluated (Figure 6), unlike evaluating near the feathered edge of the blood on the slide as is done in the 30° smearing technique.[3]

Staining

When staining the smears, Wright's or Wright's-Giemsa stains are preferred because stain quality is greater than it is with quick-stain methods. Quick-stain methods do not always stain the granules found in heterophils and basophils and may distort the blood cells. The most preferred method currently used by veterinary technicians in staining avian blood cells is the May Grünwald stain. This method produces very good results and has clarity in cell differentiation.[9]

Smear Evaluation

Differential evaluation begins when the staining is complete. Differentiating between avian heterophils and eosinophils (Figures 7 and 8) is the most difficult aspect of avian hematology because the heterophils and eosinophils are similar in color and nearly the same size. The size of the heterophils and eosinophils also varies among species of birds and among birds of the same species. The difference between the two types of cells can be determined by the shape. Most sources report that heterophils have rod-shaped granules and eosinophils have round granules; however, this is not true for all species of birds (in owls, for example, the granules of eosinophils are rod shaped and those of heterophils are round). The technician should predetermine the difference in the shape of the heterophils and eosinophils for the particular species being examined and scan the entire slide for both types of cells to ensure proper evaluation. The nucleus of both types of cells generally tends to stain the same color; staining therefore is not a reliable method of differentiating between these two types of cells.[2] A good rule of thumb to differentiate between the heterophil and eosinophil is that eosinophils will generally have a cytoplasm that stains blue.

Avian thrombocytes often appear similar to mature lymphocytes. Thrombocytes have a large nucleus and very little cytoplasm; the cytoplasm stains faint blue. The nucleus stains dark and a chromatin pattern often is not evident. A distinct feature of the cytoplasm of a thrombocyte is dark pigmented granules; only a few granules are present in the cytoplasm. Again, it is best to scan the entire slide for the species differences.

When mature, lymphocytes (Figure 9) have an eccentric nucleus and a small amount of cytoplasm. Lymphocytes are delicate and tend to smudge. The pigment of the cytoplasm stains a darker blue than does the cytoplasm of the thrombocytes. Lymphocytes contain more granules than do thrombocytes; when mature, lymphocytes are larger than thrombocytes. Less mature avian lymphocytes resemble avian monocytes.[2] The chromatin pattern in the nucleus of lymphocytes is more clumped than is the pattern in monocytes. If compared with monocytes, the cytoplasm of lymphocytes stains lavender and lymphocytes have a less distinct cell border. Lymphocytes are smaller than monocytes.

Monocytes of birds (Figure 10) resemble those of mammals. Avian monocytes have a lacy chromatin pattern. The cytoplasm stains a battleship gray color[6] and often contains vacuoles.

Basophils (Figure 11) are much more common in avian blood than they are in mammalian blood. Avian basophils stain distinctly and are relatively easy to identify. These cells, which stain dark, may superficially be mistaken for smudged cells; however, on closer examination, dark granules can be distinguished and may often appear so heavily in the cell that the nucleus may be indistinguishable. As the cell degenerates, the number of granules may diminish but present granules remain a dark, distinct blue.[1]

A unique feature of avian erythrocytes is that they contain a nucleus; mammalian erythrocytes do not. The nucleus stains an intense blue-purple; the chromatin pattern is dense when the erythrocyte is mature. The nucleus is oval shaped. The cytoplasm, which stains red-orange, contrasts with the nucleus. Immature erythrocytes have a round nucleus and bluish cytoplasm. The amount of cytoplasm in an erythrocyte diminishes as it matures. The technician must be sure not to confuse erythrocytes with monocytes; the chromatin pattern is the distinguishing feature.[7]

The two main methods of deriving total white blood cell counts is by using Natt and Herrick's solution and the eosinophil stain from the Eosinophil Unopette® 5877 System (Becton—Dickinson). Each method has advantages and disadvantages. One advantage of using a Natt and Herrick's solution is that the technician can do both the erythrocyte and leukocyte count in the same chamber. A 1:100 dilution is prepared using a 20 µl pipette with well mixed blood and added to 1,980 µl of Natt and Herrick's solution. Load the hemocytometer after discarding a few drops of solution. Allow the solution to stand at least 5 minutes before counting. This allows the cells to settle and the leukocytes to stain.[8]

For total RBC (red blood cell) count, the center 1 mm square is divided into 25 squares. Count the four corner squares and the center square as you would a mammalian

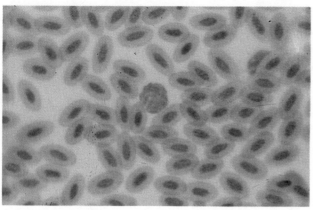

Figure 7—Heterophils of a blue and gold macaw; the granules resemble those of eosinophils.

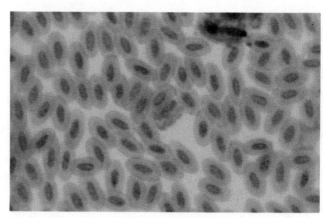

Figure 8—Eosinophils of the same bird in Figure 7; the shape of the granules varies among avian species.

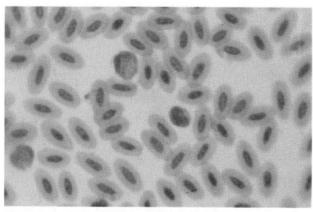

Figure 9—Avian lymphocytes (center right); the amount of cytoplasm is limited.

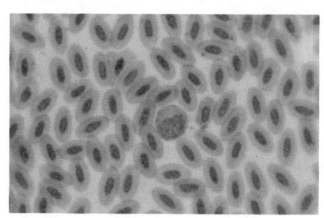

Figure 10—Avian monocytes; the cytoplasm is battleship gray in color.

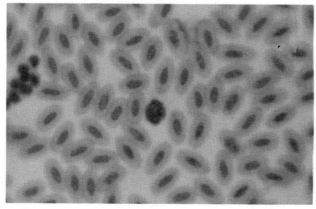

Figure 11—A cluster of avian thrombocytes (left) and a basophil (center); basophils are much more common in birds than they are in mammals.

RBC count. The calculation for RBCs is as follows:

$$\text{\# of RBCs} \times 5000 = \text{Total RBC count}[8]$$

If Natt and Herrick's solution is not available, an alterna-

tive source to count avian RBCs is by using the Unopette® test no. 5850. Follow the manufacturer's instructions to obtain a count. The erythrocytes are difficult to see using this method.

Natt and Herrick's solution stains all white cells; the solution also stains thrombocytes, which makes counting more difficult. The eosinophil stain only stains cells that contain granules; thus, heterophils and eosinophils are the only cells that can be evaluated by this method.

Both methods use a hemocytometer. Automatic cell counters, such as the Coulter Counter, count both red and white blood cells and therefore cannot be used. For the purpose of avian hematology, only heterophils and eosinophils are necessary to be counted.

The Natt and Herrick's method uses a 1:100 diluting pipette. The stain is mixed thoroughly in the blood. Each side of the hemocytometer is charged and covered and should stand for five minutes to allow proper absorption of the stain throughout the cells. All nine squares on both sides of the hemocytometer are counted by using the fol-

(continues on page 135)

Sexing of Caged Birds

Monica M. Tighe, RVT
Veterinary Technician Program
St. Clair College
Windsor, Ontario, Canada

Because of an increasing demand for pet birds, true or breeding pairs have become a popular commodity in aviculture. Accurate knowledge of a bird's sex can be important for increased sale prices and for health reasons. Hormonal problems and even neoplastic diseases occur more often in a certain sex. If an anxious client calls and gives a description of an egg-bound bird, determining the patient's sex will obviously help rule the condition in or out. Owners often are confused or mistaken about the sex of their birds. Knowledge of sexing techniques thus can be helpful to veterinary technicians from a medical standpoint and can play a role in client education.

In the past 20 years, sex determination techniques in avian medicine have progressed. Traditional methods—such as observation (i.e., nest box behavior), color or physical differences, and surgical sexing of monomorphic species (those in which males and females have no outward physical differences)—are still being used. The noninvasive method of DNA testing has, in recent years, become more common.

General Guidelines

The following methods for sexing common pet birds are intended as guidelines. There are exceptions to every rule, and young birds are difficult to sex. In general, the head and beak are larger in male birds. Many experienced handlers believe that females bite harder and more frequently.

Finches

Finches range in weight from 10 to 35 g. A breeder of finches might be able to distinguish between sexes by their song or behavior in the nest; however, color differences are the easiest method of sex determination. Some common dimorphic passerine birds are zebra, cut-throat, melba, cordon blue, gouldian, owl, star, and twin-spots finches. Common monomorphic finches include Bengalese or society, diamond sparrow, Java rice bird, black-headed nun or munia, bronze-winged mannikin, African silverbill, and spice finches. Some finches not listed in these groups have very subtle color differences or seasonal color changes. The male generally is more colorful than the drab-looking hen in dimorphic species.

Canaries

Canaries range in weight from 20 to 30 g. A mature, breeding male canary is one of the best singing birds; occasionally females also will sing. A mature male has some physical differences that experienced aviculturists can recognize. The breeding male has a vent that protrudes slightly when he is held on his back. The breeding female canary's vent is enlarged but does not extend as far as the male's.[1]

Budgerigars

Budgerigars range in weight from 30 to 35 g. Like other birds, immature budgies are hard to sex. The dark-colored bars on the forehead, which begin close to the cere, denote a bird less than four months of age. When the bird is mature, the bars recede to the top of the head. A young male budgie has a pink or bluish cere; the young female tends to have a very pale or almost white cere. A mature male's cere is bright blue. Some breeders say male budgies have nostrils that are larger or differently shaped than those of females. An adult female has a brown cere. Male budgies often have bluish gray feet; female budgies have pinkish feet. The exceptions to the rule are pied, albino, and lutino male budgies. These colored males never develop blue ceres, instead remaining pale pink or mauve. Pied, albino, and lutino females retain brown ceres at maturity (Figures 1 and 2).

Cockatiels

Cockatiels range in weight from 80 to 100 g. All young cockatiels look like females, but at the time of the first molt (approximately six months of age) the head feathers change to their true colors first. Generally, the cheek patches are brighter orange and the face is more yellow in adult male cockatiels than in females. Females over the age of one year can easily be differentiated by their distinctive wing and tail feathers, which have spots and bars. Male pied cockatiels do not always develop yellow faces except where there are spots; the head color therefore will not distinguish the sex of a pied male cockatiel—it is necessary to look at the wings and the tail. In lutino and pied female cockatiels, the lines and spots can barely be seen; a close check of the wing feathers with a strong light source should reveal these markings (Figure 3). Female pearl cockatiels have faint bars on the tail feathers; males do not.

Cockatoos

Cockatoos range in weight from 300 to 800 g. Males are generally larger. Mature female cockatoos usually have red-brown irises, and males have black-brown irises. The exceptions to this rule are immature birds, some Moluccan or salmon-crested cockatoos, and the slender-billed cockatoo. These birds are difficult to sex accurately by this method. Immature cockatoos generally have dark irises. Some species, however, such as the Giang-gang cockatoo, have obvious dimorphic coloration (Figure 4).

African Grays

African Grays range in weight from 350 to 500 g. They are among the best talking birds. It has been reported that

the feathers surrounding the vent can be more red in males.[2,3] Males are believed to have upper tail coverts (the dorsal feathers situated between the cranial gray rump feathers and the red tail feathers) that are solid red; females

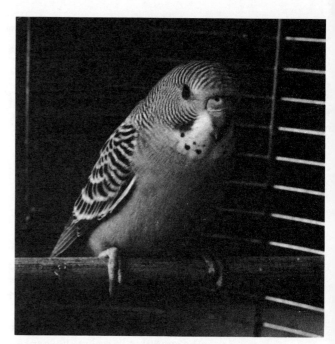

Figure 2—A 10-week-old budgie; note the bars on the forehead.

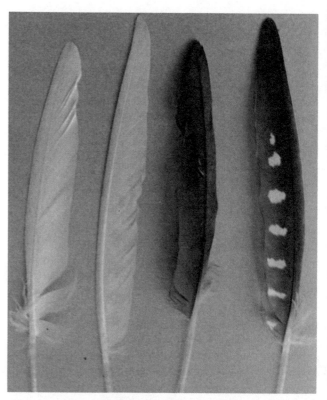

Figure 3—Cockatiel wing feathers. *Left to right*: lutino male, lutino female, normal male, and normal female.

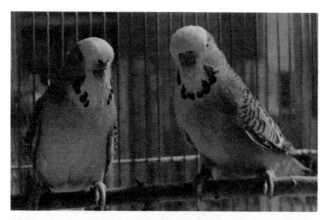

Figure 1—Two budgies. *Left*, female with brown-blue cere and pink feet; *right*, male with blue cere and gray feet.

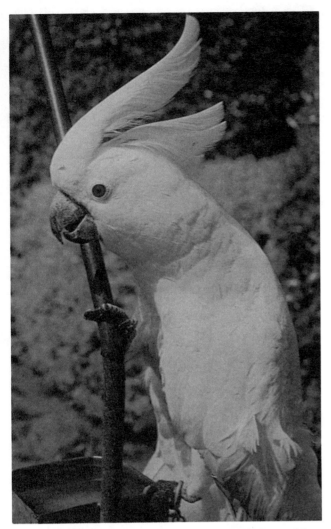

Figure 4—Sulfur-crested cockatoo female; note the brown iris.

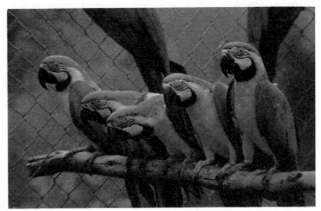

Figure 5—Blue and gold macaws with no visible differences.

can have gray borders on their coverts.[2] All of the coloration differences are recent findings and remain to be proven.

Because many larger parrots are bought after having been surgically sexed, it is advisable to check for tattoos. Alcohol can be used to part the feathers for a better look. If the bird is a female, there should be an *F* or an ink mark in the left wing webbing. If the bird is a male, there should be an *M* or an ink mark in the right wing webbing.

Almost without exception, amazons, macaws, toucans, conures, lovebirds, and grass parakeets, are monomorphic.

Laparoscopy or Surgical Sexing

Surgical sexing is a method of sex determination and a procedure used to determine the breeding condition and gonadal size of birds. Most aviculturists agree that laparoscopy is the most accurate and rapid method for sexing birds. The risk is minimal if performed by an experienced avian clinician.

Instruments used in examining the ovary or the testicle include endoscopes, laparoscopes, and otoscopes. The laparoscope consists of a trocar, a cannula, a fiber-optic cable, and a fiber-optic scope. The trocar is used to penetrate the body wall and often the air sacs. The cannula acts as a hollow sleeve or guide; after penetration, the trocar is removed from the cannula and the eyepiece is inserted. The tungsten-halogen light source makes this the preferred instrument for surgical sexing.[5,6] The difference between the laparoscope and the endoscope is that the endoscope is flexible. Veterinarians who do not have these instruments sometimes sex birds using an otoscope with the appropriate-size speculum attached[7] (generally a 700-g bird requires a size 7 to 8 speculum and a 300-g bird requires a size 4 to 5 speculum). This arrangement works well in most cases.

A patient to be surgically sexed is weighed and examined carefully. Birds often are fasted for two to four hours before surgery so that the crop is empty.[5] Anesthesia usually consists of 30 to 40 mg/kg of ketamine hydrochloride combined with 0.5 to 1.5 mg/kg of xylazine hydrochloride, injected by 27-gauge needle into the breast muscle. Isoflurane gas also is becoming popular as a sole anesthetic for surgical sexing; however, halothane is still more common and frequently is given after ketamine hydrochloride and xylazine hydrochloride. The technician's role in monitoring the patient is invaluable. A light plane of anesthesia is best for this procedure because the bird's recovery time should be minimized.

Because only the left ovary is present in female birds, patients are positioned in right lateral recumbency. Although the bird is usually taped to the table with wings extended above the back, many clinicians use manual restraint. The left leg is extended caudally while the right leg is positioned craniodorsally (Figure 6). The feathers are plucked from a small triangle cranial to the thigh muscles and caudal to the last rib (just below the back muscles).[6,7] The skin is surgically cleansed. Alcohol is used to wet the feathers surrounding the surgical site; use of clear plastic drapes is preferred.

A small, 1-cm incision is made in the skin, and blunt

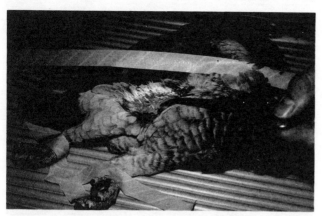

Figure 6—Surgical sexing position and surgical site.

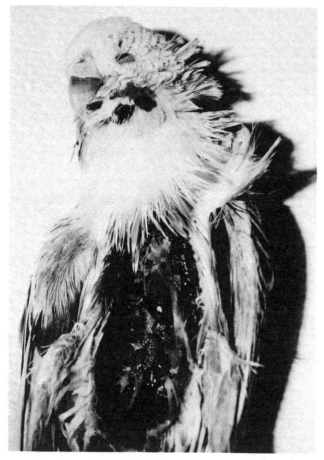

Figure 7—An inactive ovary is visible lying on the corner of the kidney (approximately 1 cm below the heart) of this young female budgie.

dissection is used to gain access to the abdominal cavity. Air sacs might obscure the view (these act as bellows to move air through the lungs; nine separate air sacs are present in most birds).[5] Various methods can be used to puncture the thoracic air sacs; alligator forceps are common. When a clear view of the viscera is achieved, the practitioner looks for the gonad lying cranial to the kidney (Figure 7). The gonad also can be located next to the adrenal gland and caudal to the lungs.

The mature avian ovary appears as a cluster of round follicles. Young birds have ovaries that are cobblestone in appearance.[5] The male has a smooth, oval testicle that usually is white in color. Male cockatoos have pigmented or black testes. Breeding males will have much larger testicles than young or inactive males. While the gonads are being examined, the veterinarian also can evaluate the air sacs, lungs, adrenal glands, spleen, intestines, and liver.[8] The body wall and the skin then can be closed with absorbable suture material and the bird tattooed according to the findings of the veterinarian. The bird is allowed to recover in a warm, padded environment.

DNA Testing

DNA testing can be done only by a cytogeneticist experienced in avian systems. The test can be used to determine the sex of ratite or parrot species. This procedure is used by breeders to determine which chicks are of the correct sex for future breedings. The advantage of DNA testing is it can be done at a young age with a noninvasive procedure.

Either through toenail clipping or venipuncture of the wing or leg vein, 0.05 mL–0.1 mL of unclotted blood is collected in plain capillary tubes or a syringe. The blood is then placed in a vial containing a preservative for rapid transportation to a lab. Sexing results are usually available in approximately 2 weeks.

Along with the determination of sex, "DNA Fingerprinting" can also be performed on the sample of blood. This procedure provides positive identification for the life of the bird in the case of theft. This test can also determine the degree of relationship to other birds of the same species, progeny/parents, or siblings, which is important for outbreeding programs. The results of DNA fingerprinting are available in approximately 6 weeks and involve a step procedure using radioactive substances.

Although the traditional methods for sexing birds have been helpful in the past, there are now testing procedures which provide parrot owners with accurate sex determination techniques.

Acknowledgment
The photographs appear through the courtesy of Louise A. Bauck, DVM, Ontario, Canada, and Yvonne Lane, ACT, RVT, AVI Diagnostics Ltd., Guelph, Ontario, Canada.

REFERENCES
1. Axelson RD: *Caring for Your Pet Bird*. Toronto, Canaviax Publications Ltd, 1981, pp 88–110.
2. Voren H: IME 672 sexual dimorphism in African Gray parrots. *AAV Newsletter* 7(1):26, 1986.
3. Rosskopf WJ: Visual sexing of African Grays. *AAV Newsletter* 6(4):110, 1985.
4. Voren H: IME 671 sexual dimorphism in Amazon parrots. *AAV Newsletter* 7(1):25–26, 1986.
5. McDonald SE: Surgical sexing. *Bird Talk* 40(7):26–32, 1986.
6. Satterfield WC: Diagnostic laparoscopy in birds, in Kirk RW (ed): *Current Veterinary Therapy VII*. Philadelphia, WB Saunders Co, 1980, pp 659–661.
7. Ingram KA: Otoscope technique for sexing birds, in Kirk RW (ed):

Current Veterinary Therapy VII. Philadelphia, WB Saunders Co, 1980, pp 656–658.
8. Satterfield WC: Diagnostic laparoscopy in birds, in Starika WA, Richardson EL (eds): *The T.F.H. Book of Parrots*. New Jersey, T.F.H. Publications Inc, 1982, pp 70–77.
9. Clubb SL: Sex determination techniques, in Harrison GJ, Harrison LR (eds): *Clinical Avian Medicine and Surgery*. Philadelphia, WB Saunders Co, 1986, pp 613–619.
10. Stavy M, Gilbert D, Martin RD, et al: Routine determination of sex in monomorphic bird species using fecal steroid analysis. *Int Zoo Yearbook* 19:209–214, 1979.
11. McDonald S: Inaccuracies in blood (serum) sexing techniques. *AAV Newsletter* 6(4):110, 1985.
12. Takeshita K: Blood feather sexing. *AAV Newsletter* 6(4):109–110, 1985.
13. Halverson J, Dvorak J, Flammer K, et al: A new method of avian sex determination—Identification of the W body by C-bonding of erythrocytes. *Proceedings of the 1985 Annual Meeting of the Association of Avian Veterinarians*. June 4–9, 1985, pp 1–6.

Avian Hematology *(continued from page 130)*

lowing equation:

$$TWBC = (\text{total white blood cells counted in nine squares} + 10\%) \times 100$$

When using the Unopette® method, the differential count is usually performed first to distinguish between the heterophils and eosinophils. The dilution factor is 1:32. Before charging the hemocytometer, the blood should stand in the eosinophil stain for a few minutes. After allowing the blood to stand, the technician charges both sides of the hemocytometer and allows it to stand for five minutes. All nine squares on both sides of the hemocytometer are then counted. The total is calculated by using the following equation:

$$(\text{hemocytometer count} + 10\%) \times 16 = \text{total heterophils and eosinophils}$$

$$\frac{\text{total heterophils/eosinophils}}{\% \text{ heterophils and eosinophils}} \times 100 = \text{total WBC}$$
(from differential)

Variables occur in the evaluation of avian blood as they do in all forms of hematology; however, this information can provide basic guidelines to technicians who are interested in developing a basic knowledge of avian hematology.

REFERENCES

1. Harrison GJ, Harrison LR: *Clinical Avian Medicine and Surgery*. Philadelphia, WB Saunders Co, 1986, pp 175–191.
2. Coles EH: *Veterinary Clinical Pathology*, ed 4. Philadelphia, WB Saunders Co, 1986, p 279–301.
3. Dein FJ: *Laboratory Manual of Avian Hematology*. Northport, NY, Association of Avian Veterinarians, 1984, pp 2–12.
4. *Pullorum Instruction Manual*. Charles City, IA, Salsbury Laboratories, 1989, p 4.
5. Campbell TW, Dein FJ: Avian hematology: The basics. Symposium on caged bird medicine. *Vet Clin North Am [Small Anim Pract]* 14(2):223–232, 1984.
6. Davidson HL: *VM 030 Laboratory Manual for Hematology, Clinical Chemistry, Urinalysis*. East Lansing, MI, Michigan State University, pp H1–H79.
7. Welty JC: *The Life of Birds*, ed 3. Emporia, KS, CBS College Publishing, 1987, p 134.
8. Arnold J: Avian hematology blood cell counting procedures. *Association of Zoo Veterinary Technicians Proceedings*, 1986, pp 1–8.
9. Wilmoth K: *Laboratory Manual of Reptilian Hematology*. Houston Zoo Publications, 1992, pp 3–4.

Bibliography

Campbell TW: *Avian Hematology and Cytology*. Ames, Iowa, Iowa State University Press, 1988.
Hawkey CM, Dennett TB: *Comparative Veterinary Hematology*. Ames, Iowa, Iowa State University Press, 1989.
Dein F: Avian Leucocyte Counting Using the Hemacytometer. *JZWAM*, 1994, in press.

Avian Chlamydiosis: A Public Health Concern

Nick Ashford, DVM
Kildaire Animal Medical Center
Cary, North Carolina

The importance of veterinary medicine lies not only in the prevention and treatment of disease in animals but also in the awareness of potential zoonotic diseases. With the increasing popularity of birds as pets, veterinary staff must be alert to and able to educate their clients about potential avian zoonoses. Chlamydiosisis is an important zoonosis associated with pet birds.

History of the Disease

Chlamydiosis was first described in humans in Europe in 1876. Numerous outbreaks were recorded in the late nineteenth century; the source was purported to be infected parrots from Argentina. The disease was pandemic in 1929 and 1930; there were approximately 1000 reported cases, and the case fatality rate exceeded 20%. During this period, English researchers isolated the causative organism, *Chlamydia psittaci*. After the epidemic, many countries prohibited the importation of psittacine birds from South America.

Commercial importation into the United States was banned by the Department of Agriculture in 1946. The ban was lifted in 1973; and birds were quarantined and tested at approved facilities for velogenic, viscerotropic Newcastle disease. During the quarantine period, the U.S. Public Health Service treatment standards for chlamydiosis were enforced by Department of Agriculture personnel.

Classification

Chlamydial organisms belong to the class Rickettsiae and the order Chlamydiales. This order consists of the single family Chlamydiaceae, which is composed of one genus—*Chlamydia*. Four species belong to the genus: *C. trachomatis* and *C. pneumonia*, which primarily infect humans; *C. pecorum*, which is proposed as a ruminant specific strain; and *C. psittaci*, which infects a wide range of avian and mammalian hosts.

Microbiology

Chlamydia are obligate intracellular parasites. Initially classified as large viruses, they are more bacterialike in that they contain RNA, DNA, ribosomes, and cell walls.

After a single infectious particle (known as an elementary body) has been phagocytized by a host cell, it undergoes binary fission and forms two daughter reticulate bodies. These particles reduce in size and in turn form elementary bodies, thus completing the life cycle. The cycle takes 48 to 72 hours.

Host Range

The host range of *Chlamydia* includes humans (chlamydiosis), cats (pneumonitis and conjunctivitis), sheep (pneumonitis, polyarthritis, placentitis-abortion, and conjunctivitis), cattle (pneumonitis, polyarthritis, placentitis-abortion, and encephalomyelitis), horses (pneumonitis), pigs (pneumonitis and polyarthritis), and birds (chlamydiosis).

Terminology

Infection of psittacine birds with *C. psittaci* is referred to as psittacosis; in other birds, the condition is known as ornithosis. The zoonotic infection of humans with *C. psittaci* has traditionally been called psittacosis or parrot fever. Because the causative agent is the same in all cases, it has been recommended that the term *chlamydiosis* be used to indicate infection with *C. psittaci*.

Originally published in Volume 10, Number 4, May 1989

Clinical Presentation and Diagnosis in Pet Birds

Feces and respiratory exudates are the primary sources of infection in birds. The clinical presentation of avian chlamydiosis varies. The patient might present with a chronic intestinal or upper respiratory infection or with an acute systemic illness; some birds can be asymptomatic carriers. Such birds pose the highest risk relative to transmission of the organism.

Clinical signs can include such nonspecific findings as respiratory and ophthalmic signs, weight loss, anorexia, and poor integumentary condition (Figures 1 and 2). Green, watery diarrhea might be present; this suggests increased bilirubin resulting from hepatocellular destruction or biliary obstruction (Figure 3). When a bird exhibits these signs, it is important to inquire where and when the bird was purchased, if the bird has been stressed recently, and if the owner's family members have had influenzalike symptoms.

Tentative diagnosis can be based on the following procedures:

- **Hematology.** Results indicate leukocytosis with a left shift and heterophilia. Monocytosis might be evident in chronic cases; anemia can also be present.
- **Serum chemistry.** There might be elevations in aspartate transferase, lactate dehydrogenase, and uric acid.
- **Radiography.** Radiographs might demonstrate hepatomegaly or splenomegaly.

Serology is the most useful tool for attaining definitive diagnosis. Direct complement fixation (DCF) has been the preferred serologic test. The test is reliable in large psittacines but not in small psittacine and passerine species. A titer ranging from 1:16 to 1:32 suggests possible chlamydial infection. A titer of 1:64 is probably positive, and a titer of 1:124 or greater indicates an active case of avian chlamydiosis.

The latex agglutination test is less sensitive than direct complement fixation, although specificity is comparable. Nonspecific agglutination can be a problem.

The microimmunofluorescence test has recently emerged as the preferred diagnostic test. It is more specific and evidently more sensitive than direct complement fixation.

Isolation and identification from fecal samples or cloacal swabs can help to confirm a diagnosis. Feces should be collected for three to five days and placed in a special transport medium.

Postmortem diagnosis can be made by impression smears of liver, spleen, or air sac. When stained with Giemsa stain, chlamydial organisms appear dark purple (Figure 4). When stained with Macchiavello's or Gimenez stain, the organisms appear red. Figure 5 exemplifies the postmortem appearance of hepatomegaly in a cockatiel.

Treatment in Pet Birds

The official treatment for avian chlamydiosis is chlortetracycline in mash (4.4 to 10 mg/g of mash) or 1% chlortetracycline pellets for 45 days in large psittacines and chlortetracycline-impregnated millet for 30 days in small psittacine and passerine species. Calcium intake should be decreased during treatment because of the binding effect of calcium on tetracycline antibiotics.

Alternative (unapproved) treatments include oral doxycycline at 30 to 50 mg/kg twice daily for 45 days. Doxycycline can be given intravenously or intramuscularly in severely ill birds; such treatment should last only one to two days because of possible thrombophlebitis or muscle necrosis. The advantages of doxycycline include long half-life, complete absorption, less calcium binding, and less effect on the intestinal flora and the kidneys.

Clients must be warned of the zoonotic potential of the condition and advised to wear gloves, mask, and protective clothing when handling the bird or infectious material. Public health officials should be informed of birds with the disease.

Clinical Presentation and Diagnosis in Humans

In humans, chlamydiosis usually manifests as a transient, mild, influenzalike illness. It sometimes occurs as a more serious pneumonic disease with high fever, chills, headache, nausea, and malaise. Complications of chlamydial infection in humans include encephalitis, pericarditis, myocarditis, endocarditis, and chronic valvular heart disease. The condition can be fatal.

Humans usually acquire chlamydiosis by inhaling aerosols from infectious droppings. Feathers and dander from infected birds can also be a source of infection. A new strain of *C. psittaci* has been identified recently and designated TWAR. The TWAR strain is transmitted by contact between humans and causes mild pneumonia.

Human chlamydiosis can be diagnosed by isolation of *C. psittaci* from sputum; however, the organism is present in sputum for only the first three to seven days after infection. Direct complement fixation is the most common serologic procedure for diagnosing chlamydiosis of avian origin in humans. In a person with appropriate symptoms, especially with a history of exposure to birds, a fourfold increase between paired serum samples confirms a diagnosis of chlamydiosis. A single or stable titer of at least 1:32 justifies a presumptive diagnosis of the condition. The microimmunofluorescence test is being used more frequently because of its high sensitivity and specificity compared with direct complement fixation.

Treatment in Humans

Chlortetracycline is the preferred treatment for human chlamydiosis. The dose is 250 mg orally four times daily for 21 days. In severely ill individuals, tetracycline is given intravenously at 10 to 15 mg/kg/day.

Control

Psittacine birds are the most important source of infection with *C. psittaci*. The control of chlamydiosis in humans thus begins with the control of chlamydial infection in psittacines.

In 1973, the U.S. Department of Agriculture adopted

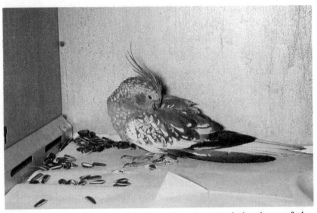

Figure 1—A cockatiel exhibiting the characteristic signs of the so-called sick-bird syndrome associated with avian chlamydiosis.

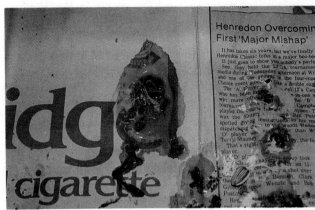

Figure 3—Watery, green diarrhea suggestive of hepatobiliary injury associated with avian chlamydiosis in a cockatiel.

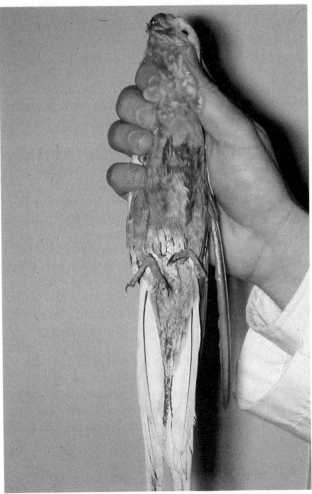

Figure 2—Signs of emaciation and a soiled vent in a patient with avian chlamydiosis.

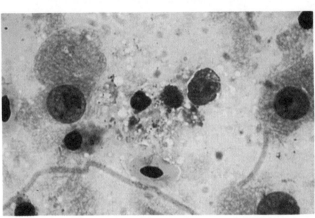

Figure 4—An impression smear of a parrot's liver illustrates the dark-purple–staining chlamydial organisms. (Giemsa)

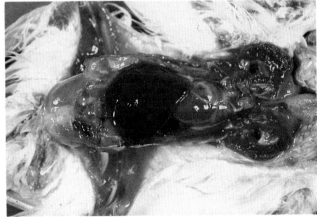

Figure 5—The postmortem appearance of hepatomegaly in a case of avian chlamydiosis.

regulations requiring all commercially imported birds to undergo a 30-day quarantine period at facilities supervised by the department. The regulations were adopted after outbreaks of velogenic, viscerotropic Newcastle disease occurred in domestic poultry and were related to imported psittacines. The U.S. Public Health Service initiated the provision of chlortetracycline treatment for psittacines with chlamydiosis during the quarantine period. For the following reasons, this provision has not entirely eliminated chlamydiosis from birds released from quarantine:

- It has been documented that 45 days of treatment is necessary to eliminate chlamydiosis in large psittacines. The 30-day period currently required is not sufficient to eliminate latent infection.
- There is too much variation in the preparation of medicated mash by quarantine station operators to ensure adequate blood levels of chlortetracycline.
- There is no monitoring of blood levels of chlortetracycline to ensure adequate treatment.
- The Department of Agriculture and the Public Health Service have not resolved the problem of which federal authority has the responsibility and authority to control chlamydiosis at the quarantine stations.

The following suggestions have been made to improve the present control program:

- Quarantine for large psittacines should be lengthened to 45 days.
- Blood levels should be monitored to determine whether adequate levels of chlortetracycline are being achieved.
- Postmortem examination of birds that die during quarantine should include diagnostic tests for chlamydiosis.
- Department of Agriculture identification leg bands should be kept on birds as long as they remain in commercial channels so that the origin of birds can be traced.
- To avoid operator variation at quarantine stations, a pelleted 1% chlortetracycline feed should be used instead of cooked mash for treating large psittacines.

The number of smuggled psittacines is increasing. In light of this fact and the ineffectiveness of the present control program, it is essential that veterinarians and veterinary technicians be aware of avian chlamydiosis and its potential as a zoonotic disease.

Acknowledgments
The author acknowledges the assistance of Keven Flammer, DVM, and John Barnes, DVM, College of Veterinary Medicine, North Carolina State University, in the preparation of the manuscript and the figures.

BIBLIOGRAPHY
Emerson JK: Psittacosis. *JAVMA* 180(6):612–613, 1982.
Grimes JE: Chlamydiosis in psittacine birds. *JAVMA* 190(4):394–397, 1987.
Hampton RJ: Chlamydiosis (psittacosis). *Can Vet J* 28:267, 1987.
Johnson FWA: Chlamydiosis. *Br Vet J* 139:93–100, 1983.
McDonald SE, Boyer EV: Psittacosis in pet birds. *California Vet* 4:6–17, 1981.
Psittacosis Surveillance. Annual Summary, 1975-1984. Atlanta, Centers for Disease Control, 1987.

UPDATE

Since this article was originally published, new polymerase chain reaction (PCR) testing has shown promise in diagnosing both avian and human chlamydiosis.

Care and Handling of Ring-Necked Pheasants

Diann L. Allee, AHT
University of Missouri
St. Louis, Missouri

Many hobbyists and serious breeders raise upland game species for their own enjoyment and for business reasons. Because of this interest, animals in these species are sometimes brought into a local veterinary clinic so that clients can consult about problems with rearing and breeding them. Various areas are of concern to breeders and thus of interest in the veterinary practices that handle wildlife clients. This article focuses on ring-necked pheasants, a wild game species that is becoming increasingly popular.

Courtship and Mating

Ring-necked pheasants court and mate in spring. It is often noted by observers as the time when males crow and fight to establish territorial boundaries. During this period, the male testes develop to full size and begin active sperm production.

Females show responsiveness by visiting the males, stopping regular activity to find nesting territories, and watching the males strut and "drum." Drumming is the fast beating of the wings of the male in a preflight stance, without the bird rising from the ground as it would in flight. The male stops crowing when a female enters his territory. He shifts his plumage to make the best display for her and may show pursuit behavior.

Actual mating occurs in early spring (April in the Midwest), about one month after the initial courtship activity has been noted. The male-female ratio is 1:3 but can be as high as 1:5. Each male establishes a harem by using territorial patrols. Some aggression occurs among males if their territories are invaded.

Nesting and Laying

Nesting and laying usually take place during the second half of April and continue into the summer or until a clutch of eggs is successfully hatched. Nests are simply dugout depressions in the soil; nest boxes containing bedding or wood chips can be provided. In the wild, or in the semi-wild atmosphere of some game farms, the birds choose light cover, such as is found at the borderline or among grasses and vegetation.

The average clutch size is about 11 eggs. Larger numbers of eggs per clutch usually mean that more than one hen is using the same nest.

Normal egg-gathering procedure is to leave the first egg and remove subsequent eggs. Hens continue to lay longer when this technique is used and are thwarted in attempts to eat their eggs if the eggs are unavailable. Eggs should be stored in a cool, moist atmosphere and turned every three to four days. Hatchability of eggs deteriorates after seven days of storage.

Incubation Time

Incubation requires between 23 and 26 days. The temperature of the incubator should be about 39.9° C (102° F) with humidity at 75%. Directions for particular brands and types of incubators should be followed closely. Incubating eggs should be turned two to three times per day until Day 20 and then left undisturbed until hatching occurs. Hobbyists usually use small chicken hens or mechanical incubators for hatching pheasant eggs. Candling is unsatisfactory because of the dark pigment in the shells. Eggs with obvious cracks or chips should be discarded during the process of incubation.

If being raised for a shooting farm, it is preferable to

leave the chicks with the pheasant hen for hatching and mothering. Chicks retain their wildness and are more natural on the hunting range when this is done.

Housing

Chicks can be housed in a brooder, or they can be kept in cardboard boxes or small batteries with heat sources. Small-breed chicks can be kept with pheasant chicks to quiet them and to aid in teaching them to eat and drink. Water sources for young chicks can be constructed from jar lids with small jars turned upside down inside, because the chicks drown using drinking fountains sized for larger chickens. Water should not be placed in corners because chicks can startle and drown while trying to hide. Dropping a few grains of food or a few green clippings on the water surface aids in teaching chicks to drink. (Caution must be used to prevent souring of the water with excess feed.)

In teaching the chicks to eat, scrambled or hard-boiled eggs can be placed on the sides of the box at head height. Bouncing the finger in the feed (simulating pecking action of the hen) increases interest; so does dropping a few grains of feed around the chick or even on other chicks' backs. Newspapers or other litter should be replaced often to provide dry, clean bedding.

The box or brooder should not have large openings or large spaces between wires, as pheasant chicks can escape through mesh even as small as one inch. Once loose, chicks are difficult to find and will not return to heat sources of their own volition.

Cannibalism occurs frequently among chicks and sporadically among adults. In the maturing adults, pulling each other's pinfeathers at the blood stage is common. "Blood feathers" have blue shafts and are blood filled; mature features have white shafts. If a feather is bleeding, the feather must be pulled in its entirety to stop further blood loss. Cannibalism also results from overcrowding, overheating, chilling, poor ventilation, intensity of light, and poor nutrition. In adult birds, debeaking, proper spacing, good nutrition, and availability of salt usually control the problem. Cannibalism among chicks is usually controlled by keeping them in semidarkness or placing a red bulb in their light source. (The red light camouflages the bleeding spots.) Chicks gang up on another chick if blood is seen. Debeaking, clipping of spurs or toes, and wing clipping can cause bleeding, which can trigger cannibalism. Semidarkness and special care are necessary after these procedures.

Nutrition

Proper nutrition begins with a game bird starter or high-quality turkey starter for the newly hatched chicks. Twenty-eight to 30 percent protein is necessary in the chick ration.[1] The nutritional requirements for rearing pheasant chicks vary according to the end product desired. For finishing the birds, more fat is included in the diet; conditioning feeds or flight feeds are needed for strong muscles and sustained flight. Maintenance feeds are given to keep breeder birds in optimum condition without unnecessary fat. Alfalfa, clover, and lawn clippings are good supplements on occasion. Grit is important as a digestive aid and as a supply of calcium for strong bones and eggshells. Oyster shell, pigeon grit, or road grit can be used as sources of grit and calcium.

Parasite Control

Control of parasites is achieved through dustings of the chicks for lice and mites. Each bird is dusted by hand or is given access to a box of sand or wood ashes in which insecticidal powder for poultry has been added and mixed according to package directions. With the latter method, birds dust themselves. The container should be large enough that the birds can get into the box, and it should be in an area where the contents cannot become wet and solid or be washed away. Hens used for incubation should be dusted before they are placed on the eggs and once during the incubation time, but eggs or newly hatched chicks should not be dusted.

Wormers can be placed in the water supply or birds can be pilled individually. Clean ground and proper waste disposal and sanitation around buildings and equipment aid in control of parasites.

After the chicks are started, housing and cages depend on the ages of the birds and the end product desired. The season of the year and the reproductive stage of the birds are also factors. Two types of housing are used in breeding colonies: *harem* and *community*.[2] Harem housing consists of a small pen containing one cock and three or four hens. Community housing requires more space but less equipment and is more commonly used by breeders. In community housing, all the adult birds are kept in the same pen in a 1:5 or 6 male-female ratio.

The main problems with community housing are fighting and aggression. Pens should allow enough room for the birds to exercise. Small-mesh wire should be used for young birds. Use of netting for a roof prevents birds from flying up into the wire and killing themselves and keeps predators from entering. If frightened, birds become hysterical and can seriously injure themselves. On a range, birds should be placed in a flight pen at the end of their sixth week.

Housing requirements are simpler for adults than for young birds. Adults require shade and some protection from more severe elements but, if given a choice, will sit out in rain and snow rather than under a building. This is apparently an instinctual escape mechanism. Standard-sized feeders and fountains are all that is required. Sanitation is important at all ages: clean feed and water, fresh litter or clean ground, and removal of debris as needed.

Care and Handling

Even the most careful and quietest handling can result in shock or injury and death of a bird. Most pheasant owners have a catching area where the birds cannot injure themselves when attempting to escape human touch. A long-handled fishing net or other safe device or trap is handy when catching birds for removal, treatment of disease, and other procedures. Adult birds kept in smaller areas huddle in one corner. Pheasants should be handled one at a time by grasping the wings and the feet and pushing down toward the ground. Unless handled knowledgeably, the birds will injure themselves, may twist off their legs, or might claw the handler in their frantic efforts to escape. For moving, birds can be put into burlap bags or darkened cages. Darkness stops the frantic attempts to escape and prevents injury. No more than three or four birds should be placed into one bag or container.

In open-topped pens, it is necessary to clip flight feathers periodically on one wing to prevent the birds from flying away. Flight feathers regrow in two to three weeks on young birds, and disasters can result if the feathers are allowed to reach full growth. Early flight of young birds may last only 75 to 100 yards, then "freezing" occurs and birds cannot be found or predators catch them at night. Young birds often run for great distances and hide.

Sexing Chicks

Determination of the sex of a chick is difficult for amateurs. Gentle and quiet handling is again crucial, because being handled can cause even day-old chicks to go into shock. Some identification can be made through coloration on the head of a day-old chick (Figure 1).

Both sexes are tannish with black striping, similar to the coloration of Brown Leghorn chicks when first hatched. Later, when beginning to feather, males and females remain brown mottled; but the roosters, or cocks, tend to develop blunt tails, while the females have longer and more tapered tails. Soon males begin to lose feathers around the eyes and form the red cheek patch visible at the rear area of each eye of an adult male (Figure 2). A few colored feathers begin to appear in the breast and neck areas. Gradually, the coloration spreads to other portions of the body.

Hens remain a mottled brown with a smooth appearance. Cocks develop distinctive ring-necked coloration and patterning. Viewed as a group, pheasants appear to be quite similar in a pen, regardless of sex; but on closer examination, there are distinctive color and pattern variations. Some pheasants have an overall golden appearance and some a more silver appearance, while some males appear only green and rust. Variation in the patterning over the body also exists. Hens appear an overall mottled brown; but on closer examination, some appear violet at the neck area, while others are strictly tannish. Egg color also varies; some eggs appear darker khaki colored than others. Coloration of both the hens and eggs is geared toward camouflage and propagation of the species, but the male coloration is for reproductive appeal.

Rules and Regulations for Wildlife Handling

Rules and regulations govern the growing of upland game birds and other wild animals in the United States. The United States also maintains wildlife agreements with some other nations. The U.S. Department of Agriculture

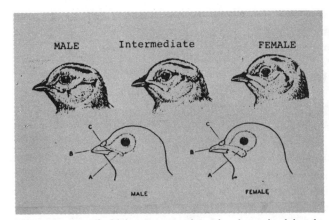

Figure 1—Sex of chicks can sometimes be determined by the head coloration. Cheek patches on day-old, ring-necked pheasant chicks are shown. *A* = strip of long down; *B* = upper mandible; *C* = cere. (Reprinted with permission from the Pennsylvania Game Commission.)

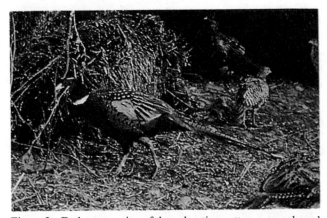

Figure 2—Early maturation of the coloration patterns on male and female birds. The cock has developed the distinctive ring-necked coloration and patterning (note the red cheek patch characteristic of adult males).

regulates the transport of live animals regarding size of containers and number of animals per container as well as humane considerations.

Most states have state-level regulations as well, and a state's department of agriculture and wildlife conservation agency should be contacted before anyone acquires game animals. As an example of one state's regulations, the Wildlife Code of Missouri has basically the following rules for possession of wild upland game. (These are included in such sections as 3CSR 10-10.750 pertaining to a wildlife breeders' permit, which can be purchased annually.) Requirements are given for recordkeeping, acquisition, species allowed, buying, selling, giving away, transportation, and all uses for a bird or an animal. A hobby permit can be acquired annually for a fee and allows keeping bobwhite quail, wild turkeys, or ring-necked pheasants but limits the number to 50. A hobby permit does not allow the selling or giving away of birds. Banded birds can be temporarily released for dog training but must be recaptured. A smaller additional fee is required on the recapture device. Some species of ducks, geese, and other wildlife would be subject to these regulations.[3]

State and federal regulations should be investigated by anyone considering upland game bird rearing. Shooting farms are regulated and, in Missouri, fall under the same general section of the Missouri wildlife code just highlighted.

Conclusion

Rearing exotic fowl is an interesting hobby or enterprise; and individuals with adequate knowledge of poultry and proper penning/housing as well as the time, energy, space, and money required can make it a profitable venture. As breeding programs become more popular, more veterinary practices are likely to become involved in consultation regarding the rearing, breeding, and care of game species.

REFERENCES

1. *Purina Game Birds Programs.* St. Louis, MO, Ralston Purina Co, 1970.
2. McAlee WL (ed): *The Ring-Necked Pheasant and Its Management in North America.* Washington, DC, American Wildlife Institute, 1945.
3. *Wildlife Code of Missouri: Rules of the Conservation Commission* (issued January 1, 1985). Jefferson City, MO, Missouri Department of Conservation, 1985.

Bibliography

Edminster FC: *American Game Birds of Field and Forest.* New York, Charles Scribner's Sons, 1954.
Spaulding CE, Spaulding J: *The Complete Care of Orphaned or Abandoned Baby Animals.* Emmaus, PA, Rodale Press, 1979.
Stromberg L: *Sexing Fowl.* Pine River, MA, Stromberg Publishing Co, 1979.

Avian Anesthesia: Part II (continued from page 120)

12. Sawyer DC, Evans AT, DeYoung DJ: *Anesthetic Principles and Techniques.* East Lansing, Dept of Small Animal Surgery and Medicine, College of Veterinary Medicine, Michigan State University, 1973, pp 1-57.
13. Soma LR: Systems and techniques for inhalation anesthesia, in Soma LR (ed): *Textbook of Veterinary Anesthesia.* Baltimore, Williams and Wilkins Co, 1971, pp 201-227.
14. Sawyer DC: The induction period. *Practice of Small Animal Anesthesia.* Philadelphia, WB Saunders Co, in press.
15. Krahwinkel DJ, Evans AT: Anesthetic equipment for small animals. *JAVMA* 161(11):1430-1434, 1972.
16. Manley SV, McDonell WN: Clinical evaluation of the Bain breathing circuit in small animal anesthesia. *JAAHA* 15(1):67-72, 1979.
17. Manley SV, McDonell WN: A new circuit for small animal anesthesia: The Bain coaxial circuit. *JAAHA* 15(1):61-65, 1979.
18. Soma LR: Vaporizers for volatile anesthetic agents, in Soma LR (ed): *Textbook of Veterinary Anesthesia.* Baltimore, Williams and Wilkins Co, 1971, pp 192-193.
19. Smith TC: Respiratory effects of general anesthesia, in Soma LR (ed): *Textbook of Veterinary Anesthesia.* Baltimore, Williams and Wilkins Co, 1971, pp 156-175.
20. Amand WB: General techniques for avian surgery, in Kirk RW (ed): *Current Veterinary Therapy VI.* Philadelphia, WB Saunders Co, 1977, pp 711-716.
21. Evans AT: Personal communcation, Michigan State University, 1980.
22. Booth NH: Introduction, in Jones LM, Booth NH, McDonald LE (eds): *Veterinary Pharmacology and Therapeutics,* ed 4. Ames, The Iowa State University Press, 1977, pp 191-207.
23. Gandal CP: Satisfactory general anesthesia in birds. *JAVMA* 128(4):332-334, 1956.
24. Harrison GJ, Harrison LR: *Clinical Avian Medicine and Surgery.* Philadelphia, WB Saunders Co, 1986, pp 543-548.
25. Sawyer DC: What's new in inhalation anesthesia? presented at conference *New developments in anesthesia and analgesia for companion animals.* Michigan State University, March 1993.
26. LeBlanc PH: Closed vs Semiclosed Anesthetic Systems, presented at conference *New developments in anesthesia and analgesia for companion animals.* Michigan State University, March 1993.
27. Goelz MF, Hahn AW, Kelley ST: Effects of halothane and isoflurane on mean arterial blood pressure, heart rate, and respiratory rate in adult Pekin ducks. *Am J Vet Res* 15(3):458–460, 1990.

Husbandry Concerns for Pet Reptiles

Terry W. Campbell, DVM, PhD
Sea World of Florida, Inc.
Orlando, Florida

Improper husbandry is the most common cause of clinical disorders of pet reptiles. Suboptimum environmental conditions and nutrition compromise the reptile's immune system and subsequently lead to infection by opportunistic bacterial and fungal pathogens. Gram-negative bacteria, especially of the genus *Pseudomonas* and *Aeromonas*, are the bacterial pathogens that most often infect reptiles. Important aspects of reptilian husbandry include nutrition, cage design, temperature, humidity, photoperiod, and water quality.

Reptiles of the order Squamata are commonly kept as pets. Pets from this order include the reticulated python (*Python reticulatus*), ball python (*P. regis*), Burmese python (*P. molurus*), boa constrictor (*Constrictor constrictor*), rat snakes (*Elaphe* species), king snakes (*Lampropeltis* species), green iguana (*Iguana iguana*), and leopard gecko (*Eublepharus macularis*). Common pet reptiles of the order Chelonia include the box turtles (*Terrapene* species), red-footed tortoise (*Geochelone carbonaria*), painted turtle (*Chrysemys picta*), and sliders (*Pseudemys* species). A common pet reptile of the order Crocodilia is the spectacled caiman (*Caiman sclerops*).

Nutrition

Reptiles fed an improper diet can become immunosuppressed and develop secondary bacterial or fungal infections. Metabolic bone disease, however, is the most common nutritionally related disorder of reptiles. Metabolic bone disease is relatively common in herbivorous reptiles (such as some species of turtles) and omnivorous reptiles (such as some species of lizards and turtles) that are fed poor-quality vegetables and fruits because the diet is often low in calcium and high in phosphorus. If fed properly, carnivorous reptiles (such as snakes) given whole prey animals seldom develop metabolic bone disease; however, carnivores fed unsupplemented all-meat diets can develop the disorder. An unbalanced calcium to phosphorus ratio and vitamin D_3 malnutrition result in secondary hyperparathyroidism and osteodystrophy.

Metabolic bone disease of lizards, especially the green iguana, results in thickening of the jaws, femur, radius, and ulna. Pathologic fractures also can occur. In the early stages of metabolic bone disease, affected lizards often lose the ability to move affected limbs.

Abnormal growth of the jaws and vertebrae can occur in other reptiles with calcium, phosphorus, and vitamin D_3 imbalances. In turtles, such imbalances result in abnormal shell growth.

Prevention and correction of metabolic bone disease in reptiles require provision of a diet with a proper calcium to phosphorus ratio (i.e., 1:1 or 2:1). The proper ratio can be achieved by supplementing the diet of herbivorous and omnivorous reptiles with moistened dog food, vitamins and minerals, and whole prey animals.

Other disorders caused by an improper diet include steatitis in carnivorous reptiles fed obese laboratory rodents and hypovitaminosis A (especially common in aquatic turtles fed all-meat diets). Hypovitaminosis A leads to squamous metaplasia of the harderian gland and secondary palpebral edema and conjunctivitis. Affected turtles often become anorexic and develop respiratory tract infections.

Environmental Conditions

As previously mentioned, poor husbandry practices cause most disorders of pet reptiles. Correction of improper environmental conditions and husbandry practices is usually part of the treatment plan of a pet reptile. Overfeeding, poor hygiene, excessive handling of nervous reptiles, and objects in cages that may lead to lacerations are other husbandry practices that frequently cause disorders in reptiles. Improper hygiene leads to bacterial and fungal infections, especially involving the skin and respiratory tract. Infectious stomatitis (a common disorder of pet snakes) is often secondary to environmental stress resulting from poor husbandry practices.

Lacerations are often caused by bites from cage mates or sharp objects in the cage. Bites from uneaten prey, such as mice and rats, are the most common cause of lacerations in pet reptiles. Prey food should be humanely killed before feeding to avoid

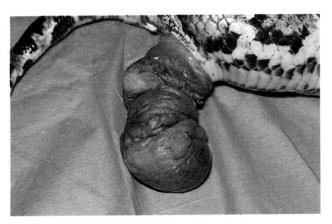

Figure 1—In this snake, intestinal prolapse resulted from fecal impaction after accidental ingestion of wood shavings (used as a cage substrate) that had combined with the food.

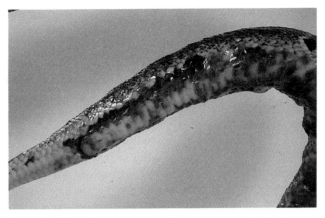

Figure 2—Clinical presentation of mycotic dermatitis. In this patient, the disorder resulted from thermal burns from a hot rock and unhygienic cage environment.

bite wounds. Freshly killed animals can be kept frozen for up to six months and thawed before feeding.

Cage Design

Cage design should minimize environmental stress. Cages that are too small make it difficult for reptiles to exercise; lack of exercise may lead to such conditions as constipation and dystocia, especially in snakes. Nose rubbing on glass is an indication of poor caging. Chronic nose rubbing results in ulceration of nostril tissue, which leads to secondary respiratory tract infection and dermatitis.

Cages should provide hiding places (i.e., hide boxes or inverted clay pots with entry holes) and branches for arboreal reptiles. Ball pythons often become anorexic if they are not given a place to hide.

Improper substrate used in the cage can lead to gastrointestinal obstruction, dehydration, and toxicity (Figure 1). The substrate should not be fine enough to adhere to food and become ingested. Hydroscopic bedding material, such as cat litter and ground corncobs, and wood shavings (which may contain toxic resins) should be avoided. Clean newspaper and indoor–outdoor carpet make adequate substrate for reptile cages.

Some disinfectants, such as phenolic compounds, are potentially toxic to reptiles. A diluted sodium hypochlorite solution (two parts per million) is an adequate disinfectant.

Temperature

Reptiles are ectothermic, and each species has an optimum temperature range that should be maintained for the animal to remain in a normal physiologic state. Suboptimum environmental temperature results in immunosuppression and disrupted digestion. Therefore, chronic hypothermia results in secondary disorders, such as pneumonia, infectious stomatitis, and septicemia. Cages should ideally be large enough to provide thermal gradients in which the reptile can find its own comfort zone. Many pet reptiles remain healthy with daytime temperatures between 26°C and 31°C (79°F and 89°F) and nighttime temperatures between 22°C and 28°C (72°F and 82°F). Obviously, specific requirements vary among species.

An out-of-the-cage radiant heat source placed over the top of the cage should provide a temperature gradient for the animal. Incandescent light bulbs are often used for this purpose. The pet reptile should not be able to come in direct contact with the heat source or thermal burns may result (Figure 2). Hot rocks and heating pads are inadequate sources of heat for reptiles.

Humidity

Relative humidity of the pet reptile's environment is another important husbandry consideration. Relative humidity of 50% to 60% evidently is adequate for many pet reptiles; however, species requirements for relative humidity vary. For example, desert reptiles require lower humidity (i.e., as low as 10%) and tropical reptiles may require higher humidity, which can be accomplished by misting the animal with warm water once or twice daily.

Relative humidity that falls below the requirement of the species often results in dehydration and secondary constipation, dysecdysis, retained spectacles, and bacterial infection. Excessive humidity often results in skin disorders, such as skin infection and blister disease. Blister disease clinically manifests as fluid-filled vesicles under the skin or within the skin. Secondary bacterial or fungal pathogens can grow within these blisters and subsequently cause severe dermatitis and/or septicemia. Excess humidity can also cause cage substrate to become wet, thereby resulting in buildup of opportunistic microorganisms.

Photoperiod

The photoperiod of lower vertebrates, including reptiles, must be optimum for them to remain healthy. Constant exposure to light results in chronic stress for the reptile. The stress subsequently results in immunosuppression, which makes the reptile susceptible to opportunistic pathogens. A natural light-to-dark cycle is ideal for pet reptiles housed indoors. If a natural light cycle cannot be achieved, then a 12-hour-light and 12-hour-dark cycle is suitable. The light source should provide a full spectrum, including ultraviolet light. Automatic timers can be used to achieve the desired photoperiod.

Water Quality

Aquatic or semiaquatic reptiles should be housed in clean water. Poor water quality leads to such conditions as severe bacterial or fungal necrotizing ulcerative dermatitis or septicemia. Middle ear infections in pet aquatic turtles are frequently seen in animals subjected to poor water quality. Open-flow systems provide the best method of maintaining a healthy aquatic environment for aquatic reptiles. Adequately filtered closed water systems also can be used to house aquatic reptiles.

Conclusion

If owners of reptiles feed a proper diet and maintain their pets in a clean, healthy environment that meets optimum requirements, then the animal will suffer from few (if any) medical problems. Many reptile owners, however, are unaware of the needs of the animal. Therefore, it is the responsibility of the veterinarian to be the source of information and to educate clients of the importance of proper husbandry in maintaining a healthy reptile pet.

BIBLIOGRAPHY

Frye FL: *Biomedical and Surgical Aspects of Captive Reptile Husbandry*. Bonner Springs, KS, Veterinary Medical Publishing, 1981, pp 6–60.

Jacobson ER: Diseases of reptiles. Part I. Noninfectious diseases, in Johnston DE (ed): *Exotic Animal Medicine in Practice*, vol I. Trenton, NJ, Veterinary Learning Systems Co, 1991, pp 125–129.

Jacobson ER: Diseases of reptiles. Part II. Infectious diseases, in Johnston DE (ed): *Exotic Animal Medicine in Practice*, vol I. Trenton, NJ, Veterinary Learning Systems Co, 1991, pp 130–134.

Jacobson ER: Evaluation of the reptile patient, in Jacobson ER, Kollias GV (ed): *Contemporary Issues in Small Animal Practice, Exotic Animals*. New York, Churchill Livingstone, 1988, pp 1–18.

Jacobson ER: Reptiles. *Vet Clin North Am [Small Anim Pract]* 17(5):1203–1225, 1987.

Jenkins JR: Medical management of reptile patients. *Compend Contin Educ Pract Vet* 13(6):980–988, 1991.

Page DC, Mautino M: Clinical management of tortoises, in Johnston DE (ed): *Exotic Animal Medicine in Practice*, vol II. Trenton, NJ, Veterinary Learning Systems Co, 1991, pp 79–88.

Russo EA: Diagnosis and treatment of lumps and bumps in snakes, in Johnston DE (ed): *Exotic Animal Medicine in Practice*, vol II. Trenton, NJ, Veterinary Learning Systems Co, 1991, pp 99–106.

Reptilian Management and Medical Care*

Sally O. Walshaw, MA, VMD
Training Coordinator and Associate Professor
University Laboratory Animal Resources
Michigan State University
East Lansing, Michigan

The popularity of reptiles as pets is increasing, especially in cities, where there are many housing restrictions on the keeping of dogs and cats. Reptiles have a relatively slow metabolic rate compared with that of birds and mammals, and this enables the reptile to survive periods of fasting for days to weeks depending on the species and environmental conditions. Reptile owners can therefore safely leave their pets unattended if they must be away from home for several days. A reptile may be one of the few pets permissible for an individual that is allergic to fur and/or feathers. Reptiles, in the eyes of many, are beautiful and interesting and can serve as a link to the natural world and thereby satisfy, as do mammalian and avian pets, one of the fundamental needs of humans in a technological society.[1,2]

This article will focus on the species of reptiles that are commonly kept as pets (Table I). Most public libraries have reference books that can provide detailed information about distinguishing characteristics and natural habitats of the various species. Some examples of useful general reference books are *Handbook of Turtles* by A. Carr, *A Field Guide to Reptiles and Amphibians of Eastern and Central North America* by R. Conant, *Living Reptiles of the World* by K. Schmidt and R. Inger, *Handbook of Lizards* by H. Smith, and *A Field Guide to Western Reptiles and Amphibians* by R. Stebbins. The management and medical care of poisonous reptiles and crocodilians are not considered in this article.

Housing of Captive Reptiles

The importance of providing a suitable environment for a captive reptile cannot be overemphasized. Proper housing, with attention to temperature and humidity requirements of each species, and good nutrition can prevent many of the diseases that shorten the lives of captive reptiles. Client education on the subjects of husbandry and nutrition should be provided to reptile-owning clients of a veterinary practice.

Housing for a reptile pet should satisfy two criteria: (1) it should simulate the natural environment of the species as much as possible,[3] and (2) it should be hygienic so as to minimize growth of infectious organisms in the environment.[3-6] It is usually necessary to compromise somewhat on the first criterion to satisfy the second. The proper environmental temperature can and should be provided for every pet reptile. However, soil, sand, and other natural bedding can be difficult to maintain in a clean dry state. Consequently, most owners of terrestrial reptiles should be advised to cover the cage floor with either paper that can be changed frequently or a synthetic turf that can be removed, washed, and dried (Figure 1). Water that is changed frequently or properly

TABLE I

CLASSIFICATION OF REPTILES
COMMONLY KEPT AS PETS

Taxonomic Group	Examples
Order Chelonia	Turtles, tortoises, terrapins
Order Squamata	
Suborder Sauria	Lizards
Suborder Serpentes	Snakes

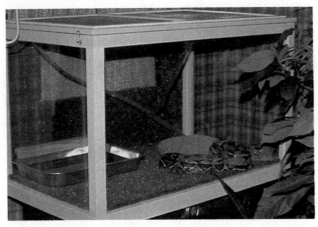

Figure 1—Excellent environment for pet boa constrictor: large, well-ventilated cage, large stone, large water pan. Cage temperature is maintained by a heat lamp outside the cage and soil-heating cables under the synthetic turf. A towel can be suspended over the branch to provide a hiding area.

filtered and circulated is essential for the survival of aquatic reptiles. Additional cage articles for reptiles are listed in Table II.

The cage and items in it should be cleaned regularly. First, droppings and other organic matter should be removed by scrubbing with a detergent solution. Disinfection is the next step. A dilute chlorine bleach solution (30 parts water to 1 part bleach) is a satisfactory disinfectant.[3,4] Finally, the items are rinsed with water and dried. Careful attention to hygiene is important for public health reasons as well as for the animal's protection.

Salmonella and other bacteria pathogenic to human beings have been isolated from many species of lizards, snakes, and turtles.[3,4] It is prudent, therefore, for individuals handling reptiles to wash their hands afterward and to refrain from using a kitchen sink to clean reptile cage items.

Reptiles are poikilotherms or ectotherms; that is, to control its body temperature, a reptile depends on its environment to a much greater extent than does a mammal or a bird. Ideally, a temperature range of 75 to 89 °F rather than a single constant temperature should

TABLE II
SPECIAL ARTICLES FOR REPTILE CAGES

Reptile	Cage Article[a]
Burrowing reptiles	Potting soil or hiding box
Tree-climbing reptiles (certain lizards and snakes)	Vines, branches
Desert-dwelling reptiles	Sand, rocks[b]
All snakes and lizards	Large rough rock (to aid in shedding)
Semiaquatic turtles	Platform or ledge

[a]Each of these items must be disinfected or changed regularly to prevent growth of pathogenic organisms within the cage.
[b]Some problems associated with ingestion of sand and rocks have been reported.[3]

be available to most pet lizards and snakes at all times so that the animal can select the most comfortable temperature for a particular part of the day.[3-5] Some turtles prefer a slightly lower temperature.[3] A range of temperatures can be established by placing the external heat source at one end of the cage and carefully monitoring the cage temperature with several thermometers.

Devices that can be used to heat a terrestrial reptile's cage include a heating pad placed underneath a slightly elevated cage, soil-heating cables buried underneath material on the cage floor, and an incandescent light bulb. The light bulb is the least satisfactory heat source because constant light is stressful for many reptiles and will interfere with reproduction.[3] If a light bulb is used to provide heat, the bulb must be placed completely outside the cage or suitably shielded. Severe thermal burns have occurred in reptiles that sought extra warmth via direct contact with a light bulb.[3,4] Aquarium heaters are suitable for aquatic species.

There is some controversy regarding optimum relative humidity recommended for terrestrial reptiles.[4] The levels advised for species from temperate zones vary from 50 to 70%[3,7] to much lower,[5] depending on the authority. Avoiding extremes and attempting to approximate the relative humidity of the animal's natural habitat are probably advisable in most cases.

Reptiles benefit from regular exposure to a light source of wide spectrum, such as direct sunlight that is not filtered through glass. Some suitable commercial lamps are available.[a] Reptiles exposed to a regular daynight schedule of wide-spectrum light are more active, feed better, and exhibit greater reproductive activity.[3,4]

Nutrition

Reptilian species may be carnivorous, insectivorous, herbivorous, or omnivorous. Good nutritional management requires knowledge of the foods consumed by the particular species in nature. Those food items or appropriate substitutes should be offered to the captive specimen. For example, thawed frozen mixed vegetables mixed with ground alfalfa pellets (guinea pig pellets) constitute a good basis for the diet of herbivorous reptiles.[3] A detailed discussion of nutrition and nutritional disorders, including several tables of food preferences by various species, is found in Reference 3.

Nutritional disorders are seen less commonly in snakes than in lizards and chelonians; this difference is probably attributable to the fact that snakes are usually fed entire animals. A diet consisting exclusively of raw meat will lead to skeletal deformities and other problems in any species (whether mammal, bird, or reptile) because of the low concentration of calcium (and high concentration of phosphorus) in meat. Other foodstuffs that if fed alone will not support life are lettuce[3,4] and commercial turtle foods composed entirely of dried insects.[4]

[a]Optima 50®, fluorescent lamp; and Vita-lite®, shielded by non-ultraviolet-transmitting plastic tube, Duro-Test Corp., North Bergen, NJ 07047; Chroma® lamp, General Electric Co., Bridgeport, CT.

Fish-eating reptiles (certain turtles and snakes) should not be fed a diet consisting exclusively of goldfish, minnows, or smelt. The large amounts of thiaminase in these fish can lead to the profound and sometimes irreversible neurologic disturbances characteristic of thiamine deficiency.[3,4]

Snakes are usually fed entire prey animals, but it is important to note that severe injuries can be inflicted on a snake by live rodents (Figure 2). Since many snakes will accept dead animals,[3,5] it is advisable to offer dead prey to a snake that feeds mainly on rodents. If the snake seems unwilling to consume the dead rodents, the owner should dangle the dead animal with tongs close to the snake to stimulate the snake's interest.[5] It is imperative to competely thaw a frozen animal before feeding it to a snake.[5] A snake that refuses food can sometimes be stimulated to eat by being exposed to direct sunlight for a few minutes[3] or by having a hiding box placed within its cage.[5] A snake, if disturbed soon after eating, may vomit its food. Table III lists some feeding tips for reptiles.

Nursing Techniques for Reptile Patients
History and Medical Records

A good history that includes information about the reptile's species, age, sex, diet, and cage environment is an essential component of a scientific, medically sound approach to the care of a reptilian patient. If the reptile is a snake or lizard, the owner should be questioned about the frequency of shedding and any problems that may have occurred. If the owner keeps more than one reptile, questions should be raised regarding housing (separate vs. group) and hygienic measures designed to prevent spread of disease from one animal to another.

The basic information, environmental history, and history of past illnesses should be carefully recorded, as well as the information about the chief complaint and the history of the present illness. A detailed medical

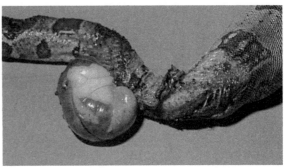

Figure 2—Massive injuries inflicted on a pet snake by a rat: extensive damage to skin, soft tissue, ribs, vertebrae, and lining of coelomic cavity with herniation of a portion of gastrointestinal tract.

record on a reptile is valuable for several reasons: (1) It is legal proof of careful treatment; (2) many illnesses in reptiles are lengthy, and good medical records are very helpful in following the course of an illness and determining response to treatment; and (3) the medical record is potentially useful for reporting new diseases and therapies in the literature.

Physical Examination and Restraint of the Reptile Pet

This article does not include information regarding the handling of poisonous reptiles or crocodilians. A variety of techniques are used by individuals experienced in restraining dangerous specimens.[3-5]

When a nonpoisonous reptile is presented for examination, ideally, it should be observed first from a distance. The reptile's attitude, coordination, and general nutritional status are assessed as well as the appearance of shell or skin. The ability of a turtle or lizard to use all four legs should be determined. Dull skin, lack of interest in its surroundings, sunken eyes, loose folds of skin, and conspicuous skeleton are indications of malnutrition and dehydration in a reptile.[3,4]

Support for the body of a snake is essential when it is

TABLE III

FEEDING TIPS

Reptile	Frequency of Feeding	Special Considerations
Turtles	Daily, if young; three times weekly if mature	Feed aquatic turtles in water
Tortoises	Daily	Feed high-fiber diet
Lizards	Daily if small or insectivorous; three times weekly if larger (e.g., mature iguana)	Provide water droplet mist on cage vegetation for species that will not lap water from a bowl
Snakes	Once or twice a week for most snakes; every two to four weeks if large, mature snake	Never leave snake unattended with aggressive live prey (e.g., mice, rats); try exposing a reluctant feeder to direct sunlight for a few minutes to stimulate appetite,[a] do not offer food during the shedding process

[a]Note: This may also stimulate aggressive behavior.

held. A nonpoisonous snake that attempts to bite can be held firmly but gently by the posterior part of the skull with one hand while the rest of the snake's body is supported with the other arm. Snapping turtles can be grasped at the base of the tail and held away from the restrainer's body; the turtle's plastron (ventral shell) should face the restrainer's body. Many turtles and tortoises tend to pull their heads into their shells while being examined; a straight obstetrical delivery forceps is useful for gently withdrawing a chelonian head for examination.

The heart rate should be recorded during the first part of the physical exam for snakes and lizards. The cardiac apex beat is palpable or observable in most specimens. In lizards the heart is located in the midline area between the forelegs, and in snakes it lies about one-fifth to one-fourth of the body length from the head. The cardiac rate on chelonian and other reptiles can be calculated from an electrocardiogram. Most pet reptiles have a cardiac rate of 25 to 50 beats per minute.[3] The respiratory rate and pattern of respiration should be noted on all reptiles if possible.

Systemic or regional examination of a reptile requires some knowledge of normal anatomy (Figure 3). There are some excellent texts dealing with reptilian medicine that contain descriptions and illustrations of reptile anatomy.[3,4] Some examples of abnormal findings on the physical exam of a reptile are listed in Table IV.

An extremely important part of the physical exam and medical record is the exact weight of the reptile. If the animal is too active to be placed directly on the scale, it can be restrained in a box or pillowcase and the weight of the restraining device subtracted from the total weight.

Blood Collection

As with domestic animals, clinical pathologic determinations contribute information that is very useful to the veterinarian in diagnosing disease, following the course of an illness, and predicting the outcome. The site used for blood collection will depend on the veterinarian's preference, the amount of blood needed, and the size and species of animal.

Small amounts of blood may be collected from a lizard or a turtle by clipping a toenail short or from the retrobulbar venous plexus in the lizard.[3,4] A capillary tube is placed directly onto the bleeding nail or is inserted and rotated in the medial ocular canthus as for blood collection from rodents. Blood can be obtained via needle puncture from the jugular vein of turtles,[3] from the dorsal tail vein of turtles,[4,8] from the ventral vessels of

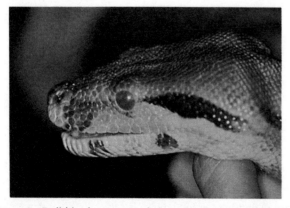

Figure 3—Dull bluish cast to snake's eyes prior to normal ecdysis (shedding).

TABLE IV

SYSTEMATIC/REGIONAL PHYSICAL EXAMINATION OF A REPTILE

System/Region	Examples of Abnormalities
Skin	Dull appearance (normal only if shedding is imminent) Longitudinal tenting Ulceration Swelling Redness Scar Ectoparasites
Shell	Abnormal curvature Flaking Softening Ulceration
Head and neck region	
Eye	Dull or bluish cast (normal only if shedding is imminent) Sunken appearance Swelling of eye and/or lid
External nare	Discharge Occlusion Scar
Tympanic membrane (present in most lizards)	Swelling Discoloration
Scales around mouth	Ulceration Scar Deformity
Oral cavity/pharynx	Ulceration Exudate around teeth or palate Parasites Discharge from tracheal opening Broken or missing teeth in snakes and lizards Deformity
Thorax	Labored and/or noisy breathing
Abdomen	Palpable mass Droppings or blood adhered to vent (cloacal opening)
Leg	Lameness Deformity Uneven wear of claws
Nervous system	Incoordination Seizure Lack of normal withdrawal and righting reflexes

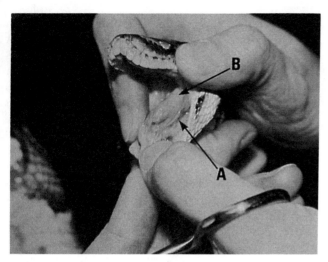

Figure 4—Ventral buccal vein *(A)*, lateral to trachea *(B)*, in snake.

the tail in lizards and snakes,[3,4,9] from the buccal veins in snakes[4,10] (Figure 4), and by cardiac puncture in all species.[3,4] The intended site for cardiac puncture should be prepared by a routine surgical scrub. In many cases, regardless of the blood collection site, capillary tubes should be placed one at a time into the needle hub to obtain necessary samples, because aspiration of blood via syringe is too traumatic for small veins or the heart. Blood collection sites are summarized in Table V.

Administration of Medication

Oral Administration Techniques—Oral medication can be mixed with a reptile's food if the animal is eating normally. Medication intended for a snake can be injected into the prey animal just before it is fed to the snake.[5]

Oral medication and nutrients can be administered via stomach tube to all reptilian species[3,4] (Figure 5). The opening to the trachea is easily visualized in the mouth of the common pet reptilian species and this opening is avoided when the lubricated stomach tube is inserted.

Parenteral Administration of Medication—An injection should be given between scales rather than directly through a scale. The main routes available for administering medication parenterally to reptiles are subcutaneous, intravenous, intramuscular, and intracoelomic. In general, the intravenous route is practical only in the larger specimens. Suitable sites for intramuscular injections are the epaxial muscles on either side of the lumbar spine in lizards and snakes and the triceps muscles in chelonians and lizards. Intramuscular injections in the tail and hindlegs should be avoided if possible because a portal renal circulation may take much of the injected drug directly to the kidney where it will be metabolized and excreted.[11] It is especially important to avoid posterior injection sites when using potentially nephrotoxic drugs such as gentamicin.[11]

Injections may be made into the body cavity, or coelom. Because reptiles do not have a diaphragm, the pleural and peritoneal cavities are continuous and are referred to collectively as the *coelom*. The skin should be prepared as for surgery prior to injection, and the needle should be inserted until it just penetrates the coelomic lining. In chelonians and lizards, intracoelomic injections are given just anterior to the rear legs in the ventrolateral quadrant.[3] Intracoelomic injections in snakes are made along the ventral midline approximately two-thirds of the body length from the head.[4]

Surgical Assisting

Anesthesia and surgical techniques for reptiles are very similar to those routinely used with other species (Figure 6). After the anesthetic agent has been administered, the surgical incision site is prepared using povidone-iodine surgical scrub and solution[b] in the same manner used with mammalian species.[3] Sterile stockinette is useful for draping the smaller specimens and snakes.[4] Surgical instruments that are used routinely in

[b]Betadine®, The Purdue Frederick Co., Norwalk, CT 06856.

TABLE V
BLOOD COLLECTION

Reptile	Possible Collection Sites
Turtle, tortoise	Toenail Jugular vein[a] Dorsal or dorsolateral tail vein[a] Heart
Lizard	Toenail Retrobulbar venous plexus Ventral tail vein[a] Heart
Snake	Buccal veins Ventral tail vein[a] Heart

[a]Unsuitable in very small specimens

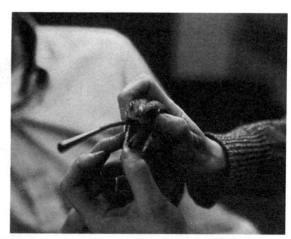

Figure 5—Stomach tube (8 French rubber urethral catheter) in place. For a longer snake, tubing designed for intravenous fluid administration can be cut in a length sufficient to reach the animal's stomach.

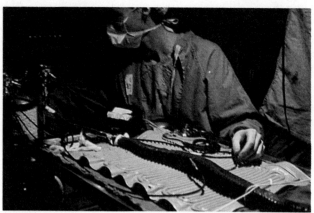

Figure 6—Snake anesthetized with halothane and monitored electrocardiographically.

small-animal surgery should be available. For surgical procedures on very small reptiles, delicate ophthalmic and dental instruments may be suitable, as well as sterile cotton swabs for sponging blood.

Intensive Care Procedures for Reptiles

Husbandry and Nutritional Support—Maintaining the optimum temperature and humidity for a particular species is vital when caring for a seriously ill reptile. This can be achieved for terrestrial species by use of a hospital incubator (Figure 7), although it may be necessary to screen the vent holes in the apparatus. Placing a hiding box within the incubator may help to reduce stress on the reptile and to diminish escape attempts.

Force-feeding may be a necessary part of the treatment regimen for a critically ill, malnourished reptile. Freshly killed small or infant mice can be lubricated with a beaten egg and gently forced down a snake's throat.[4,5] In such cases it is important to choose a mouse that is small enough to be force-fed easily to the snake and to start it down head first. A liquid diet can be given by stomach tube to any malnourished reptile. For carnivorous reptiles, the nutritional suspension can be made from meat broth mixed with egg and milk or from

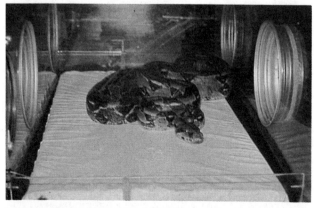

Figure 7—An incubator is suitable for providing proper environmental temperature for hospitalized reptiles.

commercially available amino acid and glucose solution used for parenteral alimentation in small animals.[4] A tube-feeding formula recommended by Frye for carnivorous reptiles consists of three parts strained meat for infants, one part beaten whole egg, one-half part of a commercial general nutritional supplement for dogs and cats,[c] and one part warm water.[3] Herbivorous and omnivorous reptiles should be fed a gruel consisting of a cooked wheat- or rice-based human breakfast cereal to which ground rabbit chow and vitamins are added.[3]

Fluid Therapy—The administration of oral, subcutaneous, and/or intracoelomic fluids is an essential part of the intensive care measures required by a reptile that is dehydrated, severely malnourished, traumatized, or critically ill from any disease process. To prevent drug-induced visceral gout in reptiles receiving aminoglycosides such as gentamicin or other potentially nephrotoxic drugs, fluids must be given daily, at a dosage of 15 to 20 ml/kg.[3]

Frye recommends lactated Ringer's solution for parenteral fluid therapy in reptiles.[3] Marcus advises an electrolyte solution prepared from 8.1 g NaCl, 0.22 g KCl, 0.20 g $NaHCO_3$, and 0.20 g $CaCl_2$ dissolved in 1000 ml sterile distilled water.[4]

Tracheal Suctioning—An advanced respiratory infection in a reptilian pet generally has an unfavorable prognosis. The lack of a functional diaphragm in these species makes coughing impossible. Inability to expel tracheal and bronchial secretions can result in rapidly fatal lung consolidation.[3]

The author has successfully treated severe respiratory infections (characterized by copious secretions) in snakes using tracheal suctioning as a adjunct to antibiotic therapy and general supportive husbandry measures.

Aseptic technique, as for tracheostomy suctioning in a dog or cat, involves use of a sterile tracheal catheter and the wearing of sterile surgical gloves by the person introducing the catheter into the snake's trachea (Figure 8). Controlled suction is applied once the catheter has been rapidly advanced as far down the trachea as possible. The catheter is removed over 5 to 10 seconds as suction is applied, the snake is permitted to take several breaths, and the process is repeated several times until the volume of secretions removed diminishes. The procedure should be repeated as needed, as often as every six to eight hours for the first 3 to 7 days and once or twice daily for another 7 to 14 days.

Clinical Pathology

The technician with experience in clinical laboratory techniques on mammalian samples can and should extend such testing services to reptilian patients. The data generated will be very useful to the veterinarian in evaluating the patient. Blood samples from lizards and snakes can be placed in standard anticoagulants.

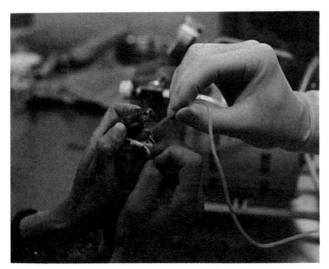

Figure 8—Tracheal suctioning of a snake with copious respiratory tract secretions.

Heparin should be used for turtle blood samples because other anticoagulants can cause hemolysis.[1]

The normal packed-cell volume (PCV) of the various reptile species ranges in general from 20 to 35%.[3] External factors that can influence the PCV include temperature, season, and stress.[3,4] Frye recommends the usual Romanowsky-type stains for blood smears, however, total erythrocyte and leukocyte counts require a different diluent than that used for mammalian blood.[3] Two main cell types in reptilian blood (nucleated erythrocytes and nucleated thrombocytes) necessitate the use of a special diluent, such as that recommended in Frye's text[3] or Shaw's avian solution,[12] and preclude the use of automated cell counters designed for analyzing mammalian samples. The color plates in Frye's textbook[3] will be helpful to the technician who is unfamiliar with reptilian blood-cell morphology. A large number of blood parasites have been identified in reptiles; many of these parasites are apparently of no clinical significance.[3,4]

Tables of reptilian blood chemistry values are provided in several texts and articles.[3,4,13-15] It is important to note that the plasma of certain species, e.g., iguanas and pythons, is normally orange or yellow because of the presence of certain pigments.[1]

Intestinal parasitism is common in reptiles. Droppings should be examined for protozoa and helminths by means of standard procedures, such as fecal flotation, wet preparations, and stained smears. It may be necessary to administer a saline enema to cause the expulsion of *Entamoeba* organisms in suspect cases with initially negative stool findings.[3] Life cycles and photographs of reptilian parasites are included in the texts by Frye and Marcus.[3,4] A good reference text is required because it can be difficult to differentiate between ova of prey species parasites and ova of reptilian parasites.

Microbiology

Reptiles are susceptible to infection by a wide variety of bacterial and fungal organisms.[3,4,16] Material for cultures and smears can be taken from skin lesions, droppings, oral cavity, trachea, and various organs during surgery or necropsy.

Routine laboratory procedures should include examination of Gram's-stained direct smears as well as smears stained for fungi. Routine procedures for bacteriologic and fungal cultures and antibiotic sensitivity testing can be used, but for some organisms special techniques are necessary for isolation and identification.[3,17,18]

A number of reptilian pathogens, e.g., *Salmonella* and *Aspergillus*, can infect humans. Therefore, when an infectious disease is suspected or a potential human pathogen has been isolated, it is advisable for persons handling the reptile or its infective secretions to wear gloves, a mask, and protective clothing.[3] Strict attention to hospital hygiene is essential to prevent the spread of contagious disease from one reptilian patient to another.

Radiography

Radiography is very important for the evaluation of bone problems.[3,19,20] In reptiles, a great deal of information about internal organs that cannot be obtained in these species by auscultation or palpation can be provided by radiographs. Radiographs have been useful in diagnosing the presence of embryos or eggs,[21,22] tumors,[3,23] thoracic trauma,[21] pneumonia,[3] visceral gout,[3] gastrointestinal foreign bodies,[3] and steatitis.[3]

A turtle can be restrained for radiography by simply tapping on its nose to induce retreat into the shell or by taping its legs inside the shell with adhesive tape. A method of immobilizing large chelonians for radiography involves placing the animal on its back in an automobile tire.[18] Gentle pressure on the eyelids usually quiets an iguana for a brief period.[3] Articles that can be used in the restraint of snakes and lizards include stockinette, cardboard tubes, and clear plastic tubes.

The average position of various internal organs for boas and pythons can be expressed as a precentage of the total length of the snake from nares to vent: 22 to 23% for the heart, 33 to 45% for the lung, 38 to 56% for the liver, 69 to 82% for the kidneys.[6]

Frye recommmends nonscreen film and exposure times of one-sixth to one-thirtieth second for most radiographic procedures on reptiles.[3] He cautions that this film is sensitive to even slight pressure, so care must be taken to avoid artifacts created by the animal's movements or during processing of the film.

Conclusion

The responsibilities of a veterinary technician with regard to a reptile and its owner are basically the same as those applicable to any animal patient. The technician should be able (1) to answer common questions about nutrition and husbandry, (2) to detect possible health problems during a telephone conversation, and (3) to provide good nursing care and laboratory services for the animal.

Because reptilian medicine is a relatively new field, the technician who desires improved skills in this area may have to spend extra time reviewing the literature and developing techniques for use in the hospital. Through enhancing the expertise of the veterinary health-care team in this area, the technician can better serve the reptile-owning clients of the practice.

Acknowledgment

The author is indebted to James Sikarskie, DVM, for his editorial assistance in the preparation of this manuscript and to Richard Walshaw, BVMS, MRCVS, Dawn Wienczkowski, LAT, and Gail Wolz, LAT, for taking the photographs that accompany this article.

REFERENCES

1. Fox M: Relationships between the human and non-human animals, in Fogle B (ed): *Interrelations between People and Pets.* Springfield, IL, Charles C Thomas, 1981, pp 23-40.
2. Levinson BM: *Pets and Human Development.* Springfield, IL, Charles C Thomas, 1972.
3. Frye FL: *Biomedical and Surgical Aspects of Captive Reptile Husbandry.* Edwardsville, KS, Veterinary Medicine Publishing Co, 1981.
4. Marcus LC: *Veterinary Biology and Medicine of Captive Amphibians and Reptiles.* Philadelphia, Lea & Febiger, 1981.
5. Kauffeld C: *Snakes: The Keeper and the Kept.* Garden City, NY, Doubleday, 1969.
6. Jackson OF: An introduction to the housing and treatment of snakes. *J Small Anim Pract* 18:479-491, 1977.
7. Jacobson ER: Diseases of reptiles. Part I. Noninfectious diseases. *Compend Contin Educ Pract Vet* 3(2):122-126, 1981.
8. Richter AG, et al: Techniques for collecting blood from Galapagos tortoises and box turtles. *VM SAC* 72:1376-1378, 1977.
9. Bush M, Smeller J: Blood collection and injection techniques in snakes. *VM SAC* 73(2):211-214, 1978.
10. Rosskopf WJ, Woerpel RW, Fudge A, Pitts BJ, Whittaker D: A practical method of performing venipuncture in snakes. *VM SAC* 77:820-821, 1982.
11. Sikarskie J: Personal communication, Michigan State University, 1982.
12. Otis VS: Leucocyte and erythrocyte diluent for reptilian blood cell counts. *Copeia* 1:252-254, March 28, 1974.
13. Gans C, Parson TS: *Biology of the Reptiles.* New York, Academic Press, 1970.
14. Rosskopf WJ, Woerpel RW, Yanoff SR: Normal hemogram and blood chemistry values for boa constrictors and pythons. *VM SAC* 77(5):822-823, 1982.
15. Chiodini RJ, Sundberg JP: Blood chemical values of the common boa constrictor *(Constrictor constrictor). Am J Vet Res* 43(9):1701-1702, 1982.
16. Jacobson ER: Diseases of reptiles. Part II. Infectious diseases. *Compend Contin Educ Pract Vet* 3(3):195-199, 1981.
17. Draper CS, Walker RD, Lawler HE: Patterns of oral bacterial infection in captive snakes. *JAVMA* 179(11):1223-1226, 1981.
18. Cambre RC, Green DE, Smith EE, Montali RJ, Bush M: Salmonellosis and arizonosis in the reptile collection at the national zoological park. *JAVMA* 177(9):800-803, 1980.
19. Crane SW, Curtis M, Jacobson ER, Webb A: Neutralization boneplating repair of a fractured humerus in a aldabra tortoise. *JAVMA* 177(9):945-948, 1980.
20. Robinson PT, Sedgwick CJ, Meier JE, Bacon JP: Internal fixation of a humeral fracture in a Komodo dragon lizard. *VM SAC* 73(5):645-649, 1978.
21. Jordan RD, Kyzar CT: Intra-abdominal removal of eggs from a gopher tortoise. *VM SAC* 73(8):1051-1054, 1978.
22. Shively MJ, Werner MB: What is your diagnosis? *JAVMA* 171(9):997-998, 1977.
23. Jacobson ER, Ackerman N: What is your diagnosis? *JAVMA* 179(11):1311-1312, 1981.
24. Robinson PT: Surgical repair of a herniated lung in a common iguana. *JAVMA* 163(6):655-656, 1973.

UPDATE

Veterinary technicians who work with or own reptiles will want to obtain more detailed information on nutrition, husbandry, and medical care from references including those listed below.

Suggested Reading

Text:
Frye FL: *Biomedical and Surgical Aspects of Captive Reptile Husbandry,* ed 2. Malabar, FL, Krieger Publishing Co, 1991.

Journal Articles:
Abrahams R: Housing reptiles in the veterinary hospital. *ARAV (Bulletin of the Association of Reptilian and Amphibian Veterinarians)* 3(1):6, 1993.
Barten SL: The medical care of iguanas and other common pet lizards. *Vet Clin North Am [Small Anim Pract]* 23(6):1213-1249, 1993.
Bennett RA: Reptilian surgery part I: basic principles. *Compend Contin Educ Pract Vet* 11(1):10-20, 1989.
Bennett RA: Reptilian surgery part II: management of surgical diseases. *Compend Contin Educ Pract Vet* 11(2):122-133, 1989.
Boyer TH: Common problems and treatment of green iguanas (Iguana iguana). *ARAV (Assoc Rept and Amph Vets)* 1(1):8-14, 1991.
Boyer TH: Common problems of box turtles (Terrapene spp) in captivity. *ARAV (Assoc Rept and Amph Vets)* 2(1):9-14, 1992.
Boyer TH: Box turtle care. *ARAV (Assoc Rept and Amph Vets)* 2(1):14-17, 1992.
Boyer TH: Clinical anesthesia of reptiles. *ARAV (Asoc Rept and Amph Vets)* 2(2):10-13, 1992.
Boyer TH, Boyer DM: Aquatic turtle care. *ARAV (Assoc Rept and Amph Vets)* 2(2):13-17, 1992.
Boyer DM, Boyer TH: Tortoise care. *ARAV (Assoc Rept and Amph Vets)* 4(1):16-28, 1994.
Innis C: Considerations in formulating captive tortoise diets. *ARAV (Assoc Rept and Amph Vets)* 4(1):8-12, 1994.
Jacobson E: Snakes. *Vet Clin North Am [Small Anim Pract]* 23(6):1179-1212, 1993.
Jenkins J: Medical management of reptile patients. *Compend Contin Educ Pract Vet* 13(6):980-988, 1991.
Johnson-Delaney CA: Potential zoonoses from nontraditional pets with particular attention to the immunosuppressed pet owner. *J Small Exotic Anim Med* 2(3):103-111, 1993.
Mader D: Cryptosporidiosis in reptiles. *J Small Exotic Anim Med* 2(3):141-142, 1993.
Mautino M, Page CD: Biology and medicine of turtles and tortoises. *Vet Clin North Am [Small Anim Pract]* 23(6):1251-1270, 1993.
Ness R: Reptilian drug dosages based on pharmacokinetic data. *J Small Exotic Anim Med* 1(3):109-110, 1992.
Russo EA: Diagnosis and treatment of lumps and bumps in snakes. *Compend Contin Educ Pract Vet* 9(8):795-806, 1987.
Smith C: Desert tortoise care. *ARAV (Assoc Rept and Amph Vets)* 4(1):12-15, 1994.
Wissman MA, Parsons B: Dermatophytosis of green iguanas (Iguana iguana). *J Small Exotic Anim Med* 2(3):137-140, 1993.
Wright KM: Captive husbandry of the Solomon Island prehensile-tailed skink. *Corucia zebrata. ARAV (Assoc Rept and Amph Vets)* 4(1):18-21, 1993.

An Introduction to Pet Iguanas

Thomas P. Ryan, DVM
Feathers, Scales and Tails Veterinary
 Hospital
Westminster, Maryland

The common iguana *(Iguana iguana)* belongs to the family of lizards called Iguanidae, of which there are about 600 species.[1] As a group, iguanas inhabit various environments ranging from the hot desert *(Callisaurus draconoides, Crotaphytus wislizenii, Uma notata)* to aquatic regions (the marine iguana *Amblyrhynchus cristatus*).[2]

Housing

Unfortunately, pet iguanas are often kept in environments totally inadequate for their needs. The housing area (usually a cage) should be spacious, with the proper amount of heat, light, and humidity. The area should be designed so that the owner can have easy access for cleaning and disinfecting.

Growth is rapid. With proper management, the growth rate is 30–60 cm/year with adult size reached in three years.[20] If an iguana is acclimated to a large cage, it can seriously injure itself if moved back into a smaller cage.

Floor Covering

The flooring of iguana cages can be constructed from many types of material. Artificial turf also has been recommended, primarily because it is pleasant in appearance and easy to clean and disinfect.[5] A disadvantage to gravel or dirtlike flooring is that the iguana may eat some of the flooring material; the substrate may provide a culture medium for pathogens. Some ingestion of grit by the iguana may be necessary, however, to enable normal digestion to occur.[5]

Habitat

The social interactions of the iguanas are perhaps the best documented of all the lizards.[6] In the wild, male iguanas (except *Phrynosoma* spp., *Anolis agassizi,* and *Crotaphytus wislizenii*) tend to be aggressive and territorial.[6] Territoriality and aggressiveness are influenced by the species, season, and geography; central portions of the home territory are defended, but tolerance of intruders may be shown at peripheral portions.[6] Defense of the home range is strongest during the breeding season.[7] In captivity, iguanas usually form dominance hierarchies, with subordinate

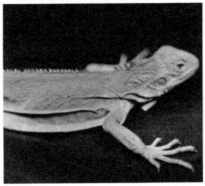

animals almost never attacking their superiors. If pet iguanas share housing, sufficient time, therefore, is necessary for adjustment to the habitat.[6] Branches and rocks for climbing should be placed in the habitat, with elevated locations for lookouts and display posts.[6,8] Iguanas, in non-breeding seasons, exhibit no defense of territories or other areas.[23]

A full spectrum light is recommended. It should produce ultraviolet B (UVB, erythemal, middlewave) in the 285nm–320nm band.[24,25] Lights that produce excessive UVB may cause fatal toxicity.[24] The Arizona-Sonoma Desert Museum uses 24″–48″ lights with one full spectrum light and one BL type *(not* BLB) black light bulb placed 8″–20″ above the animal's basking spot for 8–12 hours.[24]

Temperature

The following terminology is useful in understanding the temperature requirements of iguanas[9]:

- Activity temperature range—body temperature at which a free-ranging animal engages in its routine activities
- Critical thermal maximum—ambient temperature at which locomotor activity disintegrates and death occurs
- Critical thermal minimum—ambient temperature at which cold narcosis occurs and prevents locomotion
- Ectothermia—in cold-blooded animals, regulation of body temperature, which depends upon absorption of heat energy from the environment
- Heliothermia—solar regulation of body temperature (basking in the sun)
- Poikilothermia—variable body temperature
- Selected body temperature range—the body temperature maintained by an ectotherm in a laboratory temperature providing conditions that permit an animal

to extend its body temperature higher and lower than its mean activity temperature range.

Reptiles often voluntarily and actively seek lower ambient temperatures at night in order to lower the body temperature and rate of metabolism.[10,11] This allows iguanas to minimize the expenditure of energy at night and store energy for daily activity.[12] For captive reptiles, voluntary hypothermia and periodic inactivity may be essential for good health.[13] The mean activity temperature range for most iguanas (including *Iguana iguana*) is 30°C to 35°C.[2]

Reptiles maintain their body temperature by behavioral adaptation, such as moving between lighted areas and shade, burrowing, changing the contour of the body, and changing their orientation to the sun.[4,14] In captivity, heat can be provided by heating the rocks, installing thermal elements in the flooring, placing a heating pad underneath the cage, and installing a light (see the following discussion of photoperiod for proper use of lights).

Photoperiod

The photoperiod is the light–dark cycle. The concept of photoperiod is poorly understood by many iguana owners. Some owners depend solely upon light bulbs to serve as a source of heat and thus leave the lights on all the time. This usually results in the animal failing to thrive, which can eventually lead to death. Although light bulbs can serve as a source of heat, they must be used with caution, because light has a profound impact on the thermoregulatory behavior of iguanas.[2]

Iguanas and many other reptiles have extra optic photoreceptors, an example being the parietal eye, which is capable of sensing changes in the intensity and wavelength of incident light directly or through a modulating influence on brain centers that sense temperature.[2] The parietal-eye-pineal complex is an interrelated morphologic (and perhaps functional) set of structures developed in the roof of the diencephalon.[15]

The parietal-eye-pineal complex is important in the photosensory system of reptiles and probably is a major link between perception of light and thermoregulation,[2] with the pineal organ and parietal eye innervating different areas of the brain and thus affecting thermoregulation in different ways.[16]

If the parietal eye is damaged or covered, the reptile responds with increased thyroid activity as well as with behavioral changes, seeking higher environmental temperatures.[15] Therefore, at no time should iguanas (or other reptiles) be kept in a constantly lighted environment. Ideally, they should be exposed to light from 9:00 AM to 5:30 PM in the winter and from 8:00 AM to 9:00 PM in the summer.

Reproduction

Male iguanas can be differentiated from the females by the male's larger size, bigger head, higher dorsal crest of spines, swollen jowls, swollen tail base, 12 to 13 prominent femoral pores, and brighter overall coloration (especially during the breeding season).[3]

Behavior can be a guide to the sex of an individual. Males tend to display more than females and have slower, more pronounced head bobs often accompanied by a rolling side to side motion.

Sexing can be accomplished by probing. Individuals with a snout-to-vent length (the length of the body from the tip of the nose to the cloaca) of 100–125 mm, if a male, can be probed (use 1 mm probe) to 12 mm; females can be probed to 5 mm. Adult females can be probed to 15 mm and males up to 50 mm. In large males, the hemipenes may actually be visible as two large bulges just behind the cloaca.

Iguanas are not commonly bred in captivity.[3] Eggs reportedly hatch after 80 to 81 days in an environment of 30°C.[3,8]; other reports claim an incubation period of 90 days.[24] Forty eggs are usually laid.[24] Breeding is seasonally annual with mating taking place in the male territories 3–7 weeks before nesting.[19] Ovideposition takes place during the driest part of the season.[19] Eggs are laid in burrows and incubated at 30°C; high mortality in eggs occurs at a few degrees above and below 30°C.[19] During breeding season, male iguanas have been reported to attack their female (human) owners in an attempt to mate with them.[21] These male iguanas are usually hand-raised and imprinted on people.[21]

Iguana iguana reportedly does not feed for the first six days after hatching, although it is very active during this time.[17] During this period, the supplemental energy source is believed to be derived from the yolk before hatching occurs.[8] In reptiles, this period of yolk utilization is short and possibly allows time for the hatchling to perfect locomotive and feeding skills.[8] The juvenile growth rate of *Iguana iguana* is from 0.25 to 0.6 mm/day.[8] The life span is up to 20 years. Coprophagia is necessary in order to establish normal intestinal flora.

Communication

Social communication signals are primarily visual instead of auditory or olfactory. Head bobs, nods, pushups, extension of the dewlap and gular region, raising of the mid-dorsal crest, and movement of the tongue and tail are used for both local and long-distance communication.[8,10,19,22,23,24]

Diet

Many (if not most) of pet iguana problems seen by the practitioner can be traced directly to diet. Many pet shops and owners feed iguanas a diet of lettuce and mealworms; this is totally inadequate and can result in death. The diet of an iguana must be adequate in protein, carbohydrates, lipids, vitamins, and minerals as well as be sufficient in quantity. The food requirements differ with growth stage and age, with many juvenile iguanas eating relatively more animal matter than adult iguanas do. Generally, otogenic changes probably reflect the need of growing individuals for more protein. An iguana chow has been developed in a joint project between the Green Iguana Management Project and the National Zoo in Washington, D.C.[23]

Medical Problems

Most problems encountered in veterinary practice are related to incorrect diet and/or environment. The most common problems seen are: metabolic bone disease; parasites (especially pinworms); fractures (often diet-related); skin abscesses from wounds, running into the side of the tank or infections (bacteria, acid-fast organisms, metazoan parasites, fungi); sebaceous cysts in the tail; retained eggs; kidney disease (glomerulonephritis, gout); cystic calculi; and avascular necrosis of toes due to constriction of the toe by a strip of retained, non-molted skin.

REFERENCES

1. Pianka ER: Reptilian species diversity, in Gans C, Tinkle DW (eds): *Biology of the Reptilia. Ecology and Behavior A*, vol 7. New York, Academic Press, 1977, pp 1–34.
2. Avery RA: Field studies of body temperatures, in Gans C, Pough FH (eds): *Biology of the Reptilia. Physiology C— Physiological Ecology*, vol 12. New York, Academic Press, 1982, pp 93–166.
3. Howard CJ: Notes on the maintenance and breeding of the common iguana (*Iguana iguana*) at Twycross Zoo, in *British Herpetelogical Society Proceedings: The Care and Breeding of Captive Reptiles*. London, England, British Herpetelogical Society, 1980, pp 47–50.
4. Frye FL: *Biomedical and Surgical Aspects of Captive Reptile Husbandry*. Edwardsville, KS, Veterinary Medicine Publishing Co, 1981.
5. Sokol OM: Lithography and geography in reptiles. *J Herpetol* 5:69–70, 1971.
6. Stamps JA: Social behavior and spacing patterns in lizards, in Gans C, Tinkle DW (eds): *Biology of the Reptilia. Ecology and Behavior A*, vol 7. New York, Academic Press, 1977, pp 265–334.
7. Muller H: Okophysiologische und ethologische studien and *Iguana iguana* in Kolumbien. *Zool Beit* 18(1):109–131, 1972.
8. Licht P, Moberlý WR: Thermal requirements for embryonic development in the tropical lizard—*Iguana iguana*. *Copeia* 4:515–517, 1965.
9. Pough FH, Gans C: The vocabulary of reptilian thermoregulation, in Gans C, Pough FH (eds): *Biology of the Reptilia. Physiology C—Physiological Ecology*, vol 12. New York, Academic Press, 1982, pp 17–23.
10. Regal PJ: Voluntary hypothermia in reptiles. *Science* 155:1551–1553, 1967.
11. Cowgell J, Underwood H: Behavioral thermoregulation in lizards: A circadian rhythm. *J Exp Zool* 210:189–194, 1979.
12. Bartholomew GA: Physiological control of body temperature, in Gans C, Pough FH (eds): *Biology of the Reptilia. Physiology C—Physiological Ecology*, vol 12. New York, Academic Press, 1982, pp 167–211.
13. Huey RB: Temperature physiology and ecology of reptiles, in Gans C, Pough FH (eds): *Biology of the Reptilia. Physiology C—Physiological Ecology*, vol 12. New York, Academic Press, 1982, pp 25–91.
14. Firth BT, Turner JS: Sensory, neural and hormonal aspects of thermoregulation, in Gans C, Pough FH (eds): *Biology of the Reptilia. Physiology C—Physiological Ecology*, vol 12. New York, Academic Press, 1982, pp 213–274.
15. Quay WB: The parietal eye–pineal complex, in Gans C, Northcutt RG, Ulinski P (eds): *Biology of the Reptilia. Neurology A*, vol 9. New York, Academic Press, 1979, pp 245–406.
16. Ralph CL, Firth BT, Turner JS: The role of the pineal body in ectotherm thermoregulation. *Am J Zool* 19:273–293, 1979.
17. Andrews RM: Patterns of growth in reptiles, in Gans C, Pough FH (eds): *Biology of the Reptilia. Physiology D—Physiological Ecology*, vol 12. New York, Academic Press, 1982, pp 273–320.
18. Evans LT: Structure as related to behavior in the organization of populations in reptiles, in Blair WF (ed): *Vertebrate Speciation*. Austin, TX, University of Texas Press, 1961, pp 148–178.
19. Wiewandt TA: Evolution of nesting patterns in iguanine lizards. *Iguana Times*, 1993, 2, 4, pp 2–19.
20. Boyer TH: Green iguana care. *AARV*, 1991, 1, 1, pp 12–14.
21. Frye FL, Mader D, Centofani BV: Interspecific (lizard:human) sexual aggression in captive iguanas (*Iguana iguana*). *AARV*, 1991, 1, 1, pp 4–11.
22. Rodda G: The mating behavior of *Iguana iguana*. *Iguana Times*, 1993, 2, 2, pp 2–16.
23. Bodri MS: El manejo de la iguana verde: A look at Dr. Dagmar Werner's Breeding Project. *Vivarium*, 1993, 2, 2, pp 7–9.
24. Bodri MS: Use of full spectrum ultraviolet lighting at the Arizona-Sonoma Desert Museum. *Iguana Times*, 1994, 3, 1, p 11.
25. Gehrmann WH: Spectral characteristics of lamps commonly used in herpetoculture. *Vivarium*, 1994, 5, 5, pp 16–21.

Amphibian Husbandry and Medical Care

Terry W. Campbell, DVM, PhD
Sea World of Florida, Inc.
Orlando, Florida

The term *amphibian* is derived from the Greek word *amphibios*, which means double life—a reference to the two-stage life cycle of this class of animals. Familiar amphibians include frogs, toads, salamanders, and newts. Most adult amphibians are terrestrial; however, the eggs are laid in water and the larvae are aquatic. The larvae undergo metamorphosis, a process that involves the transformation of the body structure and most organs. During the metamorphosis, the mouth changes to adapt to different food, the gills are replaced by lungs for breathing air, and the eyes and other organs change to adapt to terrestrial life.

Terrestrial amphibians breathe in part through their skin, which is moist and contains a protective slime produced by mucous glands. In some instances, the slime may be poisonous to predators, as with the poison arrow frog of South America. Toads and frogs have special parotid glands behind the eyes that produce a milky, noxious or poisonous secretion. Secretions from the parotid gland of the marine toad (*Bufo marinus*) and the Colorado River toad (*Bufo alvarius*) contain a cardioactive glycoside (bufotoxin) that can be lethal to dogs. Amphibians periodically shed a thin layer of skin, which usually comes off in one piece and is eaten by the animal.

The collection and maintenance of amphibians are regulated by state laws; special permits may be required to possess native amphibians. Importation of amphibians into the United States is restricted by state and federal laws. Species commonly kept as pets are listed in the box.

Orders of Amphibia

The class Amphibia consists of three orders. Order Salientia (the anurans) includes frogs and toads; order Urodela (the caudates) includes salamanders, newts, and sirens; and order Gymnophiona (the apodans) includes rare legless, burrowing amphibians of the tropics. Approximately 2700 species of frogs and toads and 350 species of salamanders are known to exist worldwide.

The anurans have special skeletal adaptations that allow them to jump and hop. They have a short spine, short forelimbs, long hindlimbs, and a specialized pelvis. All adult frogs can swim. True frogs (ranids) have webbing between the toes of the hind feet; tree frogs have pads on the tips of the toes for clinging to leaves.

Most adult frogs and toads have no teeth in the lower jaw. They do, however, have large mouths and modified tongues for capturing prey. The feeding response is triggered by the prey's movement. Larval anurans (tadpoles) have mouth parts adapted for scraping algae off surfaces or for filtering water. The intestinal tract of a tadpole is long to allow digestion of vegetation.

Adult anurans have a Jacobson organ, a specialized smell–taste organ located in the nasal passages, which provides a keen sense of smell. Tadpoles, like fish, have chemoreceptors in the lateral line that are receptive to chemicals in the water. Also like fish, tadpoles have eyes that are adapted to aquatic life. Adult frogs and toads have eyes that are adapted for terrestrial life. The

Amphibian Species Commonly Kept as Pets

Bullfrog (*Rana catesbeiana*)
Clawed frogs (*Xenopus* species)
European green tree frog (*Hyla arborea*)
Green toad (*Bufo viridis*)
Green tree frog (*Hyla cinerea*)
Grey tree frog (*Hyla versicolor*)
Japanese fire-bellied newt (*Cynops pyrrhogaster*)
Northern leopard frog (*Rana pipiens*)
Red-bellied newt (*Taricha rivularis*)
Oriental fire-bellied toad (*Bombina orientalis*)
Red-spotted newt (*Notopthalmus viridescens*)
Southern toad (*Bufo terrestris*)
Tiger salamander (*Ambystoma tigrinum*)
Woodhouse's toad (*Bufo woodhousei*)

eyes are large, with slit pupils that are sensitive to light and to movement and that are effective at low light and for night vision. Adult frogs and toads also have a keen sense of hearing. The outer ear is a large, circular membrane (called a tympanum) that is located just behind the eye.

The caudates, unlike the anurans, have long bodies with numerous vertebrae. Salamanders do not have rib cages; their ribs are short and fused to the vertebrae. Specialized bones, called girdles, support the legs. The legs, which are short and extend away from the body, are too weak to lift the body during locomotion.

Salamander larvae have feather-like external gills and four legs. At several weeks of age, the larvae metamorphose into adults that have lungs rather than gills.

The senses of sight, smell, and touch are apparently well developed in salamanders. Aquatic salamanders have small eyes that do not protrude far above the skull; the small bulging eyes of terrestrial salamanders do protrude.

Adult and larval aquatic salamanders catch their prey by sucking it into the mouth. Adult salamanders usually are motionless until the prey approaches; then, stimulated by the prey's movement, the salamander grabs the food.

Care Requirements

Successfully maintaining amphibians in captivity depends on proper attention to temperature, humidity, diet, photoperiod, and housing. To ensure the best care for the pet, the owner of an amphibian should read as much as possible about the natural history of the animal before obtaining it. An attempt should be made to create a captive environment that closely resembles the animal's natural environment.

All amphibians rely on their environment and movements to regulate body temperature. Many species are active at or can tolerate temperatures of 4°C to 28°C (39.2°F to 82.4°F). The body temperature of an active amphibian tends to be lower than that of an active reptile because amphibians, which are active at night or live in microenvironments that are protected from sunlight, do not use the sun for thermoregulation. When temperatures are too low or too high, amphibians become inactive. Although some amphibians are able to change color in response to background color change, such transformation tends to occur in response to temperature: the animal becomes darker if the temperature drops or if the period of exposure to light shortens; it becomes lighter if the temperature or the period of exposure to light increases. A dull appearance to the skin may indicate an unhealthy amphibian.

Aquarium heaters can be used to maintain proper water temperature for aquatic cages; heating the terrestrial cage can be difficult unless it is kept in a room where the temperature is constant. Common methods of warming terrestrial cages include the use of heating pads, cables, or lamps. Horticultural soil-warming cables and heating pads can be used to heat the vivarium. For even heat distribution, soil warmers require sand, soil, or gravel on the cage floor; each product has a recommended depth of material to cover the heater. A barrier is suggested to prevent burrowing (fossorial) species from reaching the heat source.

High humidity is essential for the proper maintenance of amphibians. They should be housed in vivaria that provide aquatic and terrestrial environments. Clean water should be always available. With water constantly present, the humidity level is directly related to temperature and the amount of ventilation. If the temperature is held constant by a thermostat, humidity can then be regulated by the amount of ventilation provided.

The nutritional requirements of amphibians are unknown; most are fed diets based on knowledge of the animal's natural diet. Larval amphibians are herbivorous and feed primarily on algae; adult amphibians are carnivorous. Most captive adult amphibians should be fed twice weekly. Live food is usually necessary because feeding is stimu-

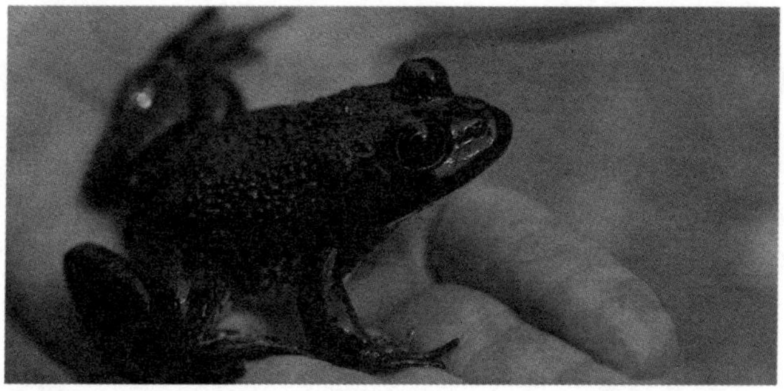

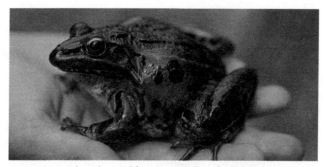
Figure 1—Bullfrog (*Rana catesbeiana*).

Figure 2—Southern leopard frog (*Rana sphenocephala*).

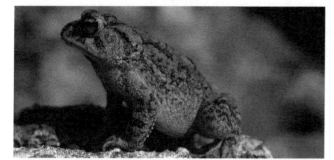
Figure 3—Southern toad (*Bufo terristris*).

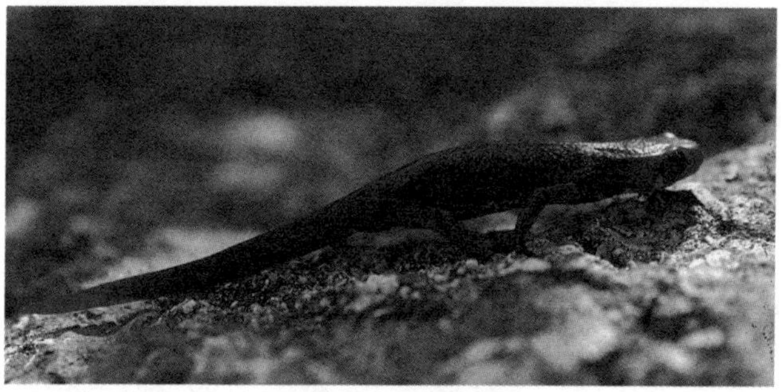

Figure 4—Red-bellied newt (*Taricha rivularis*).

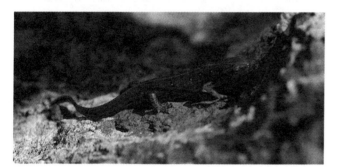
Figure 5—Eastern or red-spotted newt (*Notophthalmus viridescens*).

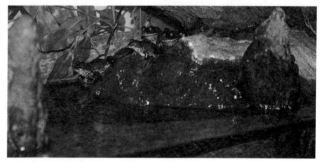
Figure 6—An amphibian habitat that provides an aquatic and terrestrial environment.

lated by the movement of the prey. Some species eventually learn to eat dead prey or prepared foods.

All frogs and toads are predators as adults and feed on invertebrates, primarily insects. Captive frogs and toads eat fruit flies, crickets, mealworms, and other live insects. Large toads eat mice. Aquatic species eat aquatic insects, earthworms, fish, and commercially prepared fish diets. Raw meat can be fed to amphibians, but it requires calcium supplementation—powdered calcium carbonate added at a ratio of 10 milligrams per gram of meat is recommended.

Adult terrestrial salamanders eat earthworms, slugs, insects, and commercially prepared fish diets. Aquatic salamanders can be fed tubifex worms, water fleas, freshwater shrimp, insect larvae, and earthworms. One species of earthworm commonly sold as fish bait is apparently toxic to salamanders. This earthworm, often referred to as a manure worm, is dark red with thin yellow bands near the caudal end.

In regard to the lighting requirements of amphibians, full-spectrum light bulbs are recommended if artificial light is used. The distance from the light source to the animals is an important consideration; for example, artificial light originating 60 centimeters from the cage floor provides only one quarter of the amount of light as the same source positioned 30 centimeters from the cage floor.

A natural photoperiod is best. Amphibians from temperate zones are accustomed to light cycles that vary from 16 hours in the summer to 8 hours in the winter.

Overcrowding should be avoided. Providing a hiding place is important; most amphibians are more likely to thrive if they can hide in or under objects in the cage or have access to soil or sand for burrowing. Aquatic amphibians should be kept in aquaria under conditions suitable for freshwater fish.

Diseases

Amphibians are subjected to a variety of diseases, the most common of which are bacterial and fungal infections, parasitic diseases, toxicities, and neoplasia. Clinical signs include dull color, lethargy, unresponsiveness to tactile stimulation, anorexia, weight loss, edematous limbs, neurologic disorders, and erosions on the head and limbs. Most of the health problems seen in pet amphibians (as with most exotic pets) result from environmental problems associated with poor husbandry practices; therefore, an assessment of the environmental conditions should always be a part of an examination.

A variety of bacteria can cause infection; *Aeromonas* species are most often isolated. Local bacterial infections can spread rapidly and result in fatal septicemia within 24 to 48 hours. Hyperemia, cutaneous hemorrhage (hemorrhage in the skin of the abdomen and appendages of frogs is known as red-leg disease), anorexia, depression, and dulling of the body color are common clinical signs.

Treatment of local and systemic bacterial infections in amphibians involves the use of a variety of antibiotics. Oral tetracycline given at a dosage of 0.16 mg/g twice a day has been recommended. One-hour dips using 50 milligrams of gentamicin per gallon of water or 250 milligrams of nifurpirinol per 10 gallons of water have also been suggested. Increasing the salinity of the water to a maximum of 0.6% may be helpful in aquatic species. Parenteral antibiotics, such as Amikacin given intramuscularly at a dose of 2.5 mg/kg every 72 hours have also been used in amphibians. The use of any medication in amphibians is dependent upon the environmental conditions. Therefore, an amphibian undergoing treatment should be housed under optimal environmental conditions to maximize the effect of the therapy.

Fungal infections often occur on wound sites and abrasions; such infections may appear as white, fluffy patches on the skin. Treatment may include a 2% malachite green bath for 30 to 60 minutes or a five-minute potassium permanganate (1:5000) bath. Systemic antifungal agents may be used on amphibians with systemic mycoses.

Aquatic amphibians are susceptible to the same cutaneous protozoa as are fish. Treatment regimens are the same as for fish. Although they may harbor a variety of internal parasites, amphibians rarely exhibit clinical signs of illness associated with such parasites. Ivermectin given orally or subcutaneously at a dose of 0.2 to 0.4 mg/kg has proven safe and effective in the treatment of nematode infestations in some amphibians. Fenbendazole used at an oral dose of 30 to 50 mg/kg is effective against intestinal nematodes in some species. Substances poisonous to amphibians include pesticides and excessive chlorine and copper in the water. Commercially available aquarium water test kits can be used to monitor the water quality of the amphibian habitat.

Conclusion

The goal of this article has been to provide the veterinarian and the veterinary technician with a general understanding of amphibians. Amphibians are kept by hobbyists, educational institutions, research facilities, and zoological parks. Although they are not a large part of the exotic animal practice, amphibians are occasionally presented for veterinary care. Veterinarians or technicians participating in wildlife rehabilitation efforts may also encounter amphibian patients. Amphibians can be cherished pets and can live for several years (adult anurans usually reach sexual maturity at one or two years of age) if proper attention is given to their environmental and nutritional needs.

BIBLIOGRAPHY

Ashton RE, Ashton PS: *Handbook of Reptiles and Amphibians of Florida. Part 3. The Amphibians.* Miami, FL, Windward Publishing, 1988.

Crawshaw GJ: Amphibian medicine, in Fowler ME (ed): *Zoo and Wild Animal Medicine, Current Therapy 3.* Philadelphia, WB Saunders Co, 1993, pp 131–139.

Fowler ME: Amphibians, in Fowler ME (ed): *Zoo and Wild Animal Medicine.* Philadelphia, WB Saunders Co, 1986, pp 100–105.

Mattison C: *The Care of Reptiles and Amphibians in Captivity.* London, Blandford Press, 1987.

Care and Handling of Pet Fish*

Gregory A. Lewbart, MS, VMD
**Department of Companion Animal
and Special Species Medicine
College of Veterinary Medicine
North Carolina State University
Raleigh, North Carolina**

The keeping of ornamental fish is a very popular hobby in the United States and abroad. Millions of dollars are spent each year on tropical fish, food, and aquarium supplies. Hundreds of species of freshwater and marine fish are currently kept by hobbyists. Some of these fish may be purchased for pennies, whereas others may be worth thousands of dollars. Regardless of cost, the need for an adequate life-sustaining aquarium system is one element that all fish have in common.

Death of recently acquired fish as a result of poor tank design, mismanaged water quality, and general ignorance of the hobbyist is all too common. Many people must learn the hard way about proper aquarium management and fish husbandry. How does the veterinary technician fit into this picture? The situation could be likened to avian medicine. Ten or fifteen years ago it was very difficult for bird owners to find a veterinarian that would treat their bird (unless it was a chicken or turkey). Now nearly every city has at least one veterinary clinic that specializes in exotic animals, many of which are psittacine birds.

Currently, many people believe that there is a promising future for veterinary care and treatment of pet tropical fish. Veterinary technicians that are familiar with aquarium management and the health requirements of ornamental fish will be very marketable. Many of today's veterinary technicians are comfortable handling birds and reptiles—trimming nails and beaks and processing laboratory samples for these animals are routine for some technicians. Very soon, it is likely that just as many technicians will be able to test aquarium water, correct aquarium flaws, give helpful advice to clients, and maintain hospitalized or boarded tropical fish.

A trained and knowledgeable veterinary technician will be able to provide knowledgeable information to inquiring clients. This information can be acquired through continuing education, hobby publications, veterinary textbooks, hands-on experience, and the local library.

Because there is no better teacher than personal experience, I encourage technicians who are seriously interested in learning more about tropical fish to set up their own home aquarium. This article highlights important considerations to enable technicians to accomplish the task. I also hope that technicians will, in turn, be better able to provide clients with information for maintaining a prosperous home aquarium.

Setting Up the Home Aquarium

A complete list of components needed to set up a home aquarium is listed in the box. The first consideration of setting up an aquarium is the size and shape of the tank as well as of what material it is constructed. Many beginning hobbyists decide to set up large aquariums after seeing similar tanks that are kept in business establishments. Such tanks are usually very costly, complex to maintain, and must be serviced by a professional aquarium maintenance company.

*This article was adapted from the 1993 TNAVC Veterinary Technician Proceedings, "Setting Up the Home Aquarium," and "Diseases of Pet Fish," and has been modified with permission.

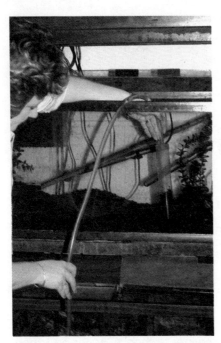

Figure 1—An aquarist is shown cleaning gravel with a special siphon that removes dirt and toxins while cleaning and redistributing the gravel bed. This practice is fast, clean, and only needs to be done every one or two months.

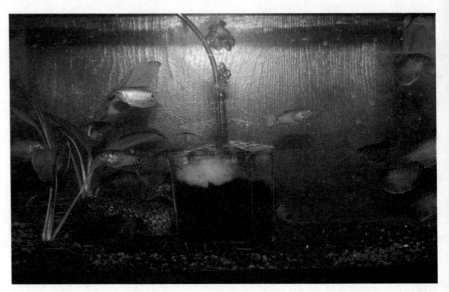

Figure 2—The filtration in this tank containing gold gouramis is accomplished by an old-fashioned box filter that contains floss to remove particulate matter and activated charcoal to remove ammonia and other toxins. State-of-the-art power filters and undergravel filters have largely replaced these unsightly yet effective filters.

The Tank

For beginning hobbyists, I recommend a rectangular glass tank that is 10 to 30 gallons in size. Such tanks are relatively inexpensive and easy to handle (one person can lift them), and the other necessary equipment (e.g., filters, pumps, and heaters) is also reasonably priced. At a retail pet store, a complete 20-gallon freshwater tank setup with high-quality components and other accessories (including a few tropical fish) costs approximately $150 to $200. Ten-gallon setups are approximately 20% less, and 30-gallon setups are approximately 30% more. Bargain specials should be avoided because components are likely to be of poor quality.

After the tank has been purchased, the aquarist should decide whether the tank needs a stand or whether it can rest on an existing piece of furniture. This is not an especially important consideration; however, regard-less of where the tank is kept, the supporting furniture must be sturdy and strong. A gallon of water weighs eight pounds; thus, a 20-gallon tank with glass, filters, hood, lights, heater, and gravel could easily weigh more than 180 pounds.

The type of filtration to be used is the next consideration. I recommend a good undergravel filter (also known as a biological filter because there are no chemicals or sponges). Such filters are rather simple in design. They consist of a perforated plastic plate that lies at the bottom of the aquarium. The filter is raised from the base by approximately $1/2$ inch to allow water to pass freely under the plastic panel. After the filter has been placed in the tank, approximately two to three inches of gravel (consisting of stones that are $1/8$ to $1/5$ inch in diameter) (Figure 1) is placed on top of the plastic grating. The plastic is usually fitted with two ports for air-lift tubes. Care should be taken to prevent gravel from entering these openings. At this point, the tank may be filled with water.

The air pump is a very important consideration because it is the life support system for the fish, and cheap ones can kill the fish. Air pumps are portable and quiet. Air is forced by means of a rubber diaphragm into small-diameter air lines that are connected to the lift tubes. Numerous air bubbles travel down the lift tubes and return to the surface, thereby drawing water from the bottom of the tank. This air bubble–water flow system establishes a circulation pattern that aerates the water and passes some of the water through the gravel filter bed. Over time (ranging from minutes to hours), all of the water in the aquarium has passed through the gravel filter. Nitrifying bacteria are special types of bacteria that colonize the small stones in the gravel. Through a two-step process, these bacteria convert toxic ammonia (produced by the animals in the tank) into a safer chemical known as nitrate. This process is similar to what happens naturally in streams and rivers.

Some aquarists like to supplement

Components of a Complete 20-Gallon Aquarium System

Twenty-gallon rectangular glass tank

Good-quality heater and air pump with two outlets

Undergravel filter

Fifteen feet of air tubing

Two to three inches of gravel to cover undergravel filter

Fluorescent light with hood

Thermometer (inside- or outside-tank variety)

Airstones for air tubing into lift tubes

Water conditioner-dechlorinator

Tank cleaning equipment (siphon hose and sponge)

Net

Fish food

Optional Components:

Real or artificial plants, tank decorations, and background paper

Aquarium stand

Outside-tank power filter

Automatic feeder

Important Questions for the Pet Fish Owner

How long have you been keeping tropical fish?

What are the problems with the fish?

When did you first notice these problems?

How long have you owned the fish? From where was it obtained?

Does the sick fish share a tank with other fish?

Have you noticed signs of illness in the other fish?

How large is the tank? How is it heated, lighted, and filtered?

Have you treated the fish with any medication?

Have you changed the water recently?

Have you tested the quality of the water? If so, what were your findings?

Could the fish have been exposed to any toxins, such as pesticides?

What and how often do you feed the fish?

an undergravel filter with a motorized power filter (Figure 2) or use a power filter alone. These filters contain a small electric motor that usually drives a magnetized propeller, thereby creating a flow of water from the tank, through the filter, and back into the tank. Power filters circulate and aerate the water while removing toxic waste materials through a chemical-absorbing substance, such as activated carbon (material similar to that used to treat dogs that have ingested various toxins). The carbon is usually housed in a spongelike matrix that helps re-move suspended particles in the water. These packets can be cleaned and reused two or three times but should eventually be replaced.

An undergravel filter alone may be sufficient for tanks containing only a few fish. Tanks with more fish may require supplemental filtration. Other types of filtration that are less frequently used (because of their cost and complexity) include ultraviolet filters, ozone filters, wet–dry biological filtration, diatom filters, and canister filters. Such intricate filtration systems are usually unnecessary in a smaller freshwater aquarium.

Lighting is important not only for aesthetic reasons but also to simulate natural photoperiods for the fish. I recommend a fluorescent lamp that is built into an attractive hood. Such hoods are easy to install and allow easy access into the aquarium for feeding, temperature adjusting, and tank cleaning. Cheap incandescent lights should be avoided, as they give off too much heat, cause stress to the fish, and burn out quickly.

A good heater with the proper wattage is essential to any aquarium. A knowledgeable employee of a local pet shop can probably recommend how strong the heater should be, based on the size of the tank. Nearly all heaters have a built-in thermostat; thermometers therefore are important for monitoring water temperature. For tropical fish, the temperature of the water should be between 76°F and 82°F.

Decorating the aquarium is a matter of personal taste, but a few suggestions should be made. Plastic plants serve as good decorations because the fish cannot eat them and they do not carry disease (unless they are transferred from one tank to another). Live plants are preferred by many aquarists and can make the aquarium very attractice. Disadvantages of live plants include the potential for disease transfer and inability to thrive with undergravel filters. Because most fish are territorial, they should be provided a place to hide within the tank.

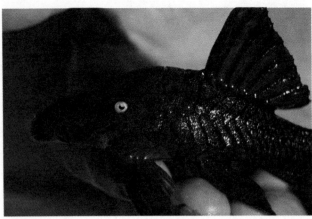

Figure 3A

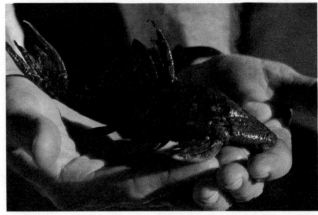

Figure 3B

Figure 3—**(A)** A healthy blue-eyed plecostomus, *Panaque suttoni*. Note the bright blue eyes, shiny moist skin, and even fin margins. **(B)** A very sick blue-eyed plecostomus. This fish has protozoal parasites and was kept in poor-quality water. Note the sunken, dull eyes; eroded dorsal and tail fins; and splotchy appearance to the skin. Fish in this condition have a poor prognosis for survival.

After the tank has been set up, the water must be prepared. I add a conditioner to the water to remove chlorine and chloramine (two toxins found in most municipal water supplies), even if the water has been left standing for several days and is supposedly free of these chemicals. A knowledgeable pet store employee can assist in selecting an adequate conditioner.

The Fish

Fish can usually be placed in the tank within minutes after the water has been conditioned. A couple of hardy fish will start the biological filter (establishment of the nitrifying bacteria usually takes three to four weeks). Patience is important—only a few fish should be added at a time after the tank has become established. Ideally, all new fish should be quarantined in a separate tank for two weeks and observed for any signs of disease before being added to the display tank.

Most commercially prepared fish foods are adequate; however, the food must be fresh for the nutrients (including fats) and vitamins to remain potent. Buying smaller cans of

fish food helps ensure that the food does not become stale; some cans may have expiration dates. It is also advisable to store fish food in the freezer to help preserve the nutrients and vitamins.

I strongly recommend that any technician interested in working with tropical fish subscribe to one of the monthly hobbyist magazines. These publications include informative articles as well as listings for books, supplies, and sources of information. Three of these publications are *Tropical Fish Hobbyist* (Neptune City, New Jersey), *Freshwater and Marine Aquarium* (Sierra Madre, California), and *Aquarium Fish Magazine* (Mission Viejo, California).

Diseases of Pet Fish

When fish are placed in an aquarium or a man-made pond, the aquarist is trying to simulate nature. The closer the man-made system comes to the natural situation, the more the fish will thrive. When dealing with the problems of fish disease, veterinary technicians must remind themselves that closed aquatic systems present special problems that may not occur with terrestrial exotic

or domesticated animals. It is far easier for humans to escape from toxins than it is for fish—fish live, breathe, eat, breed, and excrete waste into the environment that surrounds them. Some pet fish may spend their entire lives (which may be as long as 10 years) in only 10 gallons of water.

For these reasons, water quality is of utmost importance. Most commonly observed pet fish diseases can be traced directly to poor water quality or stress resulting from poor husbandry practices. The box lists important questions to ask clients with sick fish. Poor water quality may result from toxins or high levels of ammonia, improper pH, and insufficient levels of dissolved oxygen; water that is too hot or too cold will also be detrimental to the health of the fish. When fish seem to be sick or are dying, a primary water quality problem must be ruled out. Water-quality test kits that are easy to use and relatively inexpensive are commercially available.

If poor water quality is ruled out, other forms of stress must be considered. Overcrowding, incompatible species, inadequate nutrition, and excessive lighting stress pet fish.

Bacterial Disease

Bacterial diseases of pet fish are frequently encountered. Most bacterial pathogens of fish are gram negative and usually belong to one of the following genera: *Aeromonas, Pseudomonas, Flexibacter,* and *Vibrio.* Although less common, two gram-positive bacterial pathogens to be aware of are *Mycobacterium* and *Streptococcus.* Microbiological culture and sensitivity tests can be done on fish in the same manner as for terrestrial animals. One difference is that bacteria are always present in water and on the external surfaces of fish, and these bacteria are not necessarily pathogenic. In fact, some species of *Aeromonas* are facultative pathogens that only affect fish that are stressed and/or immunocompromised. Fish with bacterial diseases may have red or sloughing fins, sloughing skin, or may show no clinical signs except acute death. Sterile blood or kidney samples submitted for culture and sensitivity will provide the most informative results.

Fungal Disease

Fungal skin lesions are common on pet fish; however, diagnosis must be confirmed microscopically because parasitic and bacterial disease can grossly resemble fungal skin disease. *Saprolegnia* is a common fungal pathogen, although it is rarely the primary cause of disease. Disorders caused by this fungus usually occur when damage has been done to the mucus layer that covers the skin and fins of the fish. If the lesion is not severe, most fish recover with supportive care and the fungal tuft eventually sloughs into the water.

Parasitic Disease

A wide range of parasites affect pet fish. Some are internal (endoparasites), and others are external (ectoparasites). Many of the endoparasites are worms (helminths), and some are closely related to parasites found in dogs and cats. Many of these parasites can be treated with the same oral parasiticides used on domesticated mammals. Fecal examinations can be done on pet fish, and helminth eggs found in the stool sample aid in diagnosis and treatment.

A large number of parasites that affect pet fish are ectoparasitic and endoparasitic protozoans (Figure 3); some protozoans fall into both categories. Disease caused by protozoans is most common in wholesale fish or fish purchased from farming operations. In addition to helminths and protozoans, freshwater and marine fish are sometimes affected by crustaceans and segmented worms (leeches). In suspected cases of parasitic infection, the compound microscope is the technician's best diagnostic tool.

Conclusion

Educating clients on the best ways to control water quality and reduce stress in an aquarium is the first step toward keeping fish disease free. Through first-hand knowledge gained from setting up a home aquarium, the veterinary technician can play an important role in this area of preventive medicine.

BIBLIOGRAPHY

Beleau MB: Evaluating water problems. *Vet Clin North Am Small Anim Pract* 18(2): 293–304, 1988.

Gratzek JB: *Aquariology: The Science of Fish Health Management.* Morris Plains, NJ, Tetra Sales USA, 1992.

Hawkins AD: *Aquarium Systems.* New York, Academic Press, 1981.

Lewbart GA: Emergency care for the tropical fish patient. *J Small Exotic Anim Med* 1(1):38–42, 1991.

Lewbart GA: Medical management of disorders of freshwater tropical fish. *Compend Contin Educ Pract Vet* 13(6):969–977, 1991.

Lewbart GA: Water quality and chemistry for tropical fish. *J Small Exotic Anim Med* 1(2):79–85, 1991.

Noga EJ: Diseases and treatment of freshwater fish. *Proc North Am Vet Conf* 6:627–629, 1992.

Schneider E: *All About Aquariums.* Neptune, NJ, TFH Publications, 1982.

Spotte S: *Captive Seawater Fishes.* New York, John Wiley & Sons, Inc., 1992.

Stoskopf MK: *Fish Medicine.* Philadelphia, WB Saunders Co, 1993.

Stoskopf M: Taking the history. *Vet Clin North Am Small Anim Pract* 18(2):283–291, 1988.

Management of Tropical Fish

Tracy L. Ralston, RVT
Oakridge, North Carolina

Ten years ago, approximately 10 to 15 million people owned an aquarium,[1] and today 50% of aquarium owners regularly visit veterinarians for treatment of other pets.[2] Because a large number of fish hobbyists are accessible to veterinarians for advice, veterinary technicians should become more knowledgeable about aquatic life. The biology, management, and problems associated with an aquarium could be important sources of information to clients.

Aquariums are popular because they are quiet, clean, odorless, add aesthetic value to a room, require very little care, and are relatively inexpensive. Of the various aquarium inhabitants, goldfish are the most popular—in fact, goldfish are more popular pets than dogs and cats. In addition, statistics[3] show that aquariums now play a therapeutic role in human medicine and that fish are becoming more significant in medical research.

Biology of the Environment
Nitrogen Cycle

The aquarium's internal ecosystem is the primary concern of caring for fish. The most common cause of death in aquarium fish is an imbalance in the environment, especially in the nitrogen cycle. Fish excrete ammonia, which is lethal if allowed to accumulate in the tank. Very small amounts (anything >0.1 ppm [mg/L]) are extremely toxic.[4] This toxicity is intensified in water that has a low oxygen content, high temperature, and increased pH. Bacteria in the tank (*Nitrosomonas* spp.) convert ammonia into nitrite, which is a less toxic compound. Nitrite is further oxidized by other bacteria (*Nitrobacter* spp.) into nitrate. Although this compound is much less toxic than ammonia, it should not be allowed to accumulate in large quantities. A sign of excessive nitrate is a yellowish tint to the water.

The nitrogen cycle is the reason behind fish acquiring the "new tank syndrome." A newly assembled aquarium lacks the bacteria needed to oxidize ammonia. Because time is necessary for the nitrifying bacteria to build up in adequate

numbers, the new tank will have toxic levels of ammonia, with the highest level occurring at 7 to 10 days. Approximately 30 days are required to establish a balance, more if the tank is large. Although this process can be shortened by seeding bacteria into the new filter (adding cotton wool from an older, established tank filter or even a small piece of dead fish), it is advisable to wait 30 days before adding any new fish and thus avoid the "new tank syndrome" (Figure 1).[1]

Oxygen Cycle

Plants as well as bacteria also have roles in the ecosystem. Fish absorb oxygen through their gills and release carbon dioxide into the water. When exposed to light, plants utilize carbon dioxide during photosynthesis and release oxygen. Plants also contribute in other ways, as their roots break up solid wastes into less harmful substances and their surfaces provide areas for algae and bacteria to grow. Plants, in addition to bacteria and algae, can absorb some nitrogenous compounds and will improve water quality. It is not essential to have plants in the aquarium, however, as long as it is well aerated and filtered.

Chlorine

Chlorine, which is found in tap water, is a common cause of death in fish. If chlorine is not removed, it will burn the delicate tissue in the gills. Chlorine removal is easy by allowing the water to sit for at least 24 hours; the chlorine will escape as a gas. Filtering water through activated charcoal before adding it to the aquarium is another

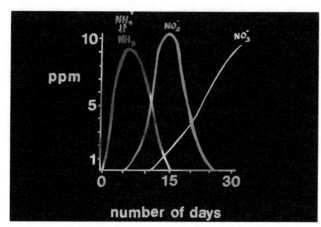

Figure 1—Graph showing time required to establish the nitrification cycle.

way to remove chlorine. In addition, commercial chemicals, such as sodium thiosulfate (Right Start®—Jungle Laboratory Corporation, Sanford, Florida; Chlorine Cure®—Aquatrol Inc., Anaheim, California), instantly combine with chlorine to remove it. Thus, although chlorine is a lethal problem, the cure can be simple.

Other Factors

Routine maintenance is necessary to keep an aquarium balanced. Partial water changes should be done about every other week, depending on the number of fish in the aquarium, or more frequently if there is a substantial biologic load. Each water change should remove 25% of the total water, and the added water must be similar in temperature and chemical makeup. Radical changes can cause stress in and possibly kill more sensitive fish. Immediate removal of dead fish keeps the aquarium free of pollutants and reduces the stress load on the biologic system. Other routine maintenance duties consist of monitoring the temperature (tanks near windows will fluctuate in temperature with the seasons), changing the cotton wool and charcoal in a box or outside filter monthly, and cleaning (with vinegar) any calcium deposits that collect on the aquarium sides. Extreme care must be taken to rinse all vinegar thoroughly,[5] particularly when soft water (low alkalinity) is used. Other duties, such as monitoring the pH, nitrite, and water hardness, are possible with the various monitoring kits that are commercially available.

Equipment
Tank

The basic equipment needed for an aquarium consists of a tank, a filtering system, an air pump, light source, and such miscellaneous items as rocks and plants (optional). The tank size and shape are dictated by the kind of fish, the number of fish, and the location of the tank. Large, more active fish need tanks that will supply sufficient room and proper aeration. The surface area of the aquarium, not the depth, dictates the number of fish a tank can accommodate. For example, a deep aquarium has a larger area for visualizing the fish than does a shallow tank, but they may have

the same surface area and can hold the same number of fish. Thus, the surface area into which the oxygen is diffused from the atmosphere into the tank is the primary criterion. Tanks made of plastic should be avoided, since with time and use they can eventually become distorted and are easily scratched.

Filtering System

Every aquarium needs a filtering system. The ideal filtering system should perform (1) mechanical filtration, which removes particulate matter, (2) chemical filtration, which removes free ions, and (3) biological filtration, which incorporates bacterial removal of nitrogenous by-products.[6] Various types of commercially available filters accomplish these three functions.

An undergravel filter consists of a screen through which water and debris are pulled. The gravel or sand acts as a filter to trap debris, after which it is broken down by bacteria. This method, however, lacks chemical filtration and toxic substances can build up. Thus, partial water changes and removal of solids are necessary.

In-tank and out-of-tank filters suck water into a container of cotton wool and activated charcoal. The cotton wool traps waste particles, and the charcoal removes some toxins by adsorption. (The most biologically important toxins in an aquarium, however, are nitrogenous wastes and hydrogen ions; and charcoal adsorption does not remove these.) Bacterial degradation also occurs in the filter; thus, when the cotton wool is changed, an old bacteria-laden piece of cotton should be seeded into the new cotton.

Undergravel filters have a much greater filtration capacity compared with that of box filters and therefore are preferred. Because nitrifying bacteria require a surface for attachment, the number of bacteria will correlate with the total surface area available. To get maximum filtration, these two types of filters can be used together.[6]

Air Pump

The air pump, which is the power source of an aquarium, pumps air through a small hose attached to an air stone. The air stone breaks up the air into small bubbles, which move water as they rise to the surface (filters also operate in this manner). By moving the water, an air pump helps in the aeration of the tank, speeding the process of oxygen exchange within the surface area.

Lighting

Natural sunlight is not generally the recommended light source, as artificial lighting allows more control of the intensity and duration of light. Tropical fish should have approximately 12 hours of light per day (imitating the natural environment). Fluorescent lighting is recommended over incandescent bulbs. Incandescent lighting gives off too much heat and is not suitable for growing plants, while fluorescent lighting is more energy efficient and can support plant life. If the tank has many plants, a fluorescent bulb(s) should be replaced at least once a year; plants can be damaged if the bulb is old.[5]

Miscellaneous Items

Miscellaneous items include plants and rocks or shells; the latter items must be specified as tank safe. A heater also may be needed, as small tanks or tanks with fish that require warmth or a given temperature range usually do better with a heater. A small tank thermometer is an easy way of determining whether the tank is sufficiently heated.

Food

The easiest and most popular method of feeding fish is use of prepared flaked or dried food, as most fish will readily eat commercial food. One advantage to using flaked food instead of dried food is that the former contains a variety of ingredients to supply the proper balance of nutrients. Not all fish, however, can eat flaked food, especially small fish that have difficulty eating the flakes because of their size (Figure 2). On the other hand, some large fish may only accept other types of food, such as live food or frozen brine shrimp. Therefore, it is advisable to rotate brands or supplement the diet with live food to provide variety.[7]

Live foods are the most natural food source of fish and thus are preferred by them (plus they enjoy chasing prey). Live food can be purchased from pet stores, although it is possible to breed such food as earthworms, fruit flies, or brine shrimp. A disadvantage to live foods, especially if caught in the wild, is that it is possible to introduce disease or predatory insects. Live food can be supplied either fresh or frozen (unnecessary to thaw before feeding). Frozen food should be packaged carefully in airtight bags.

Overfeeding is possibly the most common error in caring for fish. Excess food can quickly foul the tank water and kill the fish. Feeding fish once a day is sufficient, but it is best to feed them twice daily. Very young fish need to be fed four to six times daily but in tiny amounts. Fish can survive well without food if the owners leave for the weekend. Table I lists some of the foods preferred by various groups of fish.

Biologic Data

Fish are vertebrates (as are humans) in which anatomy and physiology are adapted to life in water. Specific anatomic adaptations include body shape, fin location, and coloring. A streamlined torpedo-shaped fish indicates a fast mover with high endurance; the caudal fin (which is responsible for locomotion) of a fast fish has sharp indentations whereas the fin of a slower fish is a softer, longer shape.[5] A fish with a thick, round body (Figure 3) moves slowly and generally has low endurance. Bottom-feeding fish have undershot mouths, flat bellies, and rounded backs; surface feeders are the opposite, with flat backs, high-set mouths, and a dorsal fin set caudally on the back to avoid surfacing above the water. Fish are dark on the dorsal surface and pale on the belly, except the upside-down catfish, which is darker on the belly (because of its strange swimming habit).

Fish that hide among plants may have darker stripes, such as angelfish. Males that compete aggressively for females may be brightly colored and can be confused with some of the fancy show specimens that have been selectively bred (such brightly colored fish with extra-long finnage would not survive long in the wild). Fish, to some

TABLE I
Food for Fish Groups[7]

Category	Type of Food
Young fish (fry)	Infusorian, egg yolk, brine shrimp, nauplii, microworms
Young cichlids	Tubifex, water fleas, bloodworms
Tooth carps (live and egg)	Dried and flaked food, tubifex, algae, water fleas, bloodworms
Characins and barbs	Dried and flaked foods, tubifex, liver daphania, bloodworms, water fleas
Labyrinths	Live and dried foods with occasional vegetable supplements; not picky
Large cichlids and piranhas	Small fish, earthworms, tadpoles, liver, shrimps, lettuce, spinach

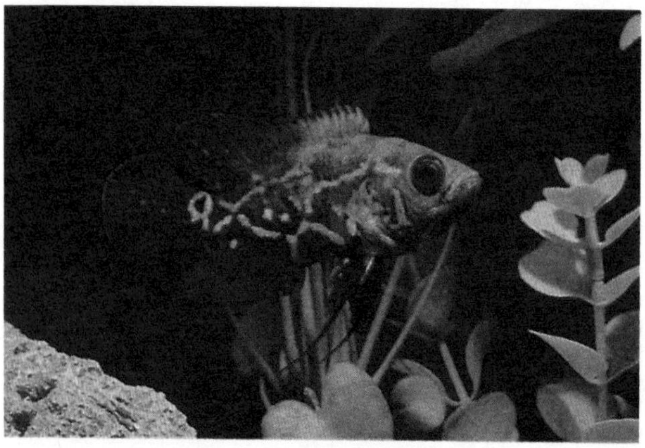

Figure 2—An oscar is an example of a fish that eats live and frozen foods. Many will reject flaked food.

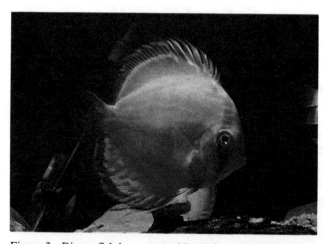

Figure 3—Discus fish have a round body for slow swimming.

extent, can change their shading to blend into light or dark surroundings. Their shading is also a clue to their health status. Vibrant shades are found in healthy fish, while sick fish are somewhat pale in comparison. Fish also become pale if pigments found in their natural diet, such as carotenoids, are not present.

Respiration

Fish primarily absorb oxygen through the gills. Water first is taken in through the mouth and then forced through the gill slits when the mouth is closed or the fish swims. The gill arches have a rakelike anterior surface to prevent foodstuff from clogging the gills. The posterior side is covered with vascular lamellae, where gas exchange takes place (Figure 4). The surface area is larger than that of the entire fish. According to Walsh:

> The respiratory rate of fishes is controlled by oxygen receptors generally found in the first functional gill arch. The monitoring of carbon dioxide is not important in fishes, since it is some 25 to 30 times more soluble in water than is oxygen.[8]

The gills are not the only site at which oxygen exchange occurs. Some fish that survive naturally in water that has low oxygen content have modified skin and organs to absorb oxygen and release carbon dioxide. Fish in the Labyrinth, or Anabantidae, family have an accessory organ called a labyrinth, which enables them to utilize atmospheric air. These fish can successfully be kept in stagnant water. The labyrinth organ is located at the fourth gill arch and consists of a folded, baglike structure that is highly vascular. In a newly hatched fish, the labyrinth is absent and develops gradually during the first month. As an adult, the fish depends on the labyrinth for additional oxygen intake and could not survive with just normal gill breathing. Other sites of oxygen absorption include the skin (especially around the lips), oral sacs, and modified swim bladders.

Integument

Fish have a dermis and an epidermis; however, they lack the protective keratin layer present on human skin. Instead, fish have two ways of protecting the body. Calcified plates, or scales, act as armor; they are imbedded in the dermis and are covered by the epidermis. There are two kinds of scales: ctenoid and cycloid. Ctenoid scales are serrated on the edge, giving the fish a rough texture; cycloid scales are not serrated and look and feel smooth. Not all fish have scales, however; some carp are completely devoid of scales, while certain catfish have bony plates for protection. Cells in the epidermis secrete mucus to provide a first line of protection. Lymphocytes and other immune cells are also present to ward off foreign invasion. Pheromones in some species are released when the skin is broken; the substance causes other fish to swim away.[8]

The beautiful coloration of fish is produced by pigment cells in the dermis. Red pigment granules are called erythrophores, yellow are xanthophores, and brown are melano-

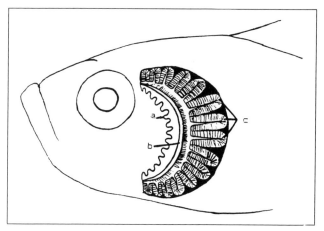

Figure 4—A fish gill and its relative location. (*a*) anterior comblike projections (gill rakers); (*b*) gill arch; (*c*) lamellae.

phores. Guanophores, which are fine crystals of guanine, cause a silvery sheen and combine with other pigments to produce iridescent colors.[9]

Circulatory System

The heart of a fish reportedly has only two chambers[10]: an atrium and a ventricle. The atrium has an enlarged chamber, positioned in front of it, that is known as the sinus venosus; here blood is collected before going into the heart. After being pumped through the heart, blood flows from the ventricle into the bulbus arteriosus, which is very elastic and aids in maintaining arterial pressure. Blood from the heart circulates first through the lamellae of the gills to collect oxygen. Capillaries regroup in two large arteries: one that leads to the head and one that goes to the body cavity. The heart rate of a fish averages 34 to 40 beats/min.

The red blood cells of fish differ considerably from human blood cells in that the former are oval in shape and are nucleated. Because fish do not have bone marrow, the blood cells are manufactured in extramedullary sites.[10]

Sensory Organs

Fish detect minute vibrations and currents in the water through a sensory organ called the lateral line, a canal that runs from the gill plate down the trunk of the body to the tail. This canal has small pits that house hairlike sensory cells that wave and bend with the flow of water. These hairlike cells are protected because they lie below the skin surface. Sensory pits may also be present on the head of a fish. On scaly fish, it is easy to see the lateral line.

The swim bladder is an "out-pouching" of the esophagus and is filled with gas received from the blood. Its primary function is that of a ballast by allowing fish to swim at any depth without constantly sinking or floating.

Fish can hear, although they do not have external or internal ear canals. Some fish on the higher end of the evolutionary scale have a membranous labyrinth in the auditory capsule of the skull. This labyrinth consists of three semicircular canals that are used for balance and three otolith

TABLE II
Specific Biologic Needs for Community Tank Fish[11,12]

Common Name	Maximum Size (in.)	Type	Water Temperature (°F)	Environment
Angelfish	6	Slow moving; do not keep with fast fish	75–80	Slightly acidic water
Archerfish	7	Individuals can be aggressive	74–85	Add salt[a] to tank
Arowana	16	Keep larger fish by themselves	76–78	Calm water
Betta	2½	No males together	75–82	Soft, acidic water
Blindfish	3¼	Good community fish; peaceful	75–80	Soft water
Bumblebee	1¾	Very aggressive; keep by themselves	75–78	Add salt[a] to tank
Cardinal tetra	1½	Peaceful in schools; have at least 6	75–78	Soft, acidic (pH <6.5) water
Clown loach	6	Good community fish	∿76	Not important
Corydoras	1–3	Good community fish; peaceful	73–83	No extreme in pH of water
Discus	8	Peaceful; does better in own group	75–83	Soft, acidic water
Giant danio	4	Will not bother anything it cannot eat	75–78	Not important
Glass cat	4	Do not keep alone or with active fish	72–82	Hard, slightly alkaline water
Glowlight tetra	2	Very peaceful	∿76	Slightly acidic, soft water
Goldfish	16	Active; do not let other fish nip their fins	50–70	Well-aerated water
Guppy	2¼	Very active; can be fin nippers	74–78	Soft, alkaline water
Hatchetfish	2½	May jump; peaceful; keep in schools	∿78	Soft, slightly acidic water
Kissing gourami	12	Large fish will pick on others	78–85	Not critical
Leopard scat	10	Peaceful; will eat plants to roots	74–78	Hard, alkaline water; add salt[a] to tank
Lyretail	2–3	Peaceful; does better with own species	∿76	Acidic, soft water
Paradise fish	3	Very quarrelsome with all fish	70–75	Any conditions
Piranha	11	Not a community fish	75–80	Soft water
Platy	3	Good community fish with other hard-water species	70–80	Hard, slightly alkaline water
Plecostomus	12	Seldom bothers other fish; needs algae	75–82	Slightly alkaline water
Puffer fish	6½	Quarrelsome, even with own species	75–80	Hard, alkaline water; add salt[a] to tank
Ram cichlid	2½	Timid; very gentle to other fish	∿80	Acidic water
Sailfin Molly	6	Peaceful in large tank with own species	78–84	Slightly alkaline water; add salt[a] to tank
Shovel-nosed catfish	12	Lazy, slow moving; will eat other fish	72–82	Soft, acidic water
Swordtail	5	Larger fish can be extremely aggressive	70–80	Hard, alkaline water; add salt[a] to tank
Tiger barb	2½	Active, fast fish; nips slower fish	70–85	Soft, slightly acidic water
Upside-down catfish	2½	Peaceful; likes to hide	76–80	Soft, slightly acidic water

[a]Salt should be added at one teaspoon per gallon.

organs that are sound detectors.[8] In carp, the gas in the swim bladder helps transmit sound waves to the labyrinth; but the sound is not directional.

Fish also have taste buds, which are mostly found on the roof and side walls of the mouth and on the floor of the pharynx. Taste buds also are found on the "whiskers" or barbels, which help locate food. Bottom feeders, on the other hand, have a unique location for the taste buds—the surface of the belly running to the tip of the tail. The whiskers of bottom fish are usually very long to help search for food among the rocks.

In fish, the sense of smell is not coupled with the mouth, as occurs in humans. Two olfactory pits located above the mouth allow a fish to smell odors. As the fish swims, water is continuously pushed into a nasal opening and exits through a posterior opening. These pits, however, do not open into the mouth. Perches have a blind sac, and water is forced in and out of the same opening instead of passing through. Fish with large olfactory pits located below the eyes have a better sense of smell.[5]

Selection of Fish

Careful consideration should be given to the kinds of fish to select. As already discussed, before buying the fish, owners should wait until the natural bacterial flora can build up to handle waste degradation in a new tank. Pet stores can measure the nitrogen content and tell when it is safe to add fish.

An important criterion of fish selection is that all fish are not compatible. Environmental needs and swimming habits vary considerably. Water pH and hardness should be compatible with all fish in the tank. Slow, peaceful fish can become stressed and easily killed by more active, fin-nipping fish. Fish can be surface swimmers, bottom feeders, or tank swimmers, according to the species. Mixing these groups uses the entire area of the tank and adds aesthetic value. Having all surface swimmers may crowd the top, however; and fin nipping may result. Another criterion is whether the fish do best in schools, such as neon tetras, or can be easily kept as solitary individuals. This decision will aid in protecting the overall health and well-being of the fish. Table II is a brief overview of the needs of common aquarium species, but there are many comprehensive books to guide in selection.[11,12] Aquarium distributors may also be a good source of information. A beginner may want to start with hardy species, like the swordtail or goldfish, and avoid sensitive fish, like the discus and angelfish.

After the species of fish to be purchased has been decided, the prospective owner should be aware of how to spot diseased fish. Tank water that is yellow, blue, or green is indicative of medicines; and fish from such a tank should be avoided.[9] The behavior of the fish, such as rocking, gasping for air at the surface, or sinking to the bottom, is a sign of disease. The swimming habits of the fish should be consistent with the species; that is, quiet fish should not be darting about and vice versa.

One of the most common diseases of pet fish is caused by *Ichthyophthirius* (commonly known as *Ich*),[2] an external parasite (protozoan) that is visible as tiny white dots on the skin (Figure 5). *Ichthyophthirius* is very communicable and can quickly infect a tank. Any lesion on the skin surface is also a sign of disease. Ulcers of the skin can be caused by mycobacteriosis or from the fish scraping its skin on a sharp object. Large parasites, such as the crustacean *Lernaea*, can be seen as well, with the hooks of the

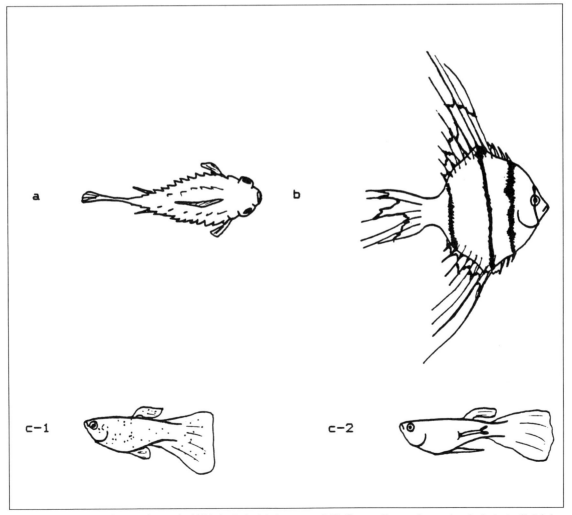

Figure 5—Common diseases in tropical fish include (*a*) dropsy and (*b*) fin rot. External parasites include (*c-1*) *Ichthyophthirius* and (*c-2*) *Lernaea*.

parasite embedded in the skin and egg sacs on the tail (Figure 5).

The fins are a great indicator of health status. Fins should be erect, not clamped down to the body. Fin rot is a common bacterial problem that leaves fins in shreds, with the bony rays jutting out (Figure 5).

Fish are also affected by a form of ascites commonly called dropsy. Fluid collects in the body cavity and causes the scales to stick out at an angle. By looking straight down on a fish, it is possible to see the scales sticking out[5] (Figure 5).

After the fish have been selected, the shop owner will probably place them in a plastic bag for transportation. Since the oxygen in the bag will last a limited time only, immediate transportation is best. If the weather is cold, the bag can be wrapped in a towel or jacket.

A common mistake on arrival is to float the bag within the tank; however, nitrite is released from the bag's surface and can pollute the tank or kill the fish. The best method is to gently empty the contents of the bag (water and fish) into a bowl and add a little water from the tank every five minutes to acclimate the fish. A half-hour is sufficient time to condition new fish to the tank water. The fish should be watched for a few moments after adding them to the tank to ensure that other fish do not nip at or chase the newcomers. Extremely territorial fish should be added smallest fish first, a practice that allows the smaller fish to establish themselves and defend themselves against larger or more aggressive fish.[5]

Anesthesia

It seems unnatural to think of a fish being sedated or anesthetized, but there are many applications of this practice. A common reason for sedation is transportation; fish can die from the stress and exhaustion of transport. The use of sedatives decreases the activity of fish and as a result decreases oxygen consumption and waste buildup. Other reasons to use anesthetics[13] include:

- Surgery for research purposes
- Surgery for therapeutic purposes
- Fish farm procedures, such as tagging and weighing
- Stress prevention
- Handling of dangerous fish, such as an electric eel or piranha
- Enhancement of colors and quieting fish for photography.

Tricaine methanesulfonate, MS 222, is the only anesthetic approved in food fishes by the FDA. It can be used as a sedative or anesthetic depending on the dose. The fish is put into a tank containing this drug and watched until it has reached the proper plane of anesthesia. The plane of anesthesia is determined by reactions to visual and vibrational stimuli, equilibrium, muscle tone, and respiratory rate. Most operations are held at stage I plane 2; at this level, there is no reaction to visual or vibrational stimuli, but the equilibrium and respiratory rate are normal.[13] Plane of an-

esthesia is maintained by dilution with water or moving the fish to a tank with less anesthetic. For short surgical procedures (less than five minutes), fish do not need a deep plane of anesthesia. They can be immediately removed from the induction tank and placed into a recovery tank. For long surgical procedures, a fish can be intubated and the gills perfused with water and anesthetic.

Extralabel anesthetics, such as quinaldine sulfate and injectable agents, are also available. Their use is dictated by the procedure and the fish species. One of the common agents is alphaxalone. Some problems associated with injectables are a prolonged recovery with pentobarbital sodium, respiratory problems with ketamine hydrochloride, and convulsions with xylazine hydrochloride.[13] The technique for administering anesthesia via syringe is to angle the needle toward the head of the fish and insert it into the muscle just above the lateral line.[14]

Role of the Veterinary Staff

Veterinarians and their staff are in a position to provide client education services and thus make people aware of the common fish diseases and how to avoid them. The technician is ideal for this job. By offering consultative advice, technicians can assist not only current clients who are primarily seeking veterinary medical treatment for their other pets but also fish dealers, researchers, and owners of fish farms.

REFERENCES

1. Janze AO: *Aquarium Techniques. 1. Care and Equipment.* New York, Universe Books Inc, 1964, pp 9–19.
2. Gorham ME: Treating sick fish can improve a veterinarian's full-service care. *DVM*:40, 1985.
3. Ford DM: The hobby of ornamental fishkeeping. *Waltham Third Annu Symp*:321, 1981.
4. Leibovitz L: Establishing and maintaining a healthy aquatic environment. *JAVMA* 176(11):1234, 1980.
5. Scheurmann I: *The New Aquarium Handbook.* Woodbury, NY, Barrons Educational Series, Inc, 1986, pp 32, 80, 86–94, 98.
6. Anders JJ, Ostrow ME: Goldfish in research—Use and maintenance. *Lab Anim* 15(5):33–41, 1986.
7. Jocher W: *Food for the Aquarium and Vivarium.* Princeton, NJ, Van Nostrand Rheinhold Co, 1966, pp 7, 62.
8. Walsh AH: Biology and diseases of fish. *Lab Anim Med*:479, 480, 483, 1984.
9. Sterba G: *Aquarium Care.* New York, EP Dutton and Co, Inc, 1967, pp 87–89, 98.
10. Wallach JD, Beaver WJ: Tropical fish, in *Diseases of Exotic Animals: Medicine and Surgical Management.* Philadelphia, WB Saunders Co, 1983, p 1051.
11. Axelrod HR: *Exotic Tropical Fishes.* Jersey City, NJ, TFH Publications, Inc, 1962, pp F1–608.
12. Gilbert J: *The Complete Aquarist's Guide to Freshwater Tropical Fishes.* New York, Golden Press, 1970, pp 55–229.
13. Stuart NC: Anesthetics in fishes. *Waltham Third Annu Symp*:379, 1981.
14. Brown L: Anaesthesia in fishes. *Waltham Third Annu Symp*:386, 1981.

Rehabilitation of Sea Turtles

Terry W. Campbell, DVM, PhD
Brendalee Philips
Sea World of Florida Inc.
Orlando, Florida

Sea turtles of the coastal areas of the United States are on the Endangered Species list. At least one species, the Kemp's ridley turtle, is near extinction. The primary known reasons for the marked decline of turtle populations worldwide include loss of nesting beaches to human development, excessive harvesting of turtles (especially green turtles) and eggs for food, and death of turtles accidentally caught in fishing nets. Attempts to protect sea turtles have included preservation of nesting beaches, development of turtle extruder devices (TEDs) that attach to the fishing nets of trawlers, and heightened public awareness through education. Several sea turtle rehabilitation centers have been created in an attempt to provide medical care to sick and injured sea turtles.

The following six species of sea turtles are found around the United States: green (*Chelonia mydas*), hawksbill (*Eretmochelys imbricata*), Kemp's ridley (*Lepidochelys kempi*), leatherback (*Dermochelys coriacea*), loggerhead (*Caretta caretta*), and olive ridley (*Lepidochelys olivacea*). Green turtles can weigh as much as 350 pounds and are distributed in tropical areas of the Atlantic, Pacific, and Indian oceans. The turtles primarily eat seagrasses and algae. Hawksbill turtles weigh up to 200 pounds; have a worldwide distribution in tropical waters; and feed primarily on sponges, tunicates, shrimp, and squid.

Kemp's and olive ridley turtles can weigh as much as 100 pounds and feed on crabs, shrimp, mollusks, jellyfish, and plants. The Kemp's ridley turtle has a limited distribution—it is found in the coastal waters of the Gulf of Mexico (off the coasts of Texas, Louisiana, and Florida). The olive ridley turtle is found in the tropical waters of the Pacific, Indian, and southeastern Atlantic oceans. Leatherback turtles can reach a maximum weight of 1900 pounds; they inhabit the Atlantic, Pacific, and Indian oceans; and they feed primarily on jellyfish, tunicates, and other soft-bodied prey. Loggerhead turtles can weigh as much as 400 pounds; they are found in temperate and tropical waters worldwide; and they feed on crabs, shrimp, mollusks, jellyfish, and plants.

Disorders

Common disorders of sea turtles presented to rehabilitation facilities include traumatic injuries, entanglement, gastrointestinal obstruction, intoxication by petroleum products, buoyancy disorders, emaciation, hypothermia, and green turtle papillomatosis. Hatching turtles are also frequently presented to rehabilitators. Occasionally, hatchlings are illegally taken from nesting beaches to be kept as pets in home aquaria; the turtles do not thrive in such an environment and are later presented to rehabilitators.

Traumatic injuries to sea turtles occur in various ways. Encounters with motorized watercraft frequently cause traumatic injury; the injury can be caused by the propeller (Figure 1) or the impact of the craft striking the turtle. Head and neck injuries may occur from fishing operations when turtles are dropped onto the decks of fishing boats as they are released from nets or from hostile fishermen who attempt to kill turtles. Traumatic injuries also occur from entrapment in dredging equipment. Shark bites are also frequently encountered in sea turtles (Figure 2). Sea turtles themselves can be aggressive and inflict bite wounds on each other, especially when held in overcrowded captive environments.

Entanglement with nets, fishing line, crab and fish traps, and plastic rings from beverage containers are examples of common causes of injury or death of sea turtles. Entangled turtles often are unable to forage and frequently die from starvation or drown if they are unable to surface

Originally published in Volume 14, Number 3, March 1993

for air. Turtles may also suffer from wounds caused by the entangling material, which constricts or lacerates tissue. Constricting material may cut off the blood supply to a limb or the neck and head.

Turtles are frequently presented in a marked state of emaciation resulting from gastrointestinal obstruction after ingestion of foreign material. The ingested material is often non-biodegradable human waste that has been dumped into the ocean. Such materials as plastic (especially plastic bags), glass, and metal may be ingested by turtles that either mistake foreign material for food or accidentally ingest such material as they forage in areas where human garbage has been dumped.

Sea turtles are occasionally presented covered with oil or tar. The turtles often swallow the petroleum products, which may result in toxicosis.

Hypothermia can occur in sea turtles (especially green turtles) that forage on plants in shallow coastal waters during the winter when water temperatures drop suddenly (Figure 3). Hypothermia causes the turtles to become inactive and predisposes them to secondary infections, especially bacterial pneumonia.

A condition of green turtles found off the Atlantic coast of Florida involves multiple, large papillomatous growths primarily affecting the skin on the head, neck, limbs, and tail. When these growths cover the eyes, the turtles are unable to forage and are presented in a severe state of emaciation. Necropsies have indicated that internal papillomatosis also occurs. The cause of this disease is currently unknown; however, a virus is suspected.

Medical Care

A sick or injured sea turtle recovered from the beach should be transported immediately to a rehabilitation facility. The turtle should be placed in ventral recumbency on a wet blanket or foam pad (Figure 4). Wet towels can be used to cover the turtle to keep it from drying during transport.

The initial diagnostic evaluation of the turtle involves a physical examination, which includes weighing the turtle and conducting a blood profile. Blood is usually collected from the dorsal venous sinuses of the neck. When collected for a complete blood cell count, the blood is placed in a tube that contains heparin (preferably lithium heparin) as the anticoagulant because EDTA causes hemolysis in the blood of sea turtles.

Whole-body radiographs are indicated in suspected cases of foreign body ingestion, gastrointestinal obstruction, and pneumonia. Debilitated sea turtles are often covered with barnacles (Figure 5), which makes interpretation of radiographs difficult. To remove barnacles from the carapace and plastron of sea turtles, the turtles are first placed in fresh water for at least 24 hours. Exposure to fresh water kills barnacles, thereby facilitating their removal. A screwdriver or wood chisel held in the same plane as the carapace or plastron (to avoid damage to the outer surface of the turtle) is used to pry off the dead barnacles.

Most sea turtles presented to rehabilitation facilities are emaciated and dehydrated. Blood profiles frequently reveal hypoglycemia, dehydration, and anemia. Rehydrating fluids can be given intraperitoneally, intravenously, or orally by means of gastric gavage. Most patients are given an oral glucose-electrolyte solution by means of a feeding tube. This is done by inserting an appropriately sized feeding tube through the mouth and into the stomach. An oral speculum (i.e., hard plastic or wooden rod) is required to keep the mouth open and to prevent the turtle from biting into the tube. The speculum should be padded (i.e., wrapped in tape) to prevent damage to the turtle's beak as it bites down (Figure 6).

Placing the turtle in a vertical position with the caudal edge of the carapace resting on a soft surface, such as a foam pad, helps to facilitate passage of the feeding tube into the stomach. The head and neck should be extended to straighten the esophagus during passage of the feeding tube into the stomach (Figure 7). After delivery of the tube-fed solution, the feeding tube is gently removed and the turtle is held in the vertical position with its head and neck extended until it swallows to prevent leakage of the fluid out of the stomach and mouth when the turtle is returned to its normal posture.

Sick and injured turtles are usually given broad-spectrum antibiotics as treatment for established bacterial infections or as a preventive measure. Antibiotics commonly used include amikacin sulfate, chloramphenicol, and trimethoprim-sulfa. Systemic antibiotics are usually given intramuscularly. Muscles of the forelimbs are chosen as the site of injection to avoid the renal portal system when such medications as aminoglycoside antibiotics, which have nephrotoxic potential, are given.

External wounds of turtles are managed in a manner similar to that of other animals. After thorough debridement and flushing of the wound (preferably with a dilute povidone-iodine solution), open wounds on the carapace, plastron, and head can be bandaged through

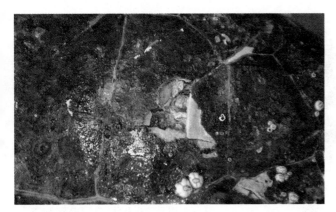

Figure 1—The carapace of a loggerhead turtle (*Caretta caretta*) showing linear fractures and wounds inflicted by a boat propeller.

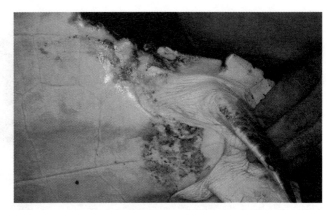

Figure 2—A green turtle (*Chelonia mydas*) with a healing shark bite wound.

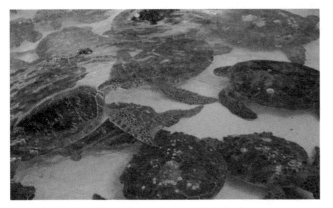

Figure 3—Green turtles with hypothermia. Their body temperatures on recovery were 7°C to 10°C (45°F to 50°F).

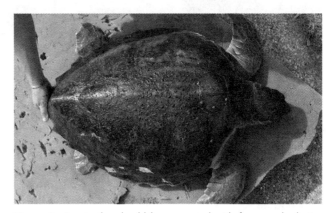

Figure 4—Sea turtles should be supported with foam pads during transportation or handling.

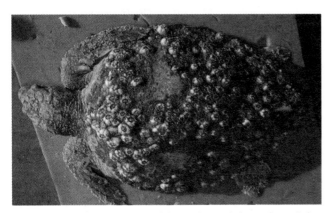

Figure 5—A sea turtle covered with barnacles and algae. The turtle has a blue identification tag on its forelimb and apparently was part of a field study.

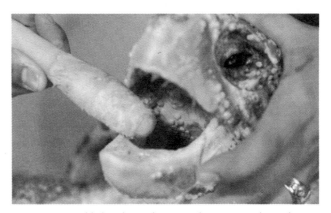

Figure 6—A padded oral speculum is used to examine the oral cavity of a sea turtle.

use of an antibiotic ointment, gauze, and tape. The antibiotic ointment and gauze are held in place by the tape, which is secured to the hard surfaces of the turtle by applying cyanoacrylate glue to the margins of the tape.

Wounds on the softer skin of the neck, limbs, tail, axilla, and inguinal areas are treated in a similar manner. If necessary, closure of wounds in these areas by suturing is possible.

Turtles coated with tar and oil can be treated in a manner similar to removal of petroleum products from the feathers of birds. Safe detergents, vegetable oil, or oil-absorbent towels can be used to remove tar and oil from turtles. To avoid toxicity, tar and oil in the oral cavity should be removed and the turtle should be given intestinal protectants, such as kaolin-pectin.

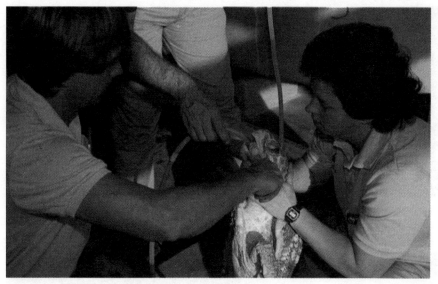

Figure 7—An emaciated green turtle is fed by means of a tube.

Short- and Long-Term Treatment and Convalescence

After the initial diagnostic evaluation and medical treatment, the sea turtle is placed in a convalescence pool. Turtles that are extremely weak and unable to raise their heads to breathe should be placed in a shower box. A shower box is a box or pool with drain holes that allow water to be continuously sprayed over the turtle but do not allow accumulation; this method protects weak turtles from drowning while keeping them wet. Turtles that are not active but are able to lift their heads to breathe can be placed in shallow water that does not cover their heads. A water spray or wet towels can be used to keep the exposed carapace wet. Weak turtles that can lift their heads to breathe and can swim should be kept in approximately two feet of water, measured from the top of the carapace as the turtle rests on the bottom of the pool. Active turtles should be placed in deep pools that provide plenty of room for swimming.

Dehydrated sea turtles as well as those covered with barnacles and algae should initially be placed in fresh water. Turtles with normal hydration that are free of barnacles should be kept in salt water with salinity equal to that of seawater (35 parts per million [ppm]). The water should be chlorinated (1.0 part per million or less) and properly filtered to maintain a healthy environment for the turtles. Chlorine levels greater than 1.0 part per million may cause irritation to the turtles' eyes. The water temperature should be maintained between 25°C and 30°C (77°F to 86°F).

Severely dehydrated and hypoglycemic turtles should be given a glucose solution by means of a feeding tube at four- to six-hour intervals during the first 24 hours. As the turtle's hydration and blood glucose levels improve, a liquid gruel can be given. The gruel is made in a blender using an oral glucose-electrolyte solution with whole fish. Small fish, such as smelt, are easily blended into the gruel. The consistency of the gruel can become thicker as the turtle's condition improves. Nutritional supplements can be included in the gruel for extremely emaciated turtles that need additional vitamins and minerals.

Feeding a fish gruel or whole fish to dehydrated turtles should be avoided because they often are unable to digest solid foods properly, and the material remains in the stomach as a result of decreased gastrointestinal motility. As the turtle's condition improves, it can be introduced to solid foods. High-protein, low-fat fish (such as smelt or mackerel) are good first choices. Depending on the size of the turtle, it may be necessary to cut the fish into smaller pieces. Squid and clams should be avoided initially because they seem to take longer to digest than fish do. Romaine lettuce or other leafy vegetables can be offered to omnivorous turtles, such as green turtles.

The amount of food fed may vary with each turtle. The amount of formula fed by stomach tube is determined by how much the turtle can hold before the formula flows back into the mouth or the turtle regurgitates. The goal is to feed approximately 7% of the turtle's body weight in grams per day. Turtles should be weighed frequently during the convalescent period. Weight gains and losses can be used as a guide for dietary management.

Hatchlings are tube-fed an oral glucose-electrolyte solution every three hours during the first 24 hours. As the hatchling's condition improves, a watery gruel can be introduced and fed at less frequent intervals. Weighing hatchling turtles daily is recommended to monitor their progress. After graduating to a thicker gruel, hatchlings can be offered solid foods, such as feeder fish and small shrimp. Hatchlings and older turtles often require the food to be held in front of their mouths to encourage intake during the introduction of new foods. When hatchlings are eating feeder fish or shrimp, introduction to cut foods (e.g., small pieces of fish) can be made.

Rehabilitating turtles should be closely monitored through blood profiles, food intake, body weights, and observation of defecation during the first few weeks of convalescence or until the turtle's condition becomes stable.

Radiographic evaluation may reveal gastrointestinal obstruction or foreign bodies (e.g., fish hooks) that may require surgical removal. Isoflurane is a safe general anesthetic for sea turtles. Isoflurane anesthesia, especially in weak turtles, can be induced by face mask and can be used as the maintenance anesthetic after intubation. The caudal half of the coelomic cavity of sea turtles can be approached through an inguinal incision. Unlike terrestrial turtles, the intestines of sea turtles are not supported by strong attachments and are easily exteriorized through the inguinal incision. Esophageal and gastric foreign bodies may be removed with endoscopic equipment; however, this procedure tends to be difficult. Recovery from general anesthesia can be prolonged in sea turtles; they should thus be put in a shower box until they have recuperated completely.

Sea turtles are often presented with buoyancy disorders. These turtles tend to float at the surface (with the caudal aspect of the carapace out of the water) and are unable to submerge. The disorder is usually caused by air that leaks from the respiratory tract and becomes trapped in the coelomic cavity. With time, some of these turtles recover spontaneously; in others, the condition is permanent. The permanent condition most likely results from large openings in the respiratory tract that cannot heal spontaneously.

Conclusion

Successful rehabilitation of sick or injured sea turtles is completed with the reintroduction of the turtles into the ocean. The location for release is usually determined by the state and federal agencies (i.e., U.S. Fish and Wildlife Service) that govern human activity associated with sea turtles. The turtles are typically released in areas where turtles of the same species and size are located. Reintroduction can be made from a boat or, more typically, by allowing the turtle to enter the ocean from the shore.

BIBLIOGRAPHY

Bjornal KA: *Biology and Conservation of Sea Turtles.* Washington, DC, Smithsonian Institute Press, 1982.

Committee on Sea Turtle Conservation: *Decline of Sea Turtles.* Washington, DC, National Academy Press, 1990.

Jacobson ER, et al: Cutaneous fibropapillomas of green turtles (*Chelonia mydas*). *J Comp Pathol* 101:39–52, 1989.

The Veterinary Technician's Role in the Rehabilitation of Sea Otters Rescued from the Oil Spill in Prince William Sound

Laura L. Kelly, LVT

Northern Lights Animal Clinic

Anchorage, Alaska

On March 24, 1989, the T/V *Exxon Valdez* ran aground on Bligh Reef in Prince William Sound, spilling 11 million gallons of crude oil. Hundreds of sea otters (*Enhydra lutris*) were incapacitated or killed by the toxic effects of the oil. In an attempt to offset the disaster, more than 300 sea otters were captured and treated at rehabilitation centers located in Alaska.

Veterinary technicians played a vital role in assisting veterinarians in the treatment of the incapacitated sea otters. Technicians were involved in clinical pathology, surgery, daily treatment, recordkeeping, and ordering of pharmaceutical supplies; that is, the responsibilities of the technicians were very similar to those of most veterinary technicians working for veterinary clinics and animal hospitals.

Rehabilitation Center Setup

The desire to rescue the sea otters endangered by the oil spill was overwhelming. Almost immediately, volunteers went to work in an attempt to help the injured otters. In Valdez, a makeshift rescue center was set up in a small dormitory building shared with the bird rehabilitation center until an improved and larger facility could be modeled from a school gymnasium. Later, as the center in Valdez became filled to capacity, an additional rehabilitation center was opened in Seward, Alaska (Figure 1).

Exxon employed a marine mammal expert who led a team of specialists in toxicology, veterinary anesthesiology, and sea otter husbandry as well as veterinarians experienced in sea otter care. Local Alaska veterinarians and veterinary technicians were also sought to assist in the rehabilitation. Volunteers from all over the United States and from as far as Germany and Australia began arriving to help.

Naturally, housing was in short supply because of the large influx of people involved with the spill and limited facilities in the small coastal towns. Although veterinarians and technicians were supplied hotel rooms or bed-and-breakfast facilities, often five were assigned to one room. Tents and cars sheltered the less fortunate.

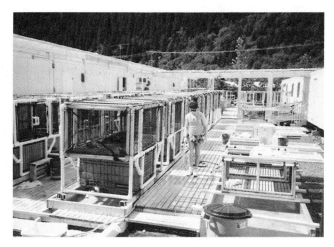

Figure 1—The Seward Otter Rehabilitation Center.

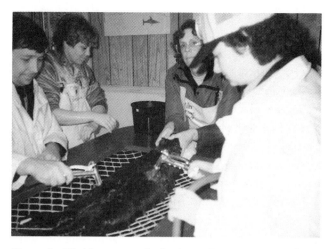

Figure 2—Washing an anesthetized otter in Seward. Dawn® detergent diluted with 16 parts water was used.

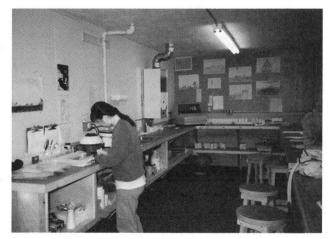

Figure 3—Veterinary technician Patty Chen processing blood in the Seward laboratory.

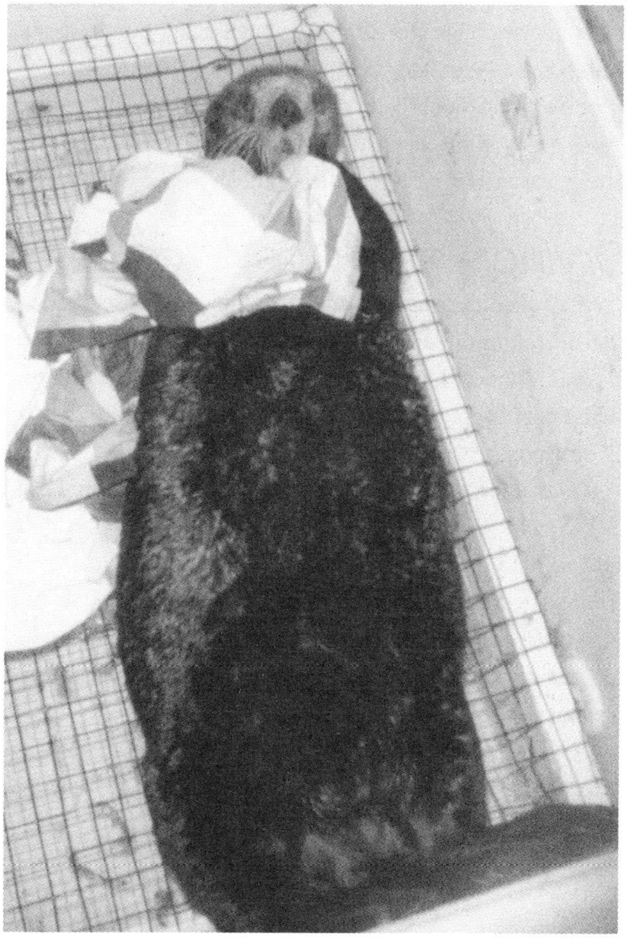

Figure 4—A recovering otter in Valdez. The otters loved to clutch towels as if they were ocean kelp.

Capture

Fishing boats, authorized by the U.S. Fish and Wildlife Service (USFWS), searched the oil-covered areas for distressed sea otters. Sea otters adversely affected by the spill were captured with nets, placed into plastic dog kennels, and flown by helicopter to the rehabilitation center in Valdez or Seward.

Arrival at Center

When each sea otter arrived at one of the centers, it was weighed and assigned a number. The animal's condition was immediately evaluated by a veterinarian. Technicians were responsible for preparing the otters to receive antibiotics, vitamins, and other fluids subcutaneously. Most of the otters required washing to rid them of the oil. Volunteers were requested to help wash the otters.

Washing Procedure

To undergo washing, each otter was transferred into a net or a wooden kennel with a sliding top designed to facilitate intramuscular administration of an anesthetic, which was necessary to approach the animal. After it was anesthetized, the otter was transferred to a wash table where an experienced otter handler restrained the animal as the volunteers washed it (Figure 2). The animals were repeatedly washed and rinsed for one to two hours. During that time, technicians monitored the otter's vital signs, including temperature and respiratory and heart rates. In addition to washing the otter's body, the volunteers used an eyewash to irrigate the otter's eyes and applied an antibiotic ophthalmic ointment.

Before the otter was released for drying, blood was taken for serum chemistry, complete blood cell count, and toxicology studies. Hair, fecal, and urine samples were also taken during this time. Initially, these samples were sent to an off-premise laboratory (a human hospital located in Anchorage) for processing. The delays, however, altered the blood values; plus, the clinical pathology results were not available for days. Eventually, the purchase and donation of laboratory equipment allowed the technicians to perform on-site blood counts, urinalyses, fecal flotation tests, and serum chemistry evaluations (Figure 3). Extra serum was archived for future studies.

Drying Procedure

After the otter was washed and completely rinsed, it was transferred to the drying table where volunteers used towels and low-heat blowdryers to dry the fur. Towels were in such short supply that a nationwide request was initiated. The response was overwhelming.

It was important to dry the otter's coat completely in order to help restore the insulating properties that the thick fur normally provides. The otters frequently required additional anesthesia, as this process could take up to two hours. When the drying process was completed, the sea otter was given the antagonist to the anesthetic and moved to a small pen for recovery.

General Husbandry

Recovering sea otters were fed and observed by volunteers and by staff (Figures 4 and 5). Any volunteer who detected signs of distress or unusual behavior displayed by a recovering otter immediately would alert a veterinarian or technician. Despite the numbers they were assigned on arrival, the recovering otters began acquiring names as the observers noted individual personality traits. ''Fat Freddie'' and ''Miss Piggy'' were hungry otters; ''Mean Lips'' tried chewing out of its cage; and ''Breaktime'' was a one-month-old pup named after the capture boat that saved her life (Figure 6).

Initially, each otter was placed in a small cage and, as the medical condition and condition of the coat improved, the animals gradually progressed to larger cages with pools. The otter's contact with humans was decreased as they neared their estimated time of release.

The diet of the otters consisted of a variety of frozen, raw seafood, including clams, shrimp, crab, squid, scallops, and (the favorite) gooeyduck.

Medical Management

Treating the critically ill otters was a difficult and often unrewarding job. In many instances, regardless of the treatment procedure or the amount of time devoted, the otter failed to respond and did not survive. Fatigue and sadness on the part of the veterinary staff and volunteers were often unavoidable. The letters of encouragement received from all over the world were greatly appreciated, as they served to increase the morale of weary workers.

On a daily basis, technicians accompanied the veterinarians on rounds and were responsible for administering the prescribed treatments with the assistance of an otter handler, who would restrain or distract the otter. Communication with the handler was of utmost importance in order to avoid the otter's crushing bite. The sea otters learned very quickly who gave them injections and would hiss as the handlers or technicians walked past them.

Hypoglycemia, hypothermia, emphysema, shock, decreased liver and kidney function, and stress were the most common conditions treated. Diarrhea and anemia were frequent complicating problems. Difficulty lay in treating the wild animals without further stressing them. Usually, oral medication could be disguised in the food.

When a radiograph was indicated, the otter was anesthetized and transferred to a local human hospital in Valdez or Seward. Several injured limbs and a broken back were studied.

Medical supplies were ordered and stocked by the technicians. Because of the remote location of the centers, it often took several days to receive the necessary supplies.

Record Keeping

Records were kept on the sea otter's food consumption, medical treatments, lab results, fur condition, behavior, and attitude. It was largely the technician's job to sort through pages of each sea otter's daily records and summarize them for the veterinarians. This information along with the veterinarian's assessment of the animal provided needed information for each sea otter's rehabilitation.

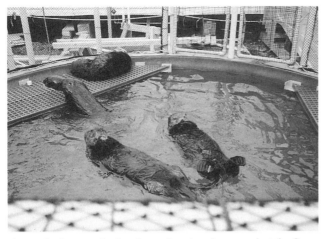

Figure 5—Otters enjoying themselves in a large pool at the Seward Otter Rehabilitation Center.

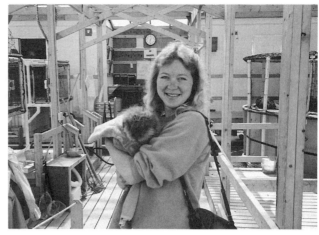

Figure 6—Volunteer Angie Grassano, MT, taking "Breaktime" from the nursery to a pool for a swim.

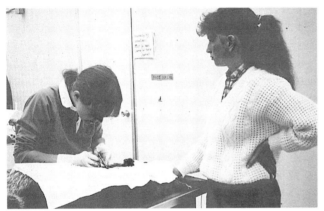

Figure 7—Veterinary technician Bonnie Miller monitoring the temperature of a sea otter while undergoing surgery performed by veterinarian Carolyn McCormick, DVM, of Eagle River, Alaska.

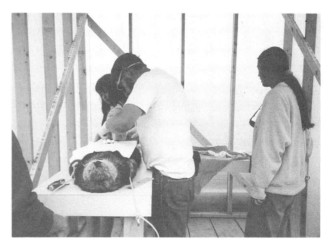

Figure 8—Veterinarian Tom Williams, DVM, of Monterey, California, surgically implants a radio transmitter into a sea otter.

Surgical Management

Surgical procedures performed at the centers included suturing wounds, ovariohysterectomy, and abdominal implantation of radio devices (Figures 7 and 8).

Implantation of transmitters was a controversial issue. The U.S. Fish and Wildlife Service wanted the ability to track some of the otters after they had been released in order to determine whether they adapted well after recovery. Many members of the veterinary staff, however, believed that the anesthesia and implantation procedure would worsen the otters' already weakened condition and add needless stress. Forty-five of the captive otters received implants.

The surgical procedure was performed by two veterinarians who have permits to operate on sea otters. Technicians were responsible for gathering and sterilizing the supplies needed for the surgery, and monitoring vital signs during anesthesia. Because of the vital insulating function of the otter's fur, no hair could be shaved in preparation for surgery. Instead, the area was saturated with sterile water-soluble lubricant mixed with povidone iodine solution and then the fur parted with a comb. The transmitter, which is about the size of a pack of cigarettes and encased in silicone plastic, was inserted into the abdominal cavity through a ventral midline incision which was then closed with absorbable sutures. The entire procedure only took about 20 minutes.

Release Procedures

The U.S. Fish and Wildlife Service required that all of the rehabilitated sea otters be quarantined in prerelease holding facilities for at least 30 days to observe the otters for any signs of contagious disease, such as canine distemper. Therefore, after an otter completely recovered, it was transferred by helicopter to a holding facility located in Valdez Harbor or Jakolof Bay near Homer, Alaska.

Several otter-inhabited areas in Prince William Sound were chosen as final release sites. Most of the sea otters were released in August 1989. Several aquariums accepted

(continues on page 189)

The Veterinary Technician's Role in a Zoologic Park or Aquarium

Joel Pond, CVT
Lincoln Park Zoo
Chicago, Illinois

The role of a veterinary technician in a zoo or an aquarium is varied and quite challenging. Veterinary medicine is becoming increasingly complex through technologic developments, and these same developments are found in zoo and aquarium medicine. The technicians of these facilities often strive for self-improvement in order to keep abreast of the latest technologic advances in veterinary medicine, just as technicians do in private practice.

Zoo veterinary technicians have widely varied educational backgrounds. Approximately 66% of the technicians are certified or licensed. Another 33% are medical technologists. A few others are keepers who have learned their craft on the job. There are a number of technicians who are both veterinary technicians and medical technologists. Many zoo veterinary technicians have bachelor's degrees in a related field.

The American Association of Zoos, Parks, and Aquariums (AAZPA) lists 154 member institutions in North America, of which approximately 40 employ one or more full-time veterinary technicians. Many of these institutions have not yet employed technicians, so it is likely that jobs will become available as funds are obtained.

The duties of zoo and aquarium veterinary technicians are similar, if not identical, to the duties of technicians in private practice. Like technicians in private practice, zoo and aquarium technicians are always under the supervision of a veterinarian.

The technicians of zoologic facilities have a 40-hour work week; however, similar to private practice, total hours worked is usually more than the scheduled number. Salaries range from $17,000 to more than $40,000 per year, with a median range of approximately $27,000. Benefits may include paid vacation, sick leave, medical and dental insurance plans, and personal days. Some technicians are members of the same local union as the zookeepers.

The responsibilities of zoo technicians vary among establishments. Some technicians only work in the laboratory, whereas others may do laboratory work, animal care, and care and feeding of the nursery animals in addition to management of the hospital and personnel.

Some of the larger zoos and aquariums in the United States have full-time technicians who are solely involved in laboratory work. Zoo clinical veterinary laboratories are equipped to do various tests in the following areas: water quality, parasitology, biochemistry, hematology, cytology, urinalysis, diagnosis of pregnancy, microbiology, serology, and sometimes histology. Other zoos may have more limited laboratory facilities and may send out their laboratory work to a veterinary or human reference laboratory. In-house laboratory support, however, provides the zoo veterinarian with nearly instantaneous results and provides a data base of normal values for the zoo animals.

Zoo technicians play a role in office management similar to that played by their peers in private practice. The telephone is as important of a tool in zoos as it is in private practice. Zoo technicians field calls from individuals who may be requesting information regarding wild animals they have found or even their own pets. The technician also deals with the zookeepers. A zookeeper plays the same role as the pet owner in private practice. Because they are in charge of day-today care of the animals, the keepers are most likely to detect veterinary problems. The zoo technician may deal with as few as 10 to as many as 150 zookeepers on a day-to-day basis by answering their questions, offering instruction on medicating an animal, or paraphrasing what the veterinarian has told the keeper. Also similar to clients in private practice, zookeepers have their own personalities, quirks, and abilities. There are zookeepers who create challenges for the technicians in a zoo just as there are clients who create challenges for the technicians in private practice.

The zookeepers alert the veterinary staff to medical problems and emergencies; if this is done by means of the telephone, the technician must triage those calls. The technician also may triage patients that are brought to the hospital. The zoo technician may play a major role in managing medical emergencies or animal escapes. Such management may include basic first aid for an injured animal or anesthetizing an escaped animal in order for it to be brought back to the zoo.

Technicians in some zoos may be responsible to care for and feed animals that are in the hospital. In addition to sick animals, the zoo hospital houses surplus animals, orphans, and social animals that have been ostracized from the group. Some technicians are responsible for the animals in the zoo nursery. The technician attends to the physical care of these animals while also providing comfort and companionship to them.

Recordkeeping

Recordkeeping is a very important task done by veterinary technicians in zoos. Weight charts, food and water intake and elimination, behav-ioral observations, and medical data are all recorded by the technician. Technicians working with fish or marine animals may be required to assess and record water quality and environmental data. Much of these data are recorded using computers.

Zoo record management is becoming more complex every day, and use of computers is increasing. Word processing is a valuable tool for communicating among zoo or aquarium technicians. Some technicians act as registrar for the facility. As a registrar, the technician is required to keep a record of acquisitions and husbandry data on all animals housed in the zoo or aquarium.

Zoos may house as few as 50 animals or as many as several thousand specimens. Each animal must be individually identified, which enables zoo personnel to track animals that are being moved to another area of the zoo or are being sent to another zoo. The International Species Inventory System (ISIS) is a recordkeeping system that is used by zoos around the world. The system inventories all animals housed by member zoos and aquariums that are members of the network. Within that system is a computer program called Animal Record Keeping System (ARKS). The ARKS program individually identifies each animal in a zoo's collection, records its ancestry and source of origin (e.g., born in another zoo or caught from the wild), and maintains the record of its reproductive history. This information allows zoos to pair genetically unrelated species in order to stir the gene pool.

Another program that a zoo technician may be responsible for maintaining is the Medical Animal Record Keeping System (MedARKS). MedARKS is capable of recording the following veterinary medical and laboratory data: parasite examinations, hematology, biochemistry, anesthesia, vaccinations, and treatments. Text medical records are being developed for this system. Many zoos use ARKS and MedARKS for all of their records. Other institutions use different data management systems.

Pharmacy control and hospital purchases may also be computerized. The technician usually is responsible for maintaining the stocks of pharmaceuticals and hospital supplies. Some establishments have computers for stock control, but most zoo or aquarium technicians use written methods for pharmacy records. The technician usually is responsible for purchasing medications, removing outdated medications from the shelves, and logging medications in and out. The controlled substances log is also maintained by the technician. Depending on the institution, the technician must be able to anticipate medical and supply orders months in advance in order for those items to go out for bid. Some technicians are actively involved in the budget-making process for the zoo or aquarium.

Radiography

Radiography is an important diagnostic modality for the zoo technician. Radiography in a zoo requires knowledge of the anatomy of many species. Although radiography of a wolf or lion is anatomically no different than that of a domestic dog or cat, respectively, radiography of more exotic species (such as tortoises [Figure 1]) is another matter. The zoo technician must be able to obtain diagnostic films of animals weighing as little 15 grams or as much as several hundred kilograms. Special procedures, such as contrast

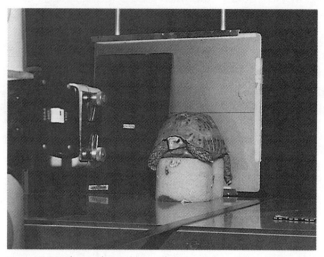

Figure 1—Radiographic technique for obtaining a skyline view of the lungs of a Greek tortoise.

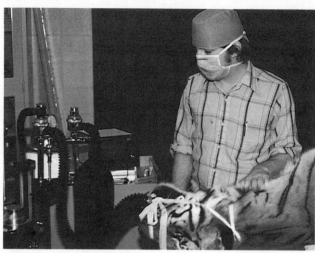

Figure 2—Inhalation anesthesia of a Bengal tiger in preparation for liver surgery.

studies and angiography, can be done on zoo animals. Ultrasonography also is being used by an increasing number of zoos. Zoo animals are sometimes taken to local animal or medical hospitals for more specialized examinations, such as computed axial tomography (CAT scan). Both stationary and portable radiography equipment are used in zoos. Rare earth films and screens are commonly used; dental film is used when tiny animals are examined or ultrafine details are required. In most cases, the animals are anesthetized before radiography or other procedures are done.

Anesthesia

Anesthesia is challenging for the zoo veterinarian and the technician. An animal may be anesthetized for several reasons. From a practical standpoint, a wild animal cannot be approached by a human if it is not anesthetized. Thus, anesthesia may be necessary for an animal to be moved from one enclosure to another or because the animal needs surgery (Figure 2).

Large and small zoo animals are anesthetized by delivery of an injectable drug via a dart. Several darts are marketed. One dart is made entirely of metal and has a relatively large bore needle. This dart uses a small explosive charge that is placed behind a rubber plunger. The charge is set off on impact with the animal, and the anesthetic is injected rapidly. These heavy darts hold between 1 and 15 milliliters of anesthetic, depending on the size of the dart barrel used.

A lightweight dart is also commercially available. The dart is made of plastic and comes in 1-, 2-, 3-, 5-, and 10-ml sizes. The special needles used are 16 to 20 gauge. The needles are soldered shut at the tip and have a small hole drilled on one side approximately three millimeters from the tip. A silicone sleeve is placed over this hole, and the needle (i.e., syringe) is placed on the dart after it has been loaded with medication. At the other end of the dart is an airspace in which a free-moving, flat bead has been placed. The airspace is pressurized using a Luer adapter on the end of an ordinary syringe. The bead acts as a one-way valve

preventing the air from leaving the dart and thus pressurizes and seals the system. The dart is fired either from a blow pipe or an air- or carbon dioxide-powered pistol or rifle. As the dart penetrates the animal's skin, it pushes the plastic sleeve away from the opening in the needle, thereby injecting the agent into the animal. Because the dart is nearly clear, the injection can be observed as it occurs. Injection by means of the lightweight dart occurs at approximately the same rate as that by a hand syringe. This method of injection is considerably less traumatic to the animal than the heavier dart method; however, because injection occurs more slowly, the animal may pull the dart out before the entire contents have been discharged. Other commercially made lightweight metal darts are available. Homemade darts also could be used.

Two injectable anesthetic agents are routinely used in zoos. Ketamine hydrochloride is readily available and seems to be safe in many species. When combined with xylazine hydrochloride, ketamine hydrochloride can be used in nearly all

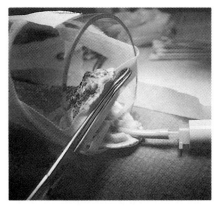

Figure 3—A venomous snake intubated for anesthesia in preparation for oral surgery. Note the forward location of the glottis.

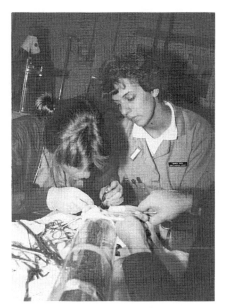

Figure 4—A rattlesnake undergoing oral surgery as a technician monitors anesthetic induction. Note the clear restraint tube.

species. Etorphine, which is a far more potent drug, is also used by zoos. This Schedule II drug is used primarily to anesthetize hoofed animals and pachyderms (e.g., elephants and rhinoceroses). Advantages of this drug include the low volume (3 to 5 milliliters) necessary to anesthetize the highly sensitive elephant and the reversibility of the drug. Diprenorphine is the antagonist used for etorphine. After an intravenous injection of diprenorphine, a large animal is able to stand normally within five minutes. The biggest danger of etorphine and diprenorphine is their toxicity to humans. One drop is lethal. Several safety precautions should be taken by the individual administering the drug. Rubber gloves and a pair of wraparound goggles should be worn, and a person familiar with cardiopulmonary resuscitation should be nearby.

Amphibians and fish are anesthetized with compounds that are administered in the water in which the animals swim. Simple surgical procedures and physical examinations can be safely done while the fish are anesthetized. Large, dangerous marine animals, such as sharks and moray eels, are immobilized in order to be handled safely. Major surgery can be done with the fish out of the water as long as it is kept wet, the gills are properly oxygenated, and a constant amount of anesthetic is delivered. If all these criteria are met, fish tolerate surgery quite well.

As soon as the animal has been anesthetized in its cage or enclosure, it can be approached for examination or treatment. Sometimes a procedure must be done at the zoo hospital instead of in the field. The animal may require supplemental anesthesia in order for the procedure to be done. The technician may place an intravenous catheter in any suitable vein with an appropriate fluid to keep the line open. The technician may give incremental doses of the original anesthetic drug to maintain anesthesia, or the animal could be intubated for administration of an inhalation anesthetic. Halothane and isoflurane are commonly used by most zoos. There are no anesthetic machines made specifically for zoo animals. Commonly, zoos have a combination anesthetic machine designed for large and small animals. Isoflurane has been found to be an excellent drug for use in all species.

There are a few considerations regarding administration of inhalant anesthetics. For example, the glottis of birds and reptiles lies forward in the mouth. Thus, these animals are intubated readily. Snakes often hold their breath for long periods and therefore require intubation followed by manual ventilation in order to be anesthetized. Venomous snakes may be restrained in a hollow acrylic tube and intubated safely for induction (Figures 3 and 4). Rodents are more difficult to intubate because of the nature of the oral anatomy. It is difficult, if not impossible, to visualize the tracheal opening in these animals.

Animals weighing less than five kilograms may be placed in an induction chamber. Small zoo patients are anesthetized with an open system (Bain breathing circuits are frequently used), and animals larger than five kilograms are anesthetized with a closed system. The zoo technician must be able to construct anesthesia masks for tiny animals (such as shrews) or very large animals (such as lions). After the patient has been successfully intubated and anesthetized, it is usually the zoo technician's responsibility to monitor the patient (Figure 5).

The principles of anesthesia are similar for all species. The technician monitors the respiratory rates and heart rates, the color of the mucous membranes, temperature, and the presence or absence of various reflexes in order to gauge the depth of anesthesia. Many zoos are equipped with sophisticated monitoring equipment.

Electrocardiography

Electrocardiography is used to monitor anesthetized patients. This includes reptiles and even fish. The zoo technician may also be required to interpret and respond to changes in the patient's electrocardiogram.

Parasitology

Zoo technicians may be responsible for the parasite control program. The technician who does the day-to-day parasitologic examinations of the animals may also be allowed to dispense the appropriate anthelmintics and initiate follow-up examinations under the supervision of the zoo veterinarian. Screening of zoo animals for internal parasites is a responsibility of the zoo technician.

Parasitology in zoos involves identification of external and internal parasites of many species. Identification of parasites can be complicated, particularly in animals taken from the wild. Individual animals may harbor several parasites, including nematodes, trematodes, cestodes, acanthocephalans (thorny headed worms), and various protozoa. The technician must attempt to identify the organisms to determine which are innocuous and which are potentially pathogenic. *Trichuris* species and roundworms are easily identified; however, there are many other parasites that have not been positively identified in exotic animals. Zoo or aquarium technicians often can classify a given organism according to its genus or perhaps only according to its class.

The zoo technician must also consider the animal's diet. Reptiles, amphibians, birds, and mammals that are fed rats or mice may pass ova of parasites that were injested along with the food. This type of infection is known as a spurious infection and does not indicate that the animal is parasitized.

Aside from spurious objects, the technician may encounter widely varied fecal artifacts. These objects are often confusing because they resemble parasite ova or cysts. Such artifacts can, however, yield information regarding the animal's diet or food quality. For example, an animal that is fed hay may have large numbers of fungal elements, such as macroconidia (spore cases) and hyphae. When these elements are passed in the feces in increased numbers, it may indicate that the hay is moldy.

Commensal organisms (i.e., those organisms that are normally found in gut flora) must also be differentiated from parasites. Equids, such as zebras or Przewalski's horses, and bovids, such as antelopes and giraffes, all normally harbor ciliate protozoa (as do their domestic counterparts); however, these large ciliates seldom are pathogenic.

The normal bacterial flora of all zoo animals must also be recognized by the zoo and aquarium technician who may be doing microbiologic examinations. Larger institutions have the capability of culturing aerobic and sometimes anaerobic bacteria and fungi. Identifying organisms may be done by use of commercially available kits, at human hospital laboratories, or at reference laboratories.

Hematology

Outside laboratories can do blood work if a zoo does not have its own laboratory. Larger zoos and aquariums have in-house hematology and blood chemistry instruments (Figure 6). Establishing normal values is necessary for each laboratory facility and is a major function of zoo laboratories throughout the United States. Normal values must be established for each species. Establishment of the normal values is a long, ongoing project. Sometimes zoos communicate with each other to obtain normal values for certain species, or a zoo may send a blood sample to another zoo for in-house analysis.

Biochemical profiles are established by each institution; however, the profiles are basically similar to those of domestic animals. Exceptions do exist, however; for example, birds, reptiles, and fish excrete nitrogenous waste in the form of uric acid instead of urea nitrogen.

There also are hematologic differences between zoo animals and animals commonly seen in private practice. All mammals have nonnucleated, round erythrocytes, although some mammals have unusually shaped erythrocytes. Deer and civet cats have sickled erythrocytes. Animals in the llama family as well as giraffes have oval-shaped erythrocytes (elliptocytes). Birds, reptiles, amphibians, and fish also have elliptocytes and nucleated erythrocytes. Because of these differences, the usual automated methods for cell counting cannot be used in these animals. Blood counts in animals with nucleated erythrocytes can be done by a number of manual methods.

Differentials of blood films of avian, reptilian, and piscine samples can be challenging. Birds and reptiles have white blood cells called heterophils. These cells, which are believed to be analogous to mammalian neutrophils, closely resemble eosinophils. Blood cells of fish seem to be more primitive in their morphology. The white blood cells of fish

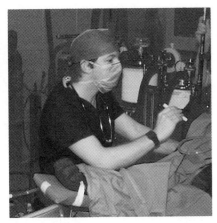

Figure 5—A technician monitors the anesthesia of a gorilla during surgery.

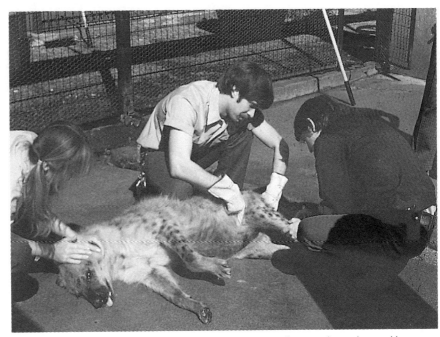

Figure 6—A blood sample is drawn from the saphenous vein of an anesthetized spotted hyena.

are classified according to the granules within them and the cell's staining characteristics. White blood cells are similar from species to species; for example, an eosinophil in a fish is similar to an eosinophil in a bird.

In addition to being familiar with the various blood cells among species, the zoo technician often finds parasites in the blood. Parasites include a variety of malarial organisms encountered in birds, reptiles, and amphibians. Many malarial organisms are considered to be pathogenic. *Haemoproteus* and *Leucocytozoon* are other protozoan parasites, which may be seen in avian blood samples. Microfilaria and trypanosomes are also occasionally seen. In general, *Haemoproteus* and *Leucocytozoon* as well as microfilaria and trypanosomes are incidental findings and are not pathogenic. Wolves and other wild canids are susceptible to heartworms. Zoos in enzootic areas administer preventive medication to susceptible animals.

Laboratory Profiles

The zoo laboratory would not be complete without the ability to do urinalysis. It is probably more difficult to obtain a clean urine specimen in a zoo situation than in private practice. Processing urine for urinalysis of zoo animals is identical to that for domestic animals.

Cytology and histology are also useful in zoos and aquariums. Cytology is done whenever possible on zoo animals in the same manner as on domestic animals. Histology is performed on many samples that have been cytologically evaluated. In addition, histopathology is the diagnostic tool of choice at necropsy. Again, it often is necessary to establish what normal tissue looks like. During necropsy, tissue in which no pathologic mechanism is noted often is taken to establish normal parameters. The zoo technician may do the cytologic sampling and examination. If histopathologic examination is done in-house, the technician may be responsible for preparing the specimens for the pathologist.

The zoo technician may be required to do serologic examinations. Zoo animals often are subject to the same diseases as domestic animals; thus, the same serologic tests are used for both types of animals. Other miscellaneous tests that can be done by zoo technicians include *Chlamydia* screening of birds, fungal screening, or testing for zoonotic parasitic disease of the keepers.

Miscellaneous Duties

Instruments that electronically monitor respiration may be available. Invasive and noninvasive blood pressure monitors and temperature probes are commonly used in zoos. The technician must be able to operate and service this equipment.

Technologic advances within the veterinary profession have resulted in the need for complex machinery, and the zoo technician may be required to maintain these machines. Larger zoos may have expensive and delicate instruments, such as laparoscopes, bronchoscopes, and arthroscopic equipment. These instruments are delicate and may be sterilized using toxic gas (ethylene oxide). A

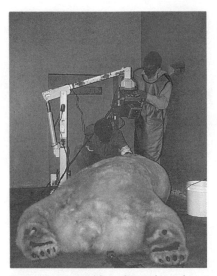

Figure 7—A portable radiograph machine is used to radiograph the upper jaw of a polar bear for an endodontic procedure. The bear has been anesthetized in its enclosure.

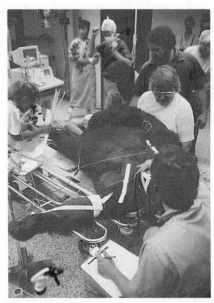

Figure 8—Reproductive soundness examination of a gorilla.

dental cart may be available and equipped to enable the zoo veterinarian to clean teeth, extract teeth, or even to fill teeth and do root canals. Electrocautery, artificial insemination apparatus, an emergency drug crash cart, defibrillator, fluid pumps, and suction apparatus also may be available. The technician may have to use these items and/or be responsible for their maintenance.

Similar to the technicians of private practice, some zoo technicians assist in surgery. This is especially true in larger establishments where there is enough technical support to have an anesthetist, scrub nurse, and surgical assistant. In addition, the zoo technician may be responsible for cleaning and sterilizing a wide variety of instrumentation.

Because zoo animals experience diverse surgical problems, no single surgical pack may be used for all species. Some zoos have a surgical pack for large animals that consists of larger, general purpose instruments. Other zoos keep individually wrapped instruments available as needs dictate. As in large animal

practices, instruments and equipment must be portable (Figure 7). It is often easier to bring the equipment and supplies to the animal than vice versa; for example, very large animals, such as elephants, rhinoceroses, camels, and walruses, cannot be transported to the zoo hospital for medical evaluation or treatment. Bringing the necessary equipment to the animal may involve a few instruments or most of the major equipment of the hospital.

Hazards to the animal as well as to the humans involved in the procedure must be considered. For example, is there a large body of water in the animal's enclosure in which it could drown during immobilization? Logistics also play a major role in what type of procedure can be done on a large animal. Is there a power source available for the equipment being used? Are supplemental generators necessary? Is a crane available to move the patient or the equipment to be used in the procedure? Will the fluids freeze during an outdoor procedure in cold climates? Zoo technicians and veteri-

narians must often adapt to these field conditions.

Necropsy is another area of responsibility for zoo technicians. During necropsy, the technician usually plays a supportive role by obtaining suitable tissue and laboratory specimens and recording data, among other duties. Some technicians are responsible for the actual prosection of the animal. Technicians also may be responsible for sending tissue for processing, or they may process the tissue themselves. Cytologic samples taken during necropsy also may be prepared and examined by the technician. The zoo technician may catalog all necropsy specimens and collate histopathology results.

Reproduction of the animals of the zoo or aquarium is a major goal. The zoo technician is often directly involved in this area in a variety of ways. Reproductive research is done at many zoos. Technicians may monitor the hormonal cycles of the animals, evaluate breeding soundness (Figure 8) via radiographic or ultrasonographic procedures, evaluate spermatozoa, and cryopreserve semen and ova. Many zoos that exhibit great apes (gorillas, chimpanzees, orangutans, and gibbons) use human pregnancy test kits that use urine for the detection of pregnancy. Most reproductive research currently being done is for endangered animals; some of these animals are extinct in the wild. Working to save a species is one of the most gratifying experiences of a zoo technician.

In addition to participation in research, zoo and aquarium technicians often are involved in a variety of educational programs. Such programs include keeper education and training, public education (including conducting educational tours of the zoo hospital), and providing additional training or instruction to veterinary technician students. Zoo technicians are often asked to speak at local allied health organization meetings. Medical technology, radiology, microbiology, and veterinary technology schools also use zoo veterinary technicians as a teaching resource.

Wildlife rehabilitation programs often involve zoo technicians. Some zoos shelter and rehabilitate injured wildlife. Other zoos stabilize injured wild animals before sending them to local rehabilitation facilities. Some technicians are responsible for comprehensive care of injured wildlife presented to the zoo.

Some zoo technicians are responsible for other veterinary and medical programs. One program may include maintaining a serum bank. Another program may involve maintaining files of the medical data of zoo employees. Obtaining a preemployment blood sample is a requirement of many zoos; therefore, if an employee becomes ill, it can then be proved or disproved that the illness was acquired in the workplace.

Another program that involves the technician is the zoo's vaccination program. The technician often administers vaccines to all animals requiring vaccinations according to a set schedule.

All zoos that house marine mammals or fish are required by law to monitor water quality. Water quality can be assessed by pH readings, measurement of dissolved solids and chemicals, and coliform bacteria counts. Water quality is obviously an issue of major importance to aquariums. Aquariums also monitor other conditions, such as water salinity, water filtration systems, algae concentration, temperature, and the presence of metallic ions (i.e, nickel, iron, copper).

Conclusion

The veterinary technician who works in a zoo or an aquarium is part of a complex management team. The professional role of these technicians is challenging and extremely rewarding, and the technician's work directly affects the welfare of the animals in the zoo or aquarium.

ACKNOWLEDGMENT

Thanks are owed to Terry W. Campbell, DVM, PhD, Sea World of Florida, Inc., Orlando, Florida, for his technical review of this article.

Sea Otters *(continued from page 181)*

the small otter pups and the injured otters that would not have survived release back into the wild.

Summary

The skills of the veterinary technicians were challenged during this rehabilitation effort. Knowledge in emergency medicine, surgical assistance, clinical pathology, and pharmaceuticals was essential to help provide the best care for the incapacitated animals.

Acknowledgments

A special thank you to all the veterinarians, veterinary technicians, sea mammal specialists, staff, and volunteers who put their lives on hold for many months in order to save these fascinating creatures of Prince William Sound.

Also, I greatly appreciate the assistance of Craig Harms, DVM, and Pam Tuomi, DVM, who reviewed this manuscript before submission for publication.

UPDATE

Out of the 45 sea otters with implants, ⅔ died or were unaccounted for 2 years after their release.[1] The surviving female sea otters exhibited a much lower reproductive rate than sea otters in the wild.[1]

Since the spill, new contingency plans and protocols for oil spills and injured wildlife have been developed. Wildlife response teams, that include veterinarians and veterinary technicians, have been formed that are able to be on the scene within 24 hours. The information gathered from the sea otter rehabilitation project strongly influenced these new wildlife contingency plans that are now in place.

REFERENCE

1. Monnet C, Rotterman LR: Mortality and Reproduction of Sea Otters Oiled and Treated as a Result of the Exxon Valdez Oil Spill NRDA Report, Marine Mammal Study No. 7. U. S. Fish and Wildlife Service, Anchorage, Alaska, 1992.

Cytodiagnosis in Exotic Animal Practice: Sample Processing

Terry W. Campbell, DVM, PhD
Sea World of Florida, Inc.
Orlando, Florida

Samples for cytologic evaluation can be collected from exotic animal patients by fine-needle aspiration techniques, washings, scrapings or swabbings, or contact smear procedures. Fine-needle aspiration techniques include paracentesis, thoracentesis, arthrocentesis, fine-needle aspiration biopsy, and aspiration of fluid-filled lesions. Fine-needle aspiration biopsy of solid tissue is performed by aspirating a small amount of tissue into the lumen of a fine-gauge needle, which is done by inserting the needle into tissue and applying negative pressure within an attached syringe using the syringe plunger. Moving the needle back and forth throughout the tissue and redirecting the needle several times obtains a larger sample, especially in tissue that exfoliates poorly. It is important to release the negative pressure from the syringe before removing the needle from the tissue to avoid aspirating the sample into the syringe rather than containing it within the lumen of the needle. The obtained specimen should immediately be applied to a microscope slide by using the air-filled syringe to force the sample onto the slide. A second microscope slide is placed on top of the first; pulling the two slides apart prepares the smear.

Fluid Samples

Samples are obtained by fine-needle aspiration of fluids (i.e., paracentesis, thoracentesis, arthrocentesis, and aspiration of fluid-filled lesions) by aspirating the fluid sample into a syringe attached to a needle. Paracentesis of exotic animals is similar to the procedure routinely used in domestic cats and dogs. A site immediately cranial to the umbilicus and slightly to the right of the midline is prepared as for surgery. After local anesthesia is given, the needle is directed through the skin and under the peritoneum; the needle must remain parallel to the body wall to avoid the intestines. The bevel of the needle should face outward toward the body wall to avoid blockage of the needle with fat or peritoneum. Abdominal fluid is aspirated into a syringe to complete the procedure.

Paracentesis of avian patients is performed in a similar manner. The needle is inserted into the ventral midline of the abdomen immediately caudal to the caudal point of the keel. The needle is directed toward the right side of the abdomen to avoid puncture of the ventriculus (gizzard). It should be noted that little, if any, fluid can be obtained from the abdomen of a normal bird. It also is difficult to enter the peritoneal space because of large abdominal air sacs; however, fluid distention of the abdomen compresses abdominal air sacs laterally, thereby allowing easy access into the peritoneal cavity.

With the exception of turtles and tortoises, paracentesis of reptiles is performed along the ventral midline in a manner similar to that of mammals. In turtles and tortoises, entry into the peritoneal cavity is made immediately cranial to the hindlimbs.

Abdominal fluid is obtained from fish by inserting the aspiration needle along the ventral midline cranial to the vent.

Thoracentesis is more commonly performed on mammals than on other vertebrates. The site of needle entry depends on the location of the fluid level in the thoracic cavity, which is determined by radiographic evaluation. The skin is prepared as for surgery, local anesthesia is given, and the needle is inserted in the intercostal space as low as possible in the thoracic wall and immediately cranial to the caudal rib to avoid puncture of nerves, arteries, or veins that lie along the caudal edge of the rib. A three-way valve and a syringe that is at least 20 cubic centimeters are required for patients with large quantities of thoracic fluid. The aspiration needle is directed under the pleural space and remains parallel to the thoracic wall with the needle bevel facing outward as suggested in paracentesis. The fluid is aspirated into the syringe.

Fluid samples can be prepared for cytologic evaluation by various techniques. Direct smears can be made from highly cellular fluids by following techniques that are used in preparing peripheral blood smears. Cellular concentration techniques facilitate cytologic evaluation of poorly cellular fluids. A convenient method of concentrating cells on a slide is to marginate the cells on the leading edge of the smear. This is done by preparing the smear in a manner similar to the method used to prepare blood smears using the wedge technique and backing slowly into the drop of fluid while holding the spreader slide at a 45° angle. The spreader slide is slowly pushed forward and quickly lifted from the surface of the bottom slide just before completing the smear.

Another method of cell concentration is by centrifugation (600 G for 10 minutes) of the fluid in a glass test tube. A smear is directly prepared from the sediment. Cellular concentration also can be achieved using special cytocentrifuge equipment (i.e., Cytospin®—Shandon Southern Instruments); however, this method generally is too expensive for use in average clinics. A less expensive cell concentration method involves a small column (i.e., small syringe barrel) that is firmly clamped to a microscope slide that uses filter paper with an 8- to 10-millimeter hole located between the column and slide. As the fluid enters the column, the fluid is absorbed by the filter paper and cells adhere to the glass slide.

Evaluating fluid samples involves describing the physical appearance of the fluid, determining a nucleated cell count (which may include erythrocytes when evaluating birds, reptiles, or fish), and estimating total protein concentration using a refractometer. Nucleated cell counts can be determined using a manual or automated counting method.

Additional tests performed on synovial fluid include mucin clot tests and viscosity tests. Because the volume of samples that are obtained from joint aspirates of small mammals, reptiles, and birds usually is very small, microtechniques are used. A simple viscosity test can be performed by placing a drop of fresh synovial fluid on a clean microscope slide and measuring the strand formed as the fluid is lifted from the surface of the slide using a wooden applicator or finger. If the strand breaks before reaching two centimeters in length, viscosity of the fluid is reduced. A micromucin clot test can be performed by mixing a few drops of synovial fluid with an equal amount of 5% acetic acid solution on a microscope slide. After one minute, the mixture should form a firm, homogenous clot that adheres to the slide if mucin quality is good. Mucin of poor quality does not clot.

Wash Samples

Wash samples frequently are used for cytodiagnosis. The procedure generally involves inserting a sterile tube into the area to be examined, infusing a small amount of sterile saline, and aspirating the fluid sample into a syringe. Tracheal washes are commonly performed on mammals, birds, and reptiles. Wash samples also are used in evaluating stomachs of reptiles and crops (ingluvies) of birds. Rectocolon washes for cytologic evaluation also are useful in evaluating the lower digestive tract of various animals.

Cytologic samples that are collected by washing are prepared for microscopic evaluation similar to the method of preparing poorly cellular fluid. Wet-mount preparations often are used in evaluating certain wash samples, such as stomach washes of reptiles (especially snakes) and crop washes from birds, especially if motile protozoa are suspected. Cell concentration techniques usually are necessary to facilitate cytologic evaluation of wash samples.

Samples Obtained by Scraping or Swabbing a Lesion

Samples obtained by scraping a lesion are applied to a microscope slide by spreading the sample across the slide in one direction or by imprinting the sample onto the slide while attempting to avoid excessive cellular rupture. Samples obtained from swabs are applied to the slide by rolling the swab across the slide in one direction only. Excessive cell rupture or a thick smear that is difficult to evaluate often results if the swab is rolled back and forth instead of in one direction.

Contact Smears or Imprints

Contact smears or imprints are made simply by touching the surface of a clean microscope slide to a freshly cut surface of an excised mass or to an exposed lesion in situ. In evaluating fish, fin and gill biopsy samples are commonly taken and examined as wet-mount preparations, although contact smears for staining can be made from biopsy samples.

Cytologic Stain for Exotic Animal Practice

Stains used in hematology are routinely used for cytologic evaluation in veterinary medicine primarily because they are uncomplicated to use, stain rapidly, and are easily applicable to clinical practice. Romanovsky's stains, such as Wright's stain, modified Wright's stain, Giemsa stain, and quick Romanovsky's stain, are commonly used in veterinary cytodiagnosis. Quick stains are especially adapted for use in clinical practice because of their simplicity and ability to stain quickly. Romanovsky's stains are used to stain air-dried cytology samples fixed in alcohol during staining.

New's methylene blue stain is a vital stain that can be used in evaluating cytologic specimens. Methylene blue stain can be used with air-dried smears or as a wet-mount stain. An advantage of this water-based stain is that it can be used immediately for evaluating a cytology specimen without previous fixation.

Special stains may be required for proper evaluation of cytology specimens. Acid-fast stains, for example, are used to identify microorganisms that stain acid-fast positive, such as tubercle bacteria. Acid-fast positive organisms stain red; acid-fast negative organisms and leukocytes stain blue.

Gram's stain is often used to identify bacteria. Gram-positive microorganisms stain deep violet; gram-negative organisms stain red. Gram's stain was developed to stain bacteria grown in pure culture on artificial media. If the stain is applied to cytology specimens, the results may be less conclusive than would be results achieved from application of the stain to smears made from pure colonies of bacteria derived from culture. Variability of material found in most cytology specimens causes the difference in results.

Macchiavellos and Gimenez stains are used to identify *Chlamydia* inclusions. Small elementary bodies (0.2 to

0.3 μm) of *Chlamydia* stain red with both types of stain. Larger initial bodies (0.9 to 1.0 μm) stain blue with Macchiavellos stain. The host tissue cells stain bluish green with Gimenez stain; therefore, red inclusion bodies contrast sharply for easier identification.

Conclusion

Materials needed to perform cytodiagnostic procedures in exotic animal practice are uncomplicated to use and are relatively inexpensive. Syringes (6 to 12 cc) and fine-gauge needles (22 to 20 gauge or 1 to 1½ inch) are needed for aspiration and fine-needle biopsy techniques. Sterile cotton swabs and scalpel blades are needed to obtain samples by scraping and swabbing. Sterile tubing and physiologic saline are needed to obtain wash samples. A microscope with a good oil immersion (100×) lens as well as clean microscope slides, coverslips, and immersion oil are essential to cytology. Cytologic stains are needed to evaluate specimens with a microscope.

BIBLIOGRAPHY

Campbell TW: *Avian Hematology and Cytology.* Ames, IA, Iowa State University Press, 1988.

Rebar AH: *Handbook of Veterinary Cytology.* St Louis, MO, Ralston Purina Co, 1978.

Rebar AH: Cytologic collection techniques and specimen handling, in *Proceeding of the Third Symposium on Veterinary Diagnostic Cytolology.* West Lafayette, IN, Veterinary Cytology Resource Center, Purdue University, 1990.

Perman V, Alsaker RD, Riis RC: *Cytology of the Dog and Cat.* Denver, CO, American Animal Hospital Association, 1979.

Cytodiagnosis in Exotic Animal Practice: Interpretation

Terry W. Campbell, DVM, PhD
Sea World of Florida, Inc.
Orlando, Florida

The primary goal in evaluating a cytologic sample is to determine cellular response, which is accomplished by examining individual cells in the smear and formulating an opinion of the cellular response based on the appearance of the majority of cells. Basic cytologic responses include inflammation, tissue hyperplasia and benign neoplasia, malignant neoplasia, mixed cytologic responses (inflammatory and noninflammatory), and normal cellularity.

Cell Types

The cytologist should attempt to classify each cell into one of four tissue groups based on whether the origin of the cell is epithelial or glandular, mesenchymal, nervous, or hemic. Cells from hemic tissue are derived from blood and hematopoietic tissue. These cells include erythrocytes, leukocytes, and thrombocytes (or platelets) and their precursors.

Epithelial cells vary in shape, depending on their origin. They tend to exfoliate easily in cellular clumps or sheets and provide a highly cellular sample. Epithelial cells typically have abundant cytoplasm and distinct cell margins. Cells from secretory epithelium often are cuboidal or columnar in shape and contain distinct cytoplasmic granules or vacuoles.

Cells of mesenchymal or connective tissue usually exfoliate poorly, thereby resulting in a sample with low cellularity. These types of cells tend to exfoliate individually instead of in cellular aggregates. Mesenchymal cells vary in shape and cytoplasmic volume. Fibroblasts of mesenchymal tissue are commonly seen in cytologic samples. Fibroblasts often are fusiform; the shape of the nucleus follows the shape of the cell. Cytoplasmic margins of mesenchymal cells often appear indistinct.

Cells originating from nervous tissue rarely are seen in cytologic samples. When present, these cells usually appear as deeply basophilic and stellate with prominent cytoplasmic projections.

Inflammatory Cytologic Responses

Inflammatory cells include neutrophils (or heterophils, depending on the species), eosinophils, lymphocytes, plasma cells, and macrophages (or monocytes). The inflammatory response can be classified as neutrophilic (or heterophilic), eosinophilic, mixed cell, or macrophagic.

Inflammatory lesions of exotic mammals resemble those of domestic mammals. Neutrophilic inflammation is identified by the predominance of neutrophils, which represent at least 70% of the inflammatory cells. Rabbits, guinea pigs, and hystricomorphic rodents (i.e., porcupines and capybaras) have neutrophils that resemble heterophils; therefore, they demonstrate a heterophiliclike inflammatory response. The neutrophils may appear degenerate and show abnormal nuclei (i.e., hyalinization, swelling, karyorrhexis, and karyolysis) and cytoplasm (i.e., increased basophilia, vacuolation, and degranulation [Figure 1]). Degenerative neutrophils suggest the presence of a toxic environment, such as bacterial toxins in septic lesions.

Mixed-cell inflammation is characterized by the presence of nearly equal numbers of neutrophils (or heterophils) and mononuclear leukocytes, such as macrophages, lymphocytes, and plasma cells (Figure 2). Macrophagic inflammation is characterized by the predominance of macrophages in the inflammatory response, in which macrophages represent more than 50% of inflammatory cells. Macrophages often contain cytoplasmic vacuoles and phagocytized material, such as cellular debris and infectious agents. Macrophages also may form multinucleated giant cells, thereby suggesting a granulomatous response (Figure 3).

Eosinophilic inflammation in exotic mammals suggests a response to degranulation of mast cells as seen in cases of immediate hypersensitivity reactions or parasitic infestation with nematodes. Eosinophils may be present in mixed-cell inflammatory responses.

Inflammatory lesions of birds resemble inflammatory lesions of mammals,

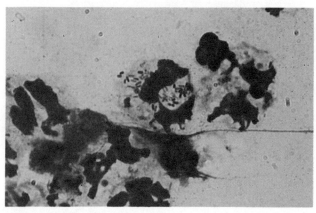

Figure 1—Septic neutrophilic inflammation in a mammal. Note the degenerate neutrophils and intracellular bacteria. (Wright's stain)

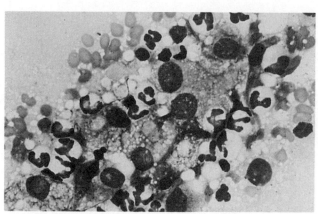

Figure 2—This example of mixed-cell inflammation in a mammal shows a mixture of macrophages and neutrophils. (Wright's stain)

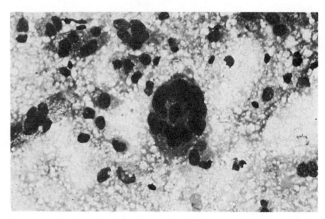

Figure 3—Macrophagic inflammation in a bird. Note the predominance of macrophages and formation of multinucleated giant cells. (Wright's stain)

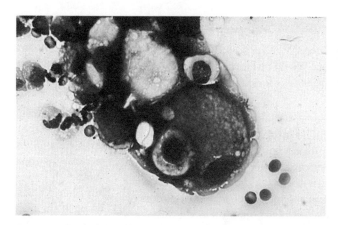

Figure 4—Epithelial cells and leukocytes appear large and abnormal in this contact smear from an adenocarcinoma in a mammal. (Wright's stain)

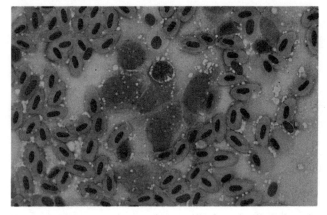

Figure 5—Numerous pleomorphic spindle-shaped cells and erythrocytes are apparent in this contact smear from a fibrosarcoma in a bird. (Wright's stain)

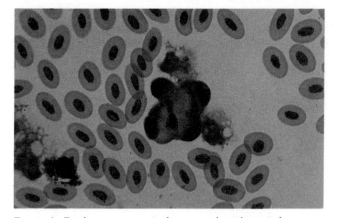

Figure 6—Erythrocytes, macrophages, and a cluster of reactive mesothelial cells in the abdominal fluid of a bird. (Wright's stain)

except that the avian heterophil replaces the neutrophil. Heterophil granules tend to lose their typical rod-shaped appearance in inflammatory lesions and become round or degranulated. As with mammalian neutrophils, avian heterophils can appear degenerate. Heterophilic inflammation in birds suggests an early stage in the inflammatory process. Macrophages appear quickly in avian inflammatory lesions; mixed-cell inflammation is therefore common. Multinucleated giant cells also are common to avian inflammation; unlike mammalian giant cell formation, avian giant cells do not necessarily indicate chronicity. In birds, lymphocytes and plasma cells also can occur with mixed-cell inflammation, even in cases of acute heterophilic granuloma formation. The presence of epithelioid cells (macrophages without cytoplasmic vacuoles or phagocytized material) and connective tissue cells (i.e., fibroblasts) suggests chronic granuloma formation in birds. Macrophagic inflammation in birds reveals predominant, large, vacuolated macrophages that frequently develop into multinucleated giant cells. This type of inflammation is common in certain avian diseases, such as chlamydiosis, tuberculosis, and cutaneous xanthomatosis.

Reptilian inflammatory lesions resemble avian inflammatory lesions. As with birds, mixed-cell inflammation is common in reptiles. Granuloma formation also is typical of the reptilian inflammatory response, and multinucleated giant cells and fibroblasts appear as the granuloma matures.

Noninflammatory Cytologic Responses

Tissue hyperplasia and benign neoplasia are indistinguishable based on cytomorphology. Tissue hyperplasia is a proliferative process involving tissue that is responding to cellular injury or to chronic stimulation, such as glandular hyperplasia. This process occurs in all species. Cells that are suggestive of tissue hyperplasia or benign neoplasia generally have a uniform appearance with increased cytoplasmic basophilia and pale, vesicular nuclei. A frequent example of tissue hyperplasia in animals is the proliferation of epithelial and mesenchymal cells adjacent to areas of chronic inflammation. Examples of tissue hyperplasia or benign neoplasia that are frequently identified during cytodiagnosis in mammals include basal epithelioma, lipoma, and lymphoid hyperplasia. Examples of tissue hyperplasia or benign neoplasia in birds include squamous cell hyperplasia associated with hypovitaminosis A, lipomas, and lymphoid hyperplasia.

The cytodiagnostic criteria of malignant neoplasia that apply to domestic mammals also apply to exotic mammals, birds, reptiles, and fish. General cellular features of malignant neoplasia include noninflammatory cells that exhibit pleomorphism, increased cellularity (especially from tissue that normally provides poorly cellular samples), and the presence of cells that are foreign to the tissue being examined. Nuclear features of malignant neoplasia are the most important criteria in cytodiagnosis of malignant neoplasia. Such features include anisokaryosis, variable nucleus-to-cytoplasm ratios, nuclear pleomorphism, abnormal nuclear chromatin, large or multiple (greater than four) nucleoli, and abnormal mitoses. Two important cytoplasmic features of malignant neoplasia include increased cytoplasmic basophilia (suggesting increased activity of ribonucleic acid) and vacuolation (small vacuoles suggest cellular degeneration, whereas large vacuoles are associated with secretory products that occur in cases of adenocarcinoma). Structural features of malignant neoplasia refer to cellular characteristics that suggest a possible origin, such as epithelial (carcinoma), mesenchymal (sarcoma), or discrete (round cell) neoplasms (Figures 4 and 5). Discrete cell neoplasms are derived from round to oval cells that lack normal cell-to-cell interaction and normally exfoliate as individual cells. A common discrete cell neoplasm of exotic animals is lymphoid neoplasia.

Effusions

Effusions of exotic mammals, birds, reptiles, and fish can be classified as transudates, modified transudates, exudates, hemorrhagic effusions, malignant effusions, or chylous effusions. Chylous effusions are primarily seen in mammals. Transudates are characterized by low cellularity (< 1000 nonerythrocytic cells/μl), low specific gravity (< 1.015), and low protein content (< 2.5 g/dl). Modified transudates resemble true transudates but have higher cellularity (< 5000 nonerythrocytic cell/μl) and protein content (2.5 to 3.0 g/dl). Mononuclear leukocytes and mesothelial cells predominate the cellularity of modified transudates (Figure 6). Exudates are characterized by high cellularity (> 5000 nonerythrocytic cells/μl), high specific gravity (> 1.020), and high protein content (> 3.0 g/dl). Inflammatory cells predominate the cellularity of exudates. Acute hemorrhagic effusions resemble peripheral blood with lower cell counts and protein content, whereas long-standing hemorrhagic effusions are characterized by leukocytes that demonstrate varying degrees of erythrocytophagy. Malignant effusions can resemble modified transudates, exudates, or hemorrhagic effusions with cells that show features of malignant neoplasia.

BIBLIOGRAPHY

Campbell TW: *Avian Hematology and Cytology.* Ames, IA, Iowa State University Press, 1988.
Montali RJ: Comparative pathology of inflammation in the higher vertebrates (reptiles, birds, and mammals). *J Comp Pathol* 99:1-26, 1988.
Perman V, Alsaker RD, Riis RC: *Cytology of the Dog and Cat.* Denver, CO, American Animal Hospital Association, 1979.
Rebar AH: *Handbook of Veterinary Cytology.* St. Louis, MO, Ralston Purina Co, 1978.

Hematology of Birds, Reptiles, and Fish

Terry W. Campbell, DVM, PhD
Sea World of Florida, Inc.
Orlando, Florida

Birds, reptiles, and fish are often presented to veterinarians for medical treatment. Hematology is often involved in the diagnostic plan of the medical evaluation of these animals. Because birds, reptiles, and fish possess erythrocytes, thrombocytes, and granulocytes that might appear different than those of mammalian blood, the evaluation of the hemogram might present a few technical problems.

ERYTHROCYTES

The laboratory evaluation of avian, reptilian, and piscine erythrocytes includes the packed cell volume (PCV), hemoglobin concentration, total erythrocyte count, and examination of the blood smear. The standard manual technique to obtain a packed cell volume by using microhematocrit capillary tubes and centrifugation (12,000 g for five minutes) can be performed on blood from these types of animals. The hemoglobin concentration is usually determined by the cyanmethemoglobin method after the free nuclei from lysed red blood cells are removed by centrifugation of the cyanmethemoglobin reagent-blood mixture. This procedure prevents an overestimation of the hemoglobin concentration before obtaining the optical density value.

The total erythrocyte count of birds, reptiles, and fish can be deter-mined by the same automated or manual methods used to determine total erythrocyte counts in mammalian blood. Formulas used to calculate the mean corpuscular values (mean corpuscular volume, MCV; mean corpuscular hemoglobin, MCH; and mean corpuscular hemoglobin concentration, MCHC) for mammalian hematologic studies can also be used for animals with nucleated erythrocytes.

The microscopic appearance of the nucleated erythrocytes in stained blood smears completes the routine evaluation of the erythron. The nucleated erythrocytes of birds, reptiles, and fish are oval shaped with centrally positioned oval-shaped nuclei. Erythrocytes from these animals are generally larger in comparison with mammalian erythrocytes. The nuclear chromatin of nucleated erythrocytes is typically clumped and becomes increasingly condensed with cellular maturity. In Wright's stain smears (Figures 1–4), the nucleus is basophilic and the cytoplasm appears orange-pink, resembling the cytoplasmic color of mammalian erythrocytes. The cytoplasm of normal reptilian and piscine red blood cells might show vacuolation. Polychromatophilic erythrocytes occur in low numbers in the peripheral blood of normal birds, reptiles, and fish.

Important abnormal erythrocyte morphology seen in the blood smears of these animals include increased polychromasia, hypochromasia, and the presence of numerous immature erythrocytes. Ruptured red blood cells and free nuclei are common artifacts seen in peripheral blood smears from animals with nucleated erythrocytes. The free nuclei often appear as amorphous, purple material throughout the smear.

The number of ruptured cells (smudge cells) in the smear can be minimized by proper blood smear preparation, such as the push-slide method using two microscope slides, a two-coverslip method, or a slide and coverslip method.

LEUKOCYTES

The presence of nucleated erythrocytes and thrombocytes in the blood of birds, reptiles, and fish precludes the use of the routine methods used to count the leukocytes of mammalian blood. The size of the erythrocytes and many of the leukocytes of birds, reptiles, and fish is very similar, as is the size of the thrombocytes and small lymphocytes; therefore, automated methods used to count the leukocytes of mammalian blood result in erroneous values if applied to the blood of these animals. Also, automated and routine manual methods of counting mammalian leukocytes depend on lysis of the erythrocytes. Lysis of the blood of birds, reptiles, and fish is often incomplete. The presence of free red blood cell nuclei might also cause confusion when counting leukocytes.

A direct manual method for obtaining total leukocyte counts in the blood of birds, reptiles, and fish involves the use of Natt and Herrick's solution (see box). A 1:200 dilution of

Natt and Herrick's Solution

Constituents

NaCl	3.88 g
Na_2SO_4	2.50 g
$[Na_2HPO_4][H_2O]_{12}$	2.91 g
KH_2PO_4	0.25 g
Formalin (37%)	7.5 ml
Gentian violet 2B	0.10 g

Preparation
The chemicals are dissolved in distilled water to make a total volume of one liter. The solution is allowed to stand overnight and is filtered through Whatman No. 2 filter paper before use.

the blood is made using Natt and Herrick's solution and a red blood cell diluting pipette. The mixture is placed in a hemocytometer and allowed to stand for five minutes or more in a humid chamber. The total leukocyte count is obtained by counting every leukocyte, which stain dark blue, in the nine large squares of the ruled area of the hemocytometer using the following formula: TWBC/µl = (Total white blood cells counted in nine squares + 10%) × 200.

A disadvantage of this method is that the differentiation between thrombocytes and small lymphocytes is often difficult, thereby creating errors in the hemocytometer chamber counts; an advantage of this method is that a total erythrocyte count can be obtained using the same charge hemocytometer and counting the four corner squares and central square of the central large square of the hemocytometer. The total erythrocyte count is calculated using the following formula: TRBC/µl = RBC counted × 10,000.

Another method that can be used to obtain a total leukocyte count in the blood of birds (not reptiles or fish) is by a semidirect manual method. This method involves the staining of heterophils and eosinophils with a phloxine B solution used as a stain and diluent. This procedure can be

simplified by using the Eosinophil Unopette 5877 System (Becton-Dickinson), which is designed to obtain total eosinophil counts in mammalian blood. The blood diluted with the phloxine B solution in the Unopette using the provided 25 µl pipette makes a 1/32 dilution. The properly charged hemocytometer is read by counting the eosin-stained cells (heterophils and eosinophils) in both sides of the chamber.

Prolonged exposure of the erythrocytes to the stain might cause difficulty in counting the leukocytes; therefore, the hemocytometer must be loaded immediately following proper mixing of the blood with the phloxine B solution to avoid staining of the erythrocytes. A total heterophil and eosinophil count per microliter of blood (Het + Eos/µl) is calculated using the formula for obtaining total eosinophil counts in mammalian blood, which is followed according to enclosed instructions. The total leukocyte count (TWBC/µl) is calculated after completing a leukocyte differential from the blood smear using the following formula:

$$\text{TWBC/µl} = \frac{(\text{Het + Eos/µl}) \times 100}{\%\text{Het and Eos}}$$

The total leukocyte count can be obtained by using the following calculation:

$$\text{TWBC/µl} = \frac{\text{Eosin-stained cells} \times 1.1 \times 16 \times 100}{\%\text{Het and Eos}}$$

where the number of eosin-stained cells are counted in both sides of the hemocytometer (18 large squares).

GRANULOCYTES

The appearance of the granulocytic leukocytes in the peripheral blood of birds, reptiles, and fish might differ greatly from those of mammalian blood; therefore, brief descriptions of the peripheral blood granulocytes from these groups of animals are provided.

Birds

Avian granulocytes are classified as

heterophils, eosinophils, and basophils. Heterophils are the most common granulocytes in the peripheral blood of birds. Normal, mature heterophils have a colorless cytoplasm that contains elongated (rod-shaped) eosinophilic granules, which might be round to oval in some species. Properly stained heterophil granules usually have a distinct, refractile central body. Heterophil granules might be affected by the staining process and appear poorly stained, partially dissolved, or fused together. Mature heterophils have lobed nuclei that usually consist of two or three lobes with coarse, clumped chromatin that stains purple. The nucleus is often partially hidden by the cytoplasmic granules.

Avian heterophils appear to exhibit toxic changes similar to those seen in mammalian neutrophils in response to severe systemic illness. Toxic heterophils exhibit increased cytoplasmic basophilia, vacuolation, abnormal granulation (degranulation, toxic granulation, and granules that appear to coalesce into larger granules), and nuclear degeneration. The degree of heterophil toxicity can be rated on a scale of 1+ to 4+. A 1+ rating is given to heterophils showing increased cytoplasmic basophilia. A 2+ toxicity is represented by heterophils with deeper cytoplasmic basophilia, vacuolation, and partial degranulation. A 3+ toxicity is given to heterophils with dark cytoplasmic basophilia, moderate degranulation, abnormal granules, and cytoplasmic vacuolation. Finally, a 4+ toxicity is represented by heterophils with deep cytoplasmic basophilia, moderate-to-marked degranulation with the presence of abnormal granules, vacuolation, and karyorrhexis or karyolysis.

Immature heterophils are occasionally found in the peripheral blood of birds with severe systemic infections. These cells are usually heterophil myelocytes and metamyelocytes. The myelocytes and metamyelocytes have a light blue cytoplasm that contains a mixture of primary and specific granules. The specific granules are the typical rod-shaped heterophil granules seen in mature heterophils. The primary granules often appear as deeply

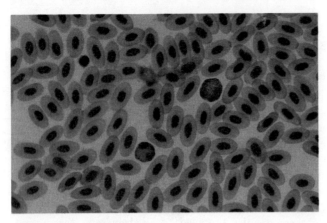

Figure 1—A heterophil, an eosinophil, and erythrocytes from a great horned owl (Wright's stain).

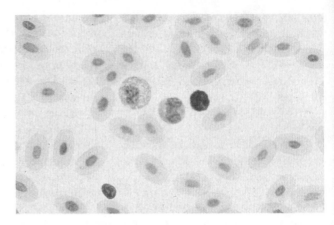

Figure 2—A monocyte, a heterophil, a basophil, and erythrocytes from a Burmese python (Wright's stain).

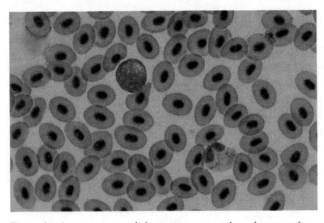

Figure 3—A toxic neutrophil, a monocyte, and erythrocytes from a teleost fish [acorna (Wright's stain)].

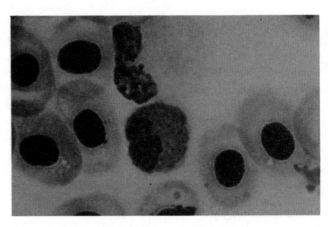

Figure 4—A Type II granulocyte, a Type III granulocyte, and erythrocytes from a cartilagenous fish [lemon shark (Wright's stain)].

basophilic or orange spheres or rings. Heterophil myelocytes have round-to-oval nuclei and possess specific rod-shaped granules that occupy less than one-half of the cytoplasmic volume. Heterophil metamyelocytes have nuclei that are slightly indented. The metamyelocytes possess specific heterophil granules that occupy greater than one-half of the cytoplasmic volume.

Normal, mature avian eosinophils have a cytoplasm that stains clear blue, in contrast with the colorless cytoplasm of normal, mature heterophils. Eosinophils typically have round, strongly eosinophilic cytoplasmic granules (a few species have elongated eosinophilic granules) that have

staining qualities differing from those of the granules found in heterophils of the same blood smear. The nuclei of avian eosinophils are lobed and usually stain darker than those of heterophils. Frequently, the cytoplasmic granules of eosinophils are affected by the staining process. Romanowsky stains might cause the cells to have large, swollen, round granules that are either colorless or blue.

Avian basophils contain deeply basophilic cytoplasmic granules that often mask the cell nucleus. The nucleus is typically nonlobed and appears round to oval. The granules are occasionally affected by alcohol-solubilized stain and might partially dissolve or appear abnormal in blood

smears stained by alcohol-solubilized stains.

Reptiles

Similar to those of birds, the granulocytic leukocytes of reptiles can be classified as heterophils, eosinophils, and basophils. Reptilian heterophils are large, round cells with nonlobed, round-to-oval nuclei (the nuclei of certain species of lizards might be lobed) and cytoplasm filled with eosinophilic, spicule- or rod-shaped granules. Reptilian heterophilic myelocytes and metamyelocytes are occasionally found in peripheral blood smears. These cells contain basophilic primary granules. Reptilian heterophils appear to undergo toxic changes similar to those described for avian heterophils. Reptilian eosinophils resemble avian eosinophils but tend to have round-to-oval nuclei. Reptilian basophils also resemble those of birds.

Fish

The nomenclature and classification of piscine granulocytes differ among classes of fish. Bony fish (class Osteichthyes) appear to have neutrophilic (heterophilic) and eosinophilic granulocytes. Whether basophilic granulocytes definitely exist in the peripheral blood of bony fish is controversial, and if they do exist, they occur in extremely low numbers. Hematologic studies of bony fish have concentrated on economically important species, such as carp, goldfish, catfish, salmon, and trout. The appearance of peripheral blood granulocytes varies between different species of fish. Goldfish and carp have neutrophils with lobed, eccentric nuclei and pale gray cytoplasm with small granules that vary from gray to pale pink. Eosinophils of goldfish tend to be round and smaller than neutrophils. The neutrophils of goldfish have round-to-bilobed nuclei and a pale blue cytoplasm that contains pale, round-to-rod-shaped granules.

Channel catfish have neutrophils (heterophils) with rod-shaped cytoplasmic granules that contain a central refractile body similar to avian heterophilic granules. Neutrophils (heterophils) are the primary granulocytes of salmon and trout; eosinophils are usually absent.

Four major types of granulocytes seem to exist in the peripheral blood of cartilaginous fish (class Chondrichthyes). The granulocyte classification used for the dogfish (*Scliorhinus canicula*) can serve as a model for this group of fish. Type I granulocytes (G1) have an eccentric, irregular, nonlobed nucleus and round-to-oval eosinophilic cytoplasmic granules. Type II granulocytes (G2) are often regarded as neutrophils because they resemble mammalian neutrophils having indented-to-lobed nuclei and a cytoplasm that lacks eosinophilic granules. Type III granulocytes (G3) have lobed nuclei and strongly eosinophilic, rod-shaped cytoplasmic granules. Type IV granulocytes (G4) differ in appearance from the other three types of granulocytes because they tend to be elongated with a nonlobed nucleus and a cytoplasm that is filled with eosinophilic granules. This cell type resembles activated thrombocytes that have an eosinophilic cytoplasm, but this cell type is larger and does not occur in clumps or clusters.

MONOCYTES, LYMPHOCYTES, AND AZUROPHILS

Birds, reptiles, and fish, like mammals, have monocytes and lymphocytes in their peripheral blood. These cells are morphologically similar to their mammalian counterparts. The monocytes typically are the largest leukocytes present in the peripheral blood of these animals. They have an abundant blue-gray cytoplasm that might contain vacuoles or tiny eosinophilic granules. The monocyte nucleus can vary in shape and has less chromatin clumping than lymphocyte nuclei.

Lymphocytes in the peripheral blood of birds, reptiles, and fish resemble mammalian lymphocytes. They are typically round but might appear irregular when they mold around adjacent cells in the blood smear. Lymphocytes have round-to-slightly indented nuclei that are usually centrally positioned in the cell. The nuclear chromatin of mature lymphocytes is heavily clumped or reticular. The cytoplasm is scant and usually appears homogenous and weakly basophilic (pale blue). Occasionally, lymphocytes contain azurophilic granules or irregular cytoplasmic projections.

Azurophils appear to be leukocytes that are present only in the blood of reptiles. They are particularly numerous in the peripheral blood of snakes. These cells resemble monocytes but have a distinct eosinophilic staining reaction to the cytoplasm with Romanowsky's stain. Like monocytes, reptilian azurophils have nuclei that vary in shape and cytoplasm that might be vacuolated. The function of these cells is unknown.

THROMBOCYTES

Birds, reptiles, and fish also possess nucleated thrombocytes. Avian and reptilian thrombocytes tend to be round to oval with round-to-oval nuclei containing densely clumped chromatin. The nucleus is large when compared with the cytoplasmic volume and is more rounded than erythrocyte nuclei. Normal, mature thrombocytes have colorless-to-pale gray cytoplasm that often has a reticulated appearance. The appearance of the cytoplasm is an important feature when differentiating between thrombocytes and lymphocytes. Thrombocytes of birds often contain distinct eosinophilic (specific) granules located in one area of the cytoplasm. The thrombocytes of fish occur as round, elongated, or fusiform, which might vary with the stage of cellular maturity or degree of reactivity. The nuclear shape follows the shape of the cell. The cytoplasm is colorless to pale blue.

Thrombocytes participate in the hemostatic process and tend to clump in blood smears. Activated thrombocytes occurring in aggregates might have indistinct cellular outlines or pseudopodia.

CONCLUSION

The hematology of birds, reptiles, and fish has yet to achieve the same degree of critical evaluation that it has in humans and domestic mammals. As veterinary clinics that treat birds, reptiles, and fish incorporate clinical hematology into their diagnostic plan, the value of this tool will increase. The hematology of birds, reptiles, and fish might also become as important as mammalian hematology.

BIBLIOGRAPHY

Campbell TW: *Avian Hematology and Cytology.* Ames, IA, Iowa State University Press, 1988, pp 3-32.
Hawkey CM, Dennett TB: *Color Atlas of Comparative Veterinary Hematology.* Ames, IA, Iowa State University Press, 1989.
Hibiya T: *An Atlas of Fish Histology. Normal and Pathological Features.* Tokyo, Kodansha Ltd, 1985, pp 64-72.
Natt MP, Herrick CA: A new blood diluent for counting the erythrocytes and leukocytes of the chicken. *Poultry Sci* 31:735-738, 1952.
Rowley AF, Ratcliffe HA: *Vertebrate Blood Cells.* New York, Cambridge University Press, 1988.

Common Parasites of Exotic Pets–Part I

Terry W. Campbell, DVM, PhD
Sea World of Florida, Inc.
Orlando, Florida

Numerous parasites can be found in or on exotic pets. The first part of this two-part presentation discusses the common parasites of pet rabbits, rodents, and birds. Part II will discuss common parasites of pet reptiles and tropical fish.

RABBITS
Ectoparasites

The rabbit ear mite, *Psoroptes cuniculi*, is one of the most commonly encountered external parasites of rabbits. Rabbits can harbor these mites and not be clinically affected by them. Those rabbits that are clinically affected develop ear infestations characterized by marked accumulation of crusts and scabs. This exudative material usually has a foul odor and contains numerous mites. Affected rabbits may frequently shake their heads and droop or scratch their ears. In rabbits with severe ear mite infestations, secondary bacterial infections may involve the inner ear, thus resulting in torticollis.

The mites are transmitted directly from rabbit to rabbit or indirectly by the contaminated material from the ear. Treatment consists of gently removing the exudate from the ear and applying ointments that contain antibiotics and antiinflammatory agents. Solutions containing an acaricide (any compound capable of killing mites) can be placed in the ear canal, and carbamate dips or dustings can be used to kill the mites in the ear and on the rabbit's body. Ivermectin (200 μg/kg) given subcutaneously or intramuscularly can also be used to kill ear mites on rabbits.

Cuterebra infection occurs in rabbits that are housed outdoors and is caused by *Cuterebra* fly larvae. The adult flies lay their eggs near rabbit hutches; and the larvae burrow into the skin of the rabbit, where they develop in subcutaneous cystic lesions. Fully developed larvae (approximately one month of age) are large, dark, and covered with distinct bands of spines. The larvae eventually leave the skin of the rabbit and pupate in the soil. They can be removed intact through the open pore in the skin.

It is important not to rupture the larva during extraction. Young (light-colored) larvae may be removed from the subcutaneous cavity by flushing hydrogen peroxide through the pore in the skin.

Endoparasites

Intestinal coccidiosis of rabbits is caused by various host-specific species of *Eimeria*. This protozoal disease is characteristically found in young rabbits (five to eight weeks of age) and associated with clinical signs that vary from acute diarrhea to sudden death.

The diagnosis is made by demonstration of the characteristic oocysts in feces. Treatment consists of symptomatic therapy for the diarrhea and administration of sulfonamides to slow the development of the coccidia (only the asexual stages are affected). Coccidiostats (i.e., sulfonamides) can be used prophylactically (0.025% in the food or 0.05% in the drinking water) for young rabbits until their immune systems mature sufficiently for them to control the coccidial parasite.

Hepatic coccidiosis, which is caused by *Eimeria stiedae*, can be fatal in rabbits, especially in weanlings housed in poor, unsanitary conditions that allow the accumulation of coccidial oocysts. Rabbits exposed to low numbers of *Eimeria stiedae* usually survive and develop lifelong immunity to the disease; however, these rabbits are often asymptomatic carriers and shed coccidial oocysts.

Rabbits that suffer from hepatic coccidiosis show clinical signs of anorexia, weakness, and ascites and may eventually die. Necropsy reveals an enlarged liver with numerous pale-yellow, irregular foci throughout the parenchyma. Control of this disease involves prevention of severe infections in weanling rabbits by providing clean housing that includes wire-bottom cages and food and water containers that prevent fecal contamination. Feeding a commercial rabbit food that contains 0.025% sulfaquinoxaline to weanling rabbits (after three weeks of age) for six to eight weeks also aids in the control of fatal hepatic coccidiosis in rabbits.

The rabbit pinworm, *Passalurus ambiguus*, can occur in enormous numbers in the cecum and colon of young rabbits but usually causes little harm. The ova of this parasite are found during routine fecal examinations or can adhere to hair in the perianal area. The ova are flattened on one side and measure 95 to 103 by 43 μm. Pinworms have a direct life cycle. Affected rabbits showing clinical signs of poor weight gain and lethargy can be treated with thiabendazole (100 mg/kg) or mebendazole (15 mg/kg).

RODENTS
Ectoparasites

With the exception of demodectic mange in hamsters, external parasite infestations are uncommon in pet rodents. *Demodex* mites are a common external parasite of hamsters; however, clinical disease usually occurs as a secondary disorder in hamsters suffering from other chronic debilitating diseases, such as renal disease. Affected hamsters develop patchy areas of alopecia in which the skin appears dry and scaly. Demodectic mange can also occur in gerbils, rats, and mice but is rare and (as in hamsters) is usually secondary to other chronic debilitating disorders. The mites can be found in skin scrapings. Treatment is usually ineffective; however, treatments used for demodicosis in dogs (e.g., amitraz [Mitaban®—Upjohn]) can be attempted.

Endoparasites

Clinical disease caused by internal parasites is rare in adult rodents, even though tapeworms, pinworms, and protozoa may occur in large numbers in the lower intestinal tract of these animals. For example, hamsters frequently carry large numbers of *Trichomonas*, *Giardia*, and *Spironucleus* organisms in their intestines but rarely suffer from clinical diseases associated with these parasites. *Giardia* and *Spironucleus*, however, occasionally cause enteric disorders in weanling hamsters or other rodents exposed to the feces of infected hamsters.

The dwarf tapeworm, *Hymenolepis nana*, is occasionally found in fecal examinations of rodents and is identified by the presence of ova with thick, irregular shells measuring 40 to 60 μm in diameter. Treatment with niclosamide (200 mg/kg) should be considered because of the zoonotic potential

even though human infections are usually derived from other humans.

Pinworms are common in rodents, but they are generally considered nonpathogenic. They are detected by the demonstration of characteristic ova in fecal examinations or microscopic examination of cellophane tape that was pressed to the perianal area. The pinworm ova are clear and banana-shaped.

BIRDS
Ectoparasites

Other than *Knemidokoptes* mites in budgerigars and canaries, external parasites are uncommon in pet birds, especially in domestically raised birds housed in proper indoor facilities. *Knemidokoptes* mange in canaries and budgerigars is one of the most common disorders of those species and is characterized by marked hyperkeratosis (a scaly, crusty appearance of the affected skin, usually involving unfeathered skin). The most commonly affected areas in budgerigars include the cere, beak, legs, and vent—hence the terms *scaly-leg* or *scaly-face* for this condition. The affected skin has a honeycombed appearance attributable to the mites tunneling into the skin. Canaries usually develop tassellike growths on the digits of the feet—hence the terms *scaly-leg* or *tassel-foot* for this condition.

The diagnosis of *Knemidokoptes* mange can usually be based on the appearance of the affected skin; however, the mites can usually be seen in skin scrapings. Adult female mites are spherical; have short, stubby legs; and are twice the size of the longer-legged males. Ivermectin (200 μg/kg) given orally or intramuscularly can provide a safe and effective treatment for *Knemidokoptes* mange; however, the condition will recur if the birds are exposed to other birds that are carriers of the mites.

Pet birds that come in contact with wild birds may suffer from fowl mite (*Ornithonyssus* species) or red mite (*Dermanyssus* species) infestations. Large numbers of these mites can parasitize birds in infested aviaries, thus causing signs of weakness, anemia, and excessive preening.

The *Dermanyssus* mites feed on the birds during the night and hide in the birds' environment (i.e., cracks and crevices in wooden perches, nest boxes, and cage structures) during the day. The mites appear as small dark-brown to red dots that move quickly when disturbed. A handheld magnifying lens is useful in the inspection of the birds' environment for red mites.

Ornithonyssus mites remain on the birds and crawl onto the handler of the infested birds. Elimination of mite infestations consists of using pyrethrins or carbaril sprays or powders to clean and treat the environment and birds. Prevention of mite infestations is accomplished by the elimination of contact between pet birds and wild birds.

Lice are rarely found on most species of pet birds; however, they are occasionally found on certain species, such as cockatiels. Lice tend to be host specific and do not survive off the avian host. The eggs (nits) can be found attached to feathers. Avian lice tend to be compressed dorsoventrally and move quickly among the feathers. Treatment for lice infestations is usually easily accomplished by using pyrethrins or carbaril sprays or powders.

Endoparasites

Internal parasites (with a few exceptions) are also rare in pet birds. Several species of wild-caught psittacines and passerines may harbor tapeworms, which are discovered as the proglottids pass in the feces or with detection of egg packets or eggs during fecal examination. Treatment for tapeworms consists of oral administration of niclosamide (200 mg/kg repeated in 10 to 14 days) or oral or parenteral administration of praziquantel (4 to 5 mg/kg). The injectable form of praziquantel, however, is toxic to some species.

Blood parasites are also commonly found in certain species of wild-caught birds. For example, microfilariae are often found in the peripheral blood of psittacines, especially African gray parrots and certain cockatoos. These parasites usually have little clinical significance, but treatment consisting of levamisole hydrochloride (15 mg/kg orally) or ivermectin (200 μg/kg) can be used.

Haemoproteus is also commonly found in the peripheral blood of wild-caught African gray parrots and certain cockatoos. This parasite is poorly pathogenic, and treatment is usually not required. *Haemoproteus* can be identified in blood smears by the presence of characteristic gametocytes within the cytoplasm of red blood cells. Only the gametocyte stage of *Haemoproteus* occurs in the peripheral blood of birds; therefore schizogony will not be found in blood smears. The mature *Haemoproteus* gametocyte occupies more than half of the cytoplasm of the host cell, forms a characteristic halter-shaped structure around the nucleus of the host cell, contains refractile pigment granules, and does not dramatically alter the position of the erythrocyte nucleus.

Plasmodium is occasionally found in the peripheral blood of pet birds, especially those housed in outdoor aviaries, where they are exposed to the mosquito vectors. In the peripheral blood of infected birds, *Plasmodium*, like *Haemoproteus*, can have erythrocytic gametocytes that contain refractile pigment granules. Unlike *Haemoproteus*, some species of *Plasmodium* can be highly pathogenic and can result in fatal hemolytic anemia.

Plasmodium can be differentiated from *Haemoproteus* by the presence of schizogony in the peripheral blood and the presence of forms of the parasite in cells other than erythrocytes. The gametocytes of some *Plasmodium* species can drastically alter the position of the erythrocyte nucleus, and mature *Plasmodium* gametocytes do not occupy more than half of the erythrocyte cytoplasm or form a halter-shaped structure around the erythrocyte nucleus. Antimalarial drugs, such as chloroquine in combination with primaquine phosphate, can be used in the treatment of *Plasmodium* infections. A commonly used regimen is 10 mg/kg initially followed by three 5 mg/kg doses given at 6, 18, and 24 hours after the first dose.

Leucocytozoon is another blood parasite that can be found in pet birds housed in outdoor aviaries but is more common in wild birds. *Leucocytozoon* is especially pathogenic to some species of passerines but is rarely seen in psittacines. *Leucocytozoon*, like *Haemoproteus*, has only the gametocyte stage of its life cycle in peripheral blood (schizogony occurs only in tissue). Gametocytes of *Leucocytozoon* lack the refractile pigment granules of *Haemoproteus* and *Plasmodium* and are large, round to elongated structures that drastically affect the host cell, thus making it unrecognizable. Antimalarial drugs can be used in an attempt to treat birds infected with *Leucocytozoon*.

Another blood parasite that is occasionally found in passerines is *Atoxoplasma*. This parasite has a direct life cycle involving *Isospora*-like oocysts. *Atoxoplasma* can be identified by the presence of pale, eosinophilic intracytoplasmic inclusions within mononuclear leukocytes, especially lymphocytes. These inclusions can be found within cells in the peripheral blood or most tissues. The *Atoxoplasma* inclusions create an indentation in the lymphocyte nucleus, thus resulting in a characteristic crescent shape to the nucleus. Atoxoplasmosis can cause high mortalities in infected passerine aviaries. No effective treatment exists.

Tracheal mites, *Sternastoma tracheacolum*, occasionally cause clinical disease in passerine birds, especially canaries and finches. Clinical signs include dyspnea and changes in vocalization. Sudden death can occur in severely affected birds, especially during the stress of handling. Diagnosis of tracheal mites is usually based on the clinical signs and demonstration of the mites by transillumination of the trachea, where they appear as small black dots that move up and down the trachea. Treatment consists of oral or intramuscular administration of ivermectin (200 μg/kg).

In pet birds, protozoal infections (e.g., trichomoniasis, giardiasis, and coccidiosis) occasionally result from the contamination of food or water.

Trichomonas infections often result in the formation of ulcers or caseous plaques in the upper alimentary tract (i.e., the oral cavity, esophagus, and ingluvies). Clinical signs include anorexia, weight loss, and frequent regurgitation.

Trichomonas organisms can be identified in scrapings from the oral lesions or in esophageal and crop swabs or aspirates. These protozoa are piriform flagellates with an anterior flagellum, an undulating membrane, and a prominent axostyle. They are best identified by their movements in a wet mount. Treatment consists of oral administration of antiflagellate drugs, such as metronidazole (25 to 50 mg/kg).

Giardia can cause a chronic mucoid diarrhea and high mortality in affected aviaries. Diagnosis of giardiasis is made by detection of oocysts or trophozoites (flagellates) in the feces. Antiflagellate drugs can be used in the treatment of this disease but often do not completely clear the infected bird of the parasite.

Coccidiosis is occasionally found in pet birds, especially softbills. Clinical signs include weight loss and mucoid or hemorrhagic diarrhea. The diagnosis is based on the detection of the coccidian oocysts in fecal smears or flotations. Treatment consists of oral medication using coccidiostats, such as sulfamethoxazole.

BIBLIOGRAPHY

Anderson LC: Guinea pig husbandry and medicine. Vet Clin North Am [Small Anim Pract] 17(5):1045–1060, 1987.

Barnes HJ: Parasites, in Harrison GJ, Harrison LR (eds): *Clinical Avian Medicine and Surgery*. Philadelphia, WB Saunders Co, 1986, pp 472–485.

Campbell TW: *Avian Hematology and Cytology*. Ames, IA, Iowa State University Press, 1988.

Harkness JE: Rabbit husbandry and medicine. Vet Clin North Am [Small Anim Pract] 17(5):1019–1044, 1987.

Harkness JE, Wagner JE: *The Biology and Medicine of Rabbits and Rodents*. Philadelphia, Lea & Febiger, 1983.

Soulsby EJL: *Helminths, Arthropods, and Protozoa of Domesticated Animals*. Philadelphia, Lea & Febiger, 1982.

Wagner JE, Farrar PL: Husbandry and medicine of small rodents. Vet Clin North Am [Small Anim Pract] 17(5):1062–1087, 1987.

Common Parasites of Exotic Pets–Part II

Terry W. Campbell, DVM, PhD
Sea World of Florida, Inc.
Orlando, Florida

Part I of Common Parasites of Exotic Pets discussed the common parasites of pet rabbits, rodents, guinea pigs, and companion birds. This segment focuses on the parasites that affect pet reptiles and fish.

REPTILES

Unless they are exposed to other reptiles with parasitic diseases (especially those with direct life cycles), captive-born reptiles that feed exclusively on domestically raised prey rarely acquire parasitic diseases. Reptilian pets obtained from the wild, however, are often parasitized by a wide variety of organisms.

Ectoparasites

Mite infestations in reptile collections can be a problem, especially in snake collections infested with the snake mite *Ophysionyssus natricis*. This species of mites can be seen as tiny gray dots moving under the scales, especially on the head of the snake. Regardless of the species, mites feed on the blood of their reptilian host and can be vectors for blood parasites (e.g., *Leucocytozoon*) or bacterial infections that may result in fatal septicemia. Mite infestation can also result in severe dermatologic disorders or anemia. Infestations can be controlled by pest strips impregnated with the organophosphate insecticide 2,2-dichlorovinyl dimethylphosphate. The insecticide strip should be prepared by hanging it outdoors for several hours before placing it in the reptile's environment. Small portions of the strip (2.5 cm²) can be suspended above the reptile's cage or placed inside a perforated plastic container within the cage for five days. Entire strips can be used to treat large rooms. The animal should never come into direct contact with the pest strips, however, because toxicity may result. Maintaining proper sanitary conditions also aids in the prevention of severe mite infestations in reptile collections.

Ticks are occasionally found on reptilian pets, especially recent acquisitions. Ticks can be mechanically removed from the reptile. Application of alcohol to the tick before removal may ease the task by relaxing the tick's mouthparts.

Aquatic or semiaquatic reptiles have various copepod, amphipod, or isopod ectoparasites. These parasites are usually found on recent acquisitions from the wild and are rare on established pets. Diluted povidone-iodine baths are usually effective in removing these organisms. Exposing marine reptiles to fresh water or freshwater reptiles to mild salt solutions is also effective in removing ectoparasites.

Endoparasites

Although reptiles can be infected with various endoparasites, protozoa and nematodes are the most common parasites found in reptilian pets. Amebiasis is one of the most clinically significant protozoan diseases of captive reptiles. A clinically important ameba is *Entamoeba invadens*, which is extremely pathogenic to snakes. Amebic infection is diagnosed when the organism is found in smears of fresh fecal samples, by colonic washes using warm sterile saline, or by colonic brush biopsies. A drop of Lugol's or Gram's iodine to the wet-mount preparation can aid in the detection of the cysts and trophozoites (15 to 20 μm) of the ameba. The motion of the ameba's pseudopodia make this parasite visible in the wet-mount preparation. The most effective treatment for reptilian amebiasis includes metronidazole or dimetridazole (both can be given at a dose of 40 to 100 mg/kg orally repeated in two weeks).

Coccidiosis, another protozoan disease of captive reptiles, usually occurs in collections maintained in suboptimum conditions. The most clinically significant genera of reptilian coccidia include *Eimeria*, *Isospora*, *Caryospora*, and *Cryptosporidium*. Clinical diagnosis of coccidiosis is based on demonstration of the characteristic sporulated oocysts in the feces. Sporulated oocysts of *Eimeria* have four sporocysts, each containing two sporozoites. Oocysts of *Isospora* have two sporocysts, each containing four sporozoites. Sporulated oocysts of *Caryospora* have only one sporocyst. *Cryptosporidium* oocysts are small (2.5 to 6.0 μm) and are best demonstrated by using special staining methods, such as Jenner-Giemsa stain. *Cryptosporidium* trophozoites can be detected in smears made from regurgitated food or gastric biopsy samples. Treatment of coccidia infections in reptiles includes the use of various sulfonamides (e.g., an oral dose of 40 mg/kg of sulfamethazine or sulfadimethoxine twice daily for the first day and 20 mg/kg twice daily for the following five to seven days). To date, no effective treatment for *Cryptosporidium* infection exists.

Blood parasites are occasionally found in the peripheral blood of reptiles. Haemosporidia, which is a group of blood-borne intracellular parasites, have been found in all major reptilian groups, except marine turtles. The Haemosporidia genera include *Haemogregarina*, *Haemoproteus*, *Plasmodium*, *Hepatozoon*, *Karyolysus*, *Schellakia*, and *Saurocytozoon*. Of this group, the haemogregarines are the most frequently encountered in clinical practice.

Haemogregarina, *Hepatozoon*, and *Karyolysus* cannot be easily distinguished by the appearance of their gametocytes within peripheral blood erythrocytes nor schizonts in host tissues. Therefore, they are usually placed under the general term haemogregarines when found in peripheral blood films of reptiles. In general, *Haemogregarina* is found in aquatic reptiles, *Hepatozoon* in terrestrial snakes, and *Karyolysus* in Old World lizards and possibly tree snakes. The

Originally published in Volume 11, Number 6, July 1990

presence of oval to elongated, basophilic, intracytoplasmic inclusions within erythrocytes identifies these organisms. Typically, these inclusions are larger than the host cell nucleus and are surrounded by a clear space in the erythrocyte cytoplasm. Haemogregarines usually distort the cell and displace the nucleus to the margins of the erythrocyte. Extraerythrocytic forms may also be found in severely infected reptiles. Schizonts of haemogregarines occur in the liver, spleen, and lungs of the reptile. Haemogregarines are transmitted by arthropod vectors, such as mosquitoes and ticks. Haemogregarines apparently have a low degree of pathogenicity to the reptile host, and no effective treatment has been found to rid reptiles of these parasites. Infections in captive reptiles, however, may be self-limiting.

Plasmodium is commonly found in the peripheral blood of semiaquatic and terrestrial chelonians and lizards. The intraerythrocytic gametocytes of *Plasmodium* contain refractile pigment granules resulting from the breakdown of hemoglobin. These refractile granules are not found in the haemogregarines.

Other types of blood parasites frequently found in reptiles include trypanosomes and microfilariae of filarial nematodes. Both types of parasite are transmitted by bites of invertebrate vectors and are considered to be poorly pathogenic to reptiles. Therefore, treatment is not indicated in most cases.

Less common blood parasites of reptiles include *Haemoproteus, Saurocytozoon, Schellakia, Leishmania,* and the piroplasmids. *Haemoproteus (Haemocystidium)* is found primarily in lizards and only the gametocyte stage is found in the peripheral blood differentiating it from *Plasmodium. Saurocytozoon* has gametocytes that lack refractile pigment granules and resemble the *Leucocytozoon* of birds. *Schellakia (Atoxoplasma)* primarily occurs in lizards and is identified by the presence of sporozoites that form round to oval inclusions within the cytoplasm of leukocytes (primarily lymphocytes). Piroplasmids, such as *Babesia, Aegyp-*

tianella (Tunetella), and *Sauroplasma (Serpentoplasma)* are rare in the peripheral blood of reptiles.

Ascarid, strongylid, and rhabdoid nematodes are occasionally found in captive reptiles. Necropsy, demonstration of adult parasites or eggs within the feces, or aspirates from the stomachs of living reptiles indicate the presence of these parasites. Ascarid eggs are typically large, thick shelled, and round to oval (80 to 100 μm by 60 to 80 μm). Strongyles (e.g., *Kalicephalus,* which is the intestinal hookworm of snakes) have thin-walled oval eggs (70 to 100 μm by 40 to 50 μm) that are often larvated. Rhabdoid eggs are smaller than strongylid eggs and are always larvated.

The feces of carnivorous reptiles, it should be noted, may contain eggs from the parasites in their prey. These eggs pass through the reptile and should be properly identified to avoid a misdiagnosis of a reptilian parasitic disease. Periodic examination of the prey for parasites may assist in the proper identification of nematode ova or parasite oocysts that are commonly found in prey animals. The common nematode infections of reptiles are usually effectively treated using mebendazole (40 to 100 mg/kg orally repeated in two weeks), thiabendazole (50 to 100 mg/kg orally repeated in two weeks), or fenbendazole (50 to 100 mg/kg orally repeated in two weeks). Unresponsive infections, especially with rhabdoid nematodes, may respond to levamisole therapy (levamisole hydrochloride at a dose of 5 mg/kg subcutaneously; 50% of the body weight of turtles and tortoises should be subtracted to allow for the weight of the shell).

FISH
Ectoparasites

Various external parasites are commonly found on the skin of tropical fish. The external protozoan parasites of fish can be classified as encysting or nonencysting. Nonencysting protozoa spend their entire life cycle on the fish host, whereas encysting protozoa reproduce off their fish host. Freshwater fish harboring external protozoa are treated topically with waterborne medications, such as formalin. Forma-

lin treatments consist of 15- to 60-minute baths using 0.4 to 0.5 ml of 37% formaldehyde per liter of water. The formalin bath should be well oxygenated; soft, acidic water should not be used to prepare the solution; and formaldehyde containing paraformaldehyde, a white precipitate, should be avoided. Copper sulfate (0.1 to 0.2 mg/L for 10 days) can be used for saltwater fish. All stages of the nonencysting protozoa are susceptible to the topical treatment, whereas the encysting protozoa are susceptible only during certain stages of their life cycle. Therefore, treatment for encysting protozoa generally requires a longer period of time than does treatment for nonencysting protozoa.

Common nonencysting external protozoa found on fish include the following trichodinids: *Epistylis, Ichthyobodo necatrix, Chilodonella,* and *Brooklynella horridus.* The trichodinids are ciliated, circular, flattened protozoa with distinct denticular rings. These parasites measure 40 to 60 nm in diameter and are commonly found on the skin and gills of pond fish, especially those living in water with a high organic load. Placing affected fish into clean water is often the only treatment necessary to rid fish of trichodinids.

Epistylis organisms are stalked, ciliated protozoa that appear as white, tufted areas on the surface of the body or fins. Goldfish and fish living in water with a high organic content are often infected with *Epistylis. Ichthyobodo necatrix* is a small (7-nm), comma-shaped, flagellate protozoan that is actively motile when viewed through a microscope. This parasite affects only freshwater fish and feeds directly on epithelial cells, thereby destroying the gill and skin epithelium. The body of the fish reacts by producing an excessive amount of mucus, which appears as a whitish film on the body surface. Fish with heavy gill infestations often exhibit respiratory distress. *Chilodonella* infestations are commonly found in cultured freshwater fish, such as goldfish and various freshwater tropical species. *Brooklynella horridus* is the saltwater counterpart of *Chilodonella.* Both types of parasites cause respiratory distress, depression, and excessive mucus production. They are flattened, ciliated protozoa (50 to 70 nm) that appear as heart or oval shaped. The cilia appear in rows. *Chilodonella* organisms move in a characteristically slow, circular manner.

The common encysting types of external protozoa found on pet fish include *Ichthyopthirus multifiliis*, *Cryptokaryon irritans*, and *Oodinium*. *Ichthyophthirus multifiliis* is the causative agent of white spot disease (which is commonly referred to as ich [pronounced ick]) to which all freshwater fish are susceptible, especially those in home aquariums. *Cryptokaryon irritans* is the saltwater counterpart. The skin of affected fish is covered with small white spots, which are the encysted stage of the protozoa or trophonts. When the trophont matures, it breaks through the epithelium, leaves the fish host, and attaches to objects on the aquarium bottom, thereby becoming a tomont. The tomont develops into hundreds of free-living ciliated theronts. The theronts penetrate the epithelium of the skin and gills and become the encysting trophonts, thus completing the life cycle.

Theronts are round to oval protozoa and are one of the few fish parasites with cilia that completely surround the organism. In addition to using the treatments described earlier (i.e., formalin treatment for freshwater fish or copper sulfate treatment for saltwater fish), elevating the water temperature several degrees above the normal aquarium temperature, which is 26°C, for a few days diminishes the number of heat-sensitive theronts. *Oodinium* is a dinoflagellate protozoan (40 to 100 μm) that contains chlorophyll and is found on the skin and gills of affected fish. Common names given to *Oodinium* infections include velvet disease, rust disease, and coral fish disease because of the color created by the chlorophyll within the parasite. *Oodinium* organisms are nonmotile and appear as pear-shaped cysts in the skin or gills. After the cysts drop off the host, numerous dinospores are released.

Monogenetic trematodes are common parasites of freshwater and marine fish and can be found on the skin or gills. Affected fish may show clinical signs of rapid respiratory movements, rubbing, or death. Treatment consists of formaldehyde baths, saltwater baths for freshwater fish, freshwater baths for marine fish, or praziquantel (10 mg/L as a three-hour bath) added to the aquarium water.

Parasitic copepods, such as *Lernaea* species, are common to fish, such as koi and goldfish, that are raised in ponds. *Lernaea* organisms are elongated copepods that attach to the skin of fish and are often referred to as anchor worms. This parasite embeds its head into the skin of the fish, leaving its elongated body with V-shaped egg sacs protruding from the surface. Affected fish may reveal cutaneous hemorrhage in areas of parasitic attachment. Treatment consists of forceps removal of the parasite or treatment of the water with organophosphates (e.g., trichlorfon at a quantity of 0.25 mg/L).

Endoparasites

Various internal parasites, including protozoa (ciliates and flagellates), sporozoans, nematodes, trematodes, and cestodes, also infect fish. *Hexamita* species are flagellate protozoans that are commonly found in the gastrointestinal tract of various species of fish. *Hexamita* organisms are small (nearly the size of an erythrocyte) and actively motile. Many fish (e.g., goldfish) can be asymptomatic carriers of this parasite, whereas other fish (e.g., angelfish, discus fish, and gouramis) often develop such clinical effects of the disease as anorexia, weight loss, unthriftiness, and death. *Hexamita* species are identified during examination of the feces of living fish or by examination of the intestinal contents during necropsy. Treatment involves the addition of metronidazole (5 mg/L) to the aquarium water and thorough cleansing of the gravel and filter.

Sporozoan diseases, such as coccidiosis, are common to fish. *Eimeria* organisms are the most commonly identified coccidia in fish. Clinical disease resulting from coccidia often causes emaciation and depression. Coccidia are detected by demonstration of oocysts in feces or intestinal scrapings. Treatment consists of an anticoccidial drug, such as sulfadiazine given as an initial oral dose of 220 mg/kg and a dose of 110 mg/kg five days later. *Plistophora hyphessobryconis* is a common microsporidian of fish and can cause clinical disease in various species, such as angelfish and neon tetras. The affected fish develop muscle necrosis and often suffer high mortalities. Diagnosis of plistophoriasis is made by the detection of cyst-like structures (pansporoblasts), which are filled with spores that have a single polar capsule. No effective treatment has been found for this disease.

Adult digenetic trematodes and tapeworms are uncommon in ornamental fishes; however, the intermediate stages of these parasites are often found encysted in the tissue of fish, especially wild-caught fish. Generally, affected fish cannot be treated.

Nematodes can also be found in pet fish. These parasites occur as adults or larvae within the intestinal lumen or coelomic cavity or as cysts within various types of tissues. These parasites rarely cause clinical disease in fish and are discovered incidentally during necropsy.

CONCLUSION

The veterinary technician caring for exotic pets should be able to identify parasites frequently found in the exotic pets that are commonly presented to veterinary hospitals or practices. The equipment and methods used for detecting parasites in exotic pets are essentially the same as those routinely used for identifying parasites in exotic animals.

BIBLIOGRAPHY

Frye FL: *Biomedical and Surgical Aspects of Captive Reptile Husbandry.* Edwardsville, KS, Veterinary Medicine Publishing Co, 1981, pp 195–227.

Gratzek JB: Parasites associated with ornamental fish, Vet Clin North Am [Small Anim Pract] 18(2):375–399, 1988.

Jacobson ER: Parasitic diseases of reptiles, in Fowler ME (ed): *Zoo and Wild Animal Medicine.* Philadelphia, WB Saunders Co, 1986, pp 162–181.

Jacobson ER: Reptiles. *Vet Clin North Am [Small Anim Pract]* 17(5):1203–1225, 1987.

Wallach JD, Boever WJ: *Diseases of Exotic Animals.* Philadelphia, WB Saunders Co, 1983, pp 1061–1067.

Physical Restraint of Exotic Patients

Terry W. Campbell, DVM, PhD
Sea World of Florida, Inc.
Orlando, Florida

Laura V. Campbell, DVM
Kissimmee, Florida

Restraining the patient properly for the clinician is an important aspect of a veterinary technician's job. Whether the technician works in a primarily exotic animal practice or a general practice that has few avian or nondomestic patients, it is imperative for the technician to have a thorough working knowledge of the proper method of physically restraining nondomestic pets for the safety of both the patient and the technician. This article discusses proper restraining techniques for birds, rodents, rabbits, ferrets, and reptiles.

Restraint of Birds

To restrain birds, the technician must remember the following key points. Any handling that prevents proper movement of the sternum (keel) inhibits respiration. Handling extremely ill or stressed avian patients should be avoided until the patient has been stabilized (e.g., maintaining hypothermic birds in an incubator). If it is absolutely necessary to handle such patients, the owner should be informed of the seriousness of the condition. Birds generally require gentle but firm handling. Removal of toys, perches, and other objects in the cage is often required to make capture of the bird easier and potentially less

traumatic. It may also be necessary to remove the top part of the cage or carrier to capture the bird. Sometimes it is helpful, especially with small birds, to dim the lights in the room. The doors and windows of the examination room should be closed. Windows should either be covered or contain a wire mesh to provide visibility to the bird; escaped birds are less likely to fly into windows if they can see them.

Small passerine or psittacine species (e.g., budgerigars) are both handled in the same manner. Capturing and holding the bird is easier with bare hands than it is with gloved hands or by using a towel. The thumb and forefinger hold the bird's head; the rest of the technician's hand cups the bird gently to restrict movement of the patient's wings and body. Medium to large passerine birds (i.e., mynah birds and crows) and medium-sized psittacines (i.e., lovebirds and cockatiels) may require using a light cloth towel (or even a paper towel) to facilitate capture. With the hand hidden by the towel, the technician grasps the bird from behind the head; the technician then places his or her thumb and forefinger underneath the patient's mandible to control its jaws. As with smaller birds, the body and wings can be restrained by wrapping the rest of the hand gently around the body. The patient's head and neck can be tilted slightly backward to maintain control. A heavier towel may be necessary to capture and restrain large passerine birds.

The same principles of head and wing restraint described for medium-

sized psittacines also apply to large psittacines, such as macaws. To facilitate restraint during examination, the bird may be wrapped in the towel; individual body parts are exposed as necessary. Skilled technicians can restrain large birds without using towels or gloves. With medium to large psittacines, it is essential to restrain the head properly because these birds can inflict serious bite wounds. Some birds learn to defend themselves against the towel capture method by rolling on their backs, making the capture more challenging for the technician. In such situations, a large wooden dowel can be used to control the mandible; as the bird bites the dowel, the technician grasps the legs and head.

Judging the temperament of the patient is helpful in capturing and restraining it. For example, a hand-raised pet often responds better to a slow approach. The technician should scratch the back of the patient's head and neck and then gently grasp the back of the head with bare hands while quickly restraining the body and wings. Untamed birds, however, require the more aggressive techniques described previously.

Birds of prey (raptors) are sometimes presented to veterinary hospitals or clinics for medical treatment. Special federal and state permits are required to treat these types of birds legally. Unlike psittacines that use their beaks for self-defense, raptors use their talons; therefore, when handling raptors, the feet must be restrained properly. These birds are captured by pinning them down using a heavy towel or gloved hands (although towels and gloves do not always provide adequate protection against talons, especially those of large birds of prey). After the bird is pinned, the feet can be controlled by inserting a finger between the legs and holding them together with the rest of the hand. When restraining large raptors, such as eagles, the technician may need both hands to hold the legs while using his or her forearms to hold the wings of the patient tightly against its body. Covering the head of the patient with a porous cloth may help to keep it calm during short-term handling and may also protect the technician from being bitten.

Restraint of Reptiles

Reptiles are another group of nondomestic pets that are presented to veterinary hospitals or clinics. Technicians would therefore be prudent to learn the proper methods of restraint of turtles, tortoises, lizards, and snakes. To restrain turtles or tortoises, the technician should hold the plastron (lower shell) and carapace (upper shell) with both hands and roll the patient into ventral or sternal recumbency. Turtles, especially snapping turtles, are often more aggressive than are tortoises and may be picked up by the tail. Lizards (such as iguanas), however, should not be picked up by the tail because it detaches as a defense mechanism. When restraining large lizards, the technician uses one hand to grasp the area behind the patient's head while the fingers of the same hand are controlling the front legs; the technician's other hand is placed around the patient's abdomen, using his or her fingers to control the hindlimbs. Gloves may be worn to restrain large, aggressive lizards.

Constrictor snakes are restrained by grasping the area behind the head firmly with one hand and supporting the body with the other. Depending on the size and demeanor of the snake, constrictors may require more than one technician for restraint.

Venomous snakes should only be handled by experienced personnel. A snake hook or noose may be used to pin the head (which should be facing away from the technician). Care must be taken when using the hook; if the technician is too forceful, the patient may be injured. The technician's middle finger and thumb are placed on the sides of the snake's head with his or her index finger on top. The technician's free hand supports the snake's body.

Another means of restraining both nonpoisonous and venomous snakes is by the use of a clear plastic tube with a diameter just large enough for the snake to fit through (the snake should not be able to turn around in the tube) and capped at one end. These tubes have slits along the sides to facilitate examination or treatment. After the snake has entered the tube a desired length or distance, the snake is grasped at the location where its body emerges from the tube to prevent the snake from backing out. If a venomous snake is being handled in this manner, the tube should be held with long forceps or tongs until the snake is inside the tube.

Restraint of Other Exotics

Nondomestic mammals, such as rabbits, ferrets, and rodents, are often presented to veterinary hospitals or clinics for medical care. When handling rabbits, the technician should keep in mind that rabbits kick and scratch with their powerful hindlimbs to defend themselves; they also have a relatively weak back or lumbar area. Improper handling of rabbits may potentially result in fracture or luxation of the patient's lumbar vertebrae. Rabbits should be picked up by the scruff of the neck (using the loose skin over their shoulders) with one hand, and the other hand should be placed under the rabbit's body and hindquarters to support its back. The technician may also hold the rabbit in an upright sitting position by grasping the scruff of the neck with one hand and supporting the rear end with the other. The rabbit should be held facing away from the technician and close to his or her body. As an alternative method, the rabbit's head (while the technician supports the rabbit with his or her forearm) can be held between the technician's body and bent elbow; the scruff of the neck is held with the technician's opposite hand. Rabbits should always be held close to the handler's body. Rabbits may also be wrapped in a towel (just as a cat would be wrapped for restraint) and held by the scruff of the neck for control. Protective long sleeves can be worn by technicians to avoid painful scratches often caused by the rear claws of fractious rabbits.

Restraint of ferrets is accomplished by grasping the patient around the thorax (behind the forelegs) with one hand, while the technician's opposite hand controls the patient's head. Gloves are not usually required but can be worn to protect the technician from bites.

Rats, mice, and gerbils should be grasped by the base of the tail to elevate the rear legs at a 45° angle. The technician grasps the scruff of the patient's neck with his or her opposite hand to control the patient's head. The patient should have a rough surface or wire mesh to grip with its forefeet. The technician should be aware that rats and mice, even while being restrained in this manner, are able to turn around and bite. This behavior can be avoided if the technician grabs an adequate amount of loose skin on the scruff of the neck to control the patient's head and neck. Gerbils generally do not bite; however, if gerbils are held improperly, the skin on the tail may slip off and thus leave exposed vertebrae. Rats can be restrained in the manner described for ferrets.

Guinea pigs should be grasped around the thorax and lifted; care must be taken to support the rear end (especially if the patient is pregnant or large) with the opposite hand. Guinea pigs are generally not aggressive and seldom bite.

Hamsters have short, stubby tails and cannot be approached in the same manner as other rodents. Hamsters bite notoriously, especially if they are disturbed while sleeping. To capture and restrain a hamster, the technician grasps the scruff of the neck with one hand and supports the body with his or her other hand. Hamsters have abundant loose skin on the neck scruff and can bite suddenly if the technician does not gather enough of this skin to control the head and neck movements.

Conclusion

Restraint of patients for examination or treatment is an important task because the safety of the patient, the technician, and the examiner may be at risk. Nearly all veterinary practices, regardless of the type, are presented with occasional nondomestic pets. Knowledge of proper handling techniques is essential.

BIBLIOGRAPHY

Almandarz E: Physical restraint of reptiles, in Fowler ME (ed): *Zoo and Wild Animal Medicine*, ed 2. Philadelphia, WB Saunders Co, 1986, pp 151–152.

Boever WJ: The restraint of nondomestic pets. *Vet Clin North Am [Small Anim Pract]* 9:392–394, 1979.

Brooks DL: Rabbits, hares, and pikas (Lagamorpha), in Fowler ME (ed): *Zoo and Wild Animal Medicine*, ed 2. Philadelphia, WB Saunders Co, 1986, pp 716–717.

Burke TJ: Rats, mice, hamsters, and gerbils. *Vet Clin North Am [Small Anim Pract]* 9:473–475, 1979.

Clark JD, Olfert ED: Rodents (Rodentia), in Fowler ME (ed): *Zoo and Wild Animal Medicine*, ed 2. Philadelphia, WB Saunders Co, 1986, pp 735–737.

Harrison GJ, Harrison LR, Fudge AM: Preliminary evaluation of a case, in Harrison GJ, Harrison LR (eds): *Clinical Avian Medicine and Surgery*. Philadelphia, WB Saunders Co, 1986, pp 104–107.

Kock N, Kock M: Physical restraint and sexing techniques in small mammals and reptiles, in Kirk RW (ed): *Current Veterinary Therapy. IX. Small Animal Practice*. Philadelphia, WB Saunders Co, 1986, pp 764–771.

Williams CF: Guinea pigs and rabbits. *Vet Clin North Am [Small Anim Pract]* 9:487–488, 1979.